Where The Wild Things Grow
A Foraging and Field Guide to 109 Healing Plants of the American Northwest
Jessica Freeborn

Copyright © [2025] Jessica Freeborn

All rights reserved.

No part of this publication may be reproduced, distributed, or transmitted in any form or by any means—electronic, mechanical, photocopying, recording, or otherwise—without the prior written permission of the author, except in the case of brief quotations embodied in critical reviews and certain other noncommercial uses permitted by copyright law.

Cover Design by Matthew Lawler

Photography by Jessica Freeborn and contributing forest friends (used with permission)

This book is intended as an educational and informational resource. The author is not a licensed medical practitioner. The statements made in this book are not intended to diagnose, treat, or cure any disease. Always consult a qualified professional before using any plant for medicinal purposes.

First Edition

Printed in the United States of America

For more information, visit: *[www.freebornfamilyfarms.com]*

ISBN: 979-8-218-82587-4

Contents

Introduction	1
How To Use This Guide	5
Foraging Ethics	7
What Is In A Plant Name?	8
Acknowledgements	10
Dedication	12
Reclaimer	14
Collecting and Preserving	15
Wild Versus Domesticated	17
Dosages	18
The Doctrine Of Signatures	20
Herbs and Flowers	22
1. Alumroot	23
2. Amaranth	25
3. Angelica	27
4. Arnica	29
5. Arrowleaf Balsamroot	31
6. Bee Balm	34

7.	Black Medic	36
8.	Broadleaf Dock	39
9.	Bluebells	41
10.	Broadleaf Plantain	43
11.	Bunchberry Dogwood	46
12.	Burdock	49
13.	Camas	51
14.	Cat's Ear	54
15.	Cattail	56
16.	Chickweed	58
17.	Chicory	61
18.	Cleavers (Bedstraw)	64
19.	Coltsfoot	67
20.	Comfrey	69
21.	Dandelion	72
22.	False Solomon's Seal	75
23.	Filaree	78
24.	Fireweed	80
25.	Gentian	82
26.	Geranium	85
27.	Ghost Pipe	87
28.	Glacier Lily	90
29.	Goldenrod	92

30.	Henbit	95
31.	Honeysuckle	97
32.	Horsetail	99
33.	Knapweed	101
34.	Lamb's Quarters	103
35.	Lanceleaf Plantain	105
36.	Lomatium	107
37.	Mallow	110
38.	Milk Thistle	112
39.	Miner's Lettuce	114
40.	Mountain Mint	116
41.	Mugwort	119
42.	Mullein	122
43.	Oxeye Daisy	125
44.	Pearly Everlasting	127
45.	Pipsissewa	129
46.	Purple Dead Nettle	132
47.	Purslane	134
48.	Rattlesnake Plantain	136
49.	Red Clover	138
50.	Salsify	141
51.	Sedum	143
52.	Self-Heal	145

53. Sheep Sorrel	148
54. Shepherd's Purse	150
55. Silverweed	153
56. Skullcap	155
57. Skunk Cabbage	157
58. Spreading Dogbane	159
59. Spring Beauty	161
60. Stinging Nettle	163
61. St. John's Wort	166
62. Sweet Cicely	169
63. Tiger Lily	171
64. Toadflax	173
65. Trillium	175
66. Violet	178
67. Usnea Lichen	181
68. White Clover	184
69. Wild Ginger	187
70. Wild Chamomile	189
71. Wild Lettuce	191
72. Wild Strawberry	193
73. Yarrow	195
74. Yellow Dock	198
75. Yellow Pond Lily	201

76.	Yerba Buena	204
Trees and Shrubs		206
77.	Alder	207
78.	Apple	210
79.	Aspen	213
80.	Birch	215
81.	Ceanothus	218
82.	Chokecherry	221
83.	Crampbark	223
84.	Cottonwood	225
85.	Devil's Club	228
86.	Dogwood	231
87.	Elderberry	233
88.	Hawthorn	237
89.	Huckleberry	240
90.	Juniper	243
91.	Kinnikinnick	246
92.	Lewis' Mock Orange	248
93.	Linden	250
94.	Lodgepole Pine	252
95.	Mountain Ash	255
96.	Ocean Spray	257
97.	Oregon Grape Root	259

98. Ponderosa Pine	262
99. Red Raspberry	264
100. Ribes	267
101. Serviceberry	269
102. Spruce	271
103. Tamarack	274
104. Thimbleberry	276
105. Western Hemlock	278
106. Western Red Cedar	281
107. Western White Pine	284
108. White Willow	287
109. Wild Rose	289
Afterword	291
About the author	292
Bibliography	293
Index	296

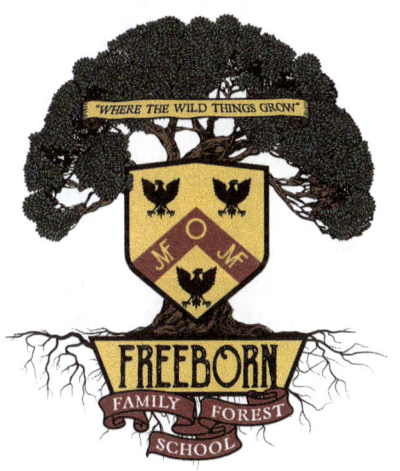

Introduction

Follow Me Where The Wild Things Grow

It is with great joy and reverence that I offer you this collection of 109 wild, edible, and medicinal plants—companions, teachers, and plant allies that have woven their way through my life and through the land I have wandered and explored. These plant profiles are more than just descriptions; they are stories gathered from my years of walking the forest paths, riversides, meadows, and mountains, learning the land, harvesting, preparing, and honoring the medicine that grows all around us. Lessons learned from the wildlife that called me home.

The birth of this book, when I first started writing down the herbal allies growing around me, began when my family and I took a bold leap into a simpler way of life. When we first moved onto Hoo Doo Mountain, we called home a Cabela's Ultimate Alaknak tent with a wood-burning stove, nestled in the old-growth forest. It was there, through the quiet mornings and star-filled nights, that I began to truly hear the voices of the plants. Eventually, we moved into my father's historical off-grid cabin, where the rhythms of nature shaped our days. It was in this sacred slowness—without electricity, surrounded by wilderness—that I studied these plants, worked with them, lived close to them. They became more than subjects of study; they became allies. They offered us nourishment, healing, connection, and a way forward—gifts that continue to sustain our family's spirit and livelihood. They kept us healthy and resilient through the hardships that came with living off-grid on a mountain in untamed terrain.

In this book, you will meet trees that have stood for centuries, shrubs that feed the body, flowers that soothe the heart and renew the spirit, and roots that heal deep within. You will find plants that have long been revered by Indigenous peoples, honored in American folk traditions, rooted in ancient cultures worldwide, and cherished by modern herbalists. Each plant profile carries both ancient wisdom and my personal experiences and lessons—a blend of traditional uses, modern understandings, and the intimate moments I have shared with these plants in the wild and at home. Most importantly, you will be submerged in the land where the wild things grow.

I have chosen to include not only common plants that many know and love, but also those often overlooked, forgotten, or misunderstood—plants that deserve to have their voices heard once again. Many of them, I believe, are calling us back into right relationship with the earth, asking us to remember how to live in harmony with the natural world.

I hope that this book serves as a trusted guide for your own foraging journeys and herbal explorations. More importantly, I hope it sparks a sense of wonder, curiosity, and respect for the wild plants that surround us. Learn their names. Spend time with them. Listen to their stories. And always harvest with care, respect, and gratitude.

May these plants bring healing to your life, to your loved ones, and to the land we share and call home. Without further ado, follow me where the wild things grow!

Forest TEAcher,☐
Jessica Freeborn

My mission is to connect people to wild plants to help heal the planet.

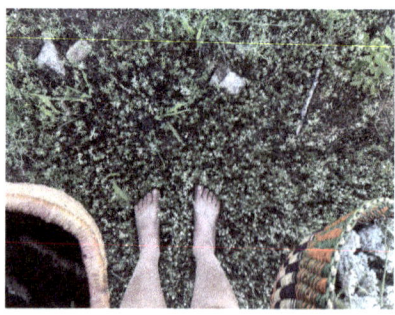

Why Forage and Harvest Wild Plants?

"The physician treats, but nature heals." -Hippocrates

Many of us are returning to the wild. As we navigate uncertain economic and political times, more people are choosing to hunt, gather, grow, and preserve their own food. Why wouldn't you be drawn to wild harvesting your own medicine and meals? A treasure trove of easily absorbed vitamins, minerals, polyphenols, and antioxidants awaits the forager. Everything you need to survive—and thrive—often grows in the very environment in which you live.

Studies have shown that wild plants are more nutrient-dense and contain higher levels of essential oils, vitamins, and minerals than those grown in monoculture crops (Duguma, 2020). This makes sense—wild plants endure the extremes of nature. They develop deep roots and form symbiotic relationships with the mycelial networks beneath the forest floor, stretching for miles.

Harvesting your own medicine and nourishment is both a sacred and spiritual act. It feels like receiving God's own medicine. It strengthens your physical body and renews your spirit.

Simply walking in nature is medicine. "Forest bathing" (Shinrin-Yoku) has become a popular topic among Japanese researchers. In one study, city dwellers took part in a weekend forest retreat. Afterward, their blood pressure decreased and white blood cell counts increased—benefits that lasted up to four weeks (Furuyashiki et al., 2019). The forest is a place for rest—a balm for the weary soul.

Take forest bathing one step further—try forest foraging. Here, you are not just walking—you are grazing and gathering living medicine from ancient soil. Then, you share it with your family or a loved one as a meal or a tea ceremony. This creates a beautiful, meaningful life—one rooted in wild wisdom. You feel you belong to the world you are in.

Many people feel disconnected from the earth. They have forgotten to take time to listen, breathe, and reconnect. Thus, chronic disease and depression attempt to take root in our modern lives. However, I see hope. We are at a crossroads in this young country: down one path lies Smart Cities and government overreach; down the other, self-sustaining communities that remember how to care for each other.

Many of us are waking up, as though we have been asleep. A new generation of modern-day pioneers are returning to the old ways. Herbalism was the first medicine. Wild plants were the tools in every healer's pouch.

When we reconnect with these ancient traditions—when we grow, gather, and prepare our own plant medicine—we honor our Creator and our ancestors. I come from a long line of teachers on both sides of my family. Teaching sustainable foraging and forest gardening is both a gift and a great responsibility.

So come—follow me where the wild things grow.

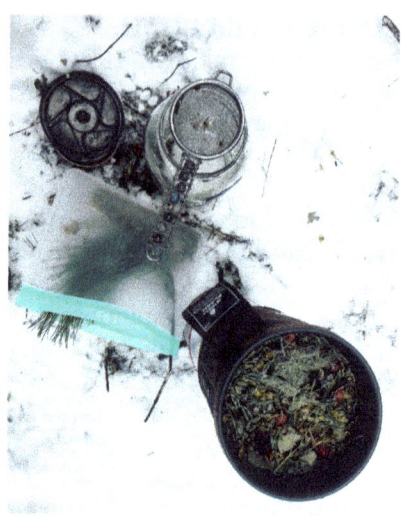

Foraging with the Seasons

There is a rhythm to the Northern forests—a cycle that teaches us how and when to gather. Sustainable foraging is about learning this seasonal flow and moving in harmony with it.

In early spring, we find edible flowers and microgreens—plants that help flush away the stagnation of winter. As summer begins, we gather nourishing herbs and restorative berries. In the fall, when the days shorten and plants return to the earth, we harvest roots to store in our winter pantry.

Winter may seem sparse, but there is still medicine to be found. Evergreen trees offer vitamin C-rich needles. Cottonwood buds are thick with resin to protect them from frost—this is the perfect time to craft your Balm of Gilead.

This seasonal cycle is sacred and awe-inspiring. Each year, a divine miracle occurs: the plants return. Like old friends, they greet us once again—ready to nourish, heal, and teach.

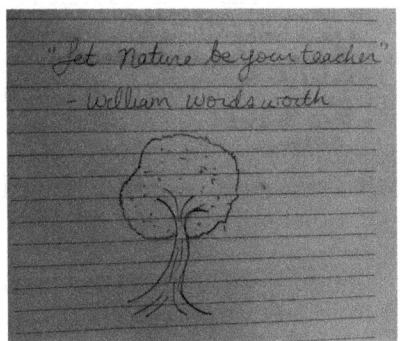

How To Use This Guide

Each plant profile in this guide follows a consistent format to help you identify, understand, and build a relationship with 109 edible and medicinal plants of the Northwest. This layout is designed to be both practical for field use and rich in ancestral and herbal knowledge.

Common Name(s): These are the names I am most familiar with—often the ones you will hear in casual conversation or find in folk herbalism. Many plants have multiple common names, and I have included the most recognized ones.

Botanical Name: The scientific name, written in Latin and italicized, is used universally by taxonomists and herbalists. It ensures clarity in plant identification, especially when common names vary by region.

Plant Family: Each plant's family is included to show its relationship to other forest flora. Recognizing plant families can deepen your understanding of shared traits and medicinal properties.

Description: Here you will find a detailed botanical description to support accurate identification. I have used specific botanical terms where helpful and always aim to make visual recognition easier in the field.

Where It Grows: This section describes the terrain and ecological conditions in which the plant commonly thrives. Knowing a plant's preferred environment will help you locate it and gain a deeper understanding of its nature.

When and How to Harvest: Learn the best time of year to gather each plant, and how to do so with respect and sustainability. I also note which specific parts to harvest and how to work in harmony with the seasons and cycles.

How to Work with It / Medicinal Use: This is the heart of each entry. I share my own methods for working with these plants to create nourishing and healing remedies, drawing from folk traditions, ancient wisdom, and the teachings of incredible herbalists I have studied from.

Healing Constituents / Therapeutic Actions: This section includes the plant's known vitamins, minerals, phytochemicals, and medicinal properties. These are the tools behind the plant's healing power, grounded in herbalism, science, and tradition.

Historical Connections: Here, we journey into the past to discover how our ancestors worked with these plants. This includes traditional uses, folklore, etymology (the origins of plant names), and fascinating tales from history.

Jessica's Notes: Includes personal stories, field experiences, or heartfelt reflections from my time working with specific plants. These notes bring the plants to life through a lived relationship.

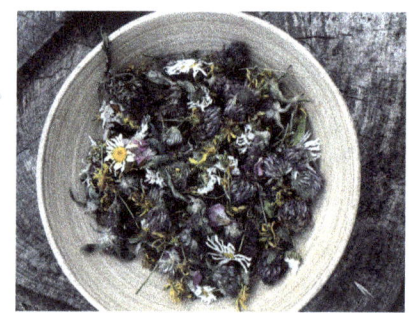

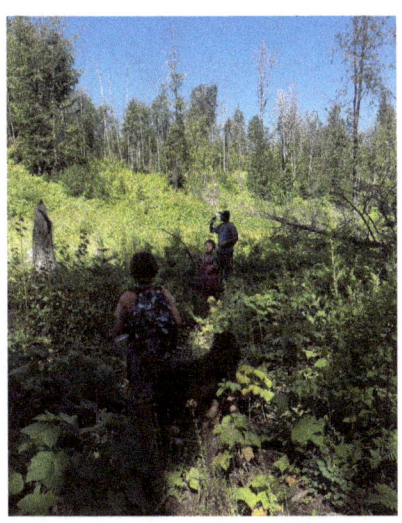

Foraging Ethics

- Always ask for permission—whether from the landowner or through required permits. It is illegal to harvest in state parks, but it is often legal (with some exceptions) in national forests. Also, ask the plants for permission and observe closely. Are they healthy? Are they thriving?

- Only harvest what you need. Leave plenty behind for other forest creatures—birds, bees, and unseen beings who also rely on the wild.

- Harvest during the appropriate season. Know the right time for each plant's gift.

- Ensure the area is not polluted or sprayed with chemicals.

- Be 100% certain of the plant you are harvesting.

- Leave no trace. Pick up any trash you find—the land will thank you.

What Is In A Plant Name?

Etymology and Taxonomy

Each plant has many common names. To simplify, I have chosen the ones most relevant to me and my local community. Many of these names are steeped in folklore and ancient history, helping us connect with and better remember each plant. We are wired to learn through stories and word of mouth, and plant names often carry these oral traditions forward.

I have also included each plant's scientific name and its classification within the plant kingdom. Because of the confusion that arises from multiple common names, Swedish botanist Carl Linnaeus (1707–1778) developed the system of botanical classification in Latin (influenced by Greek roots). Known as the father of taxonomy, Linnaeus created a system we still use today, though it has evolved. Latin names are always italicized. Each plant's binomial (two-part) name consists of a genus and a species. The genus is capitalized, the species is not. Think of it like a first and last name: for example, I come from the genus *Freeborn*, previously classified under *Ballew*, and I am the *jessica* species.

Scientific names are important because they enable us to be precise about the plants we are working with, especially when harvesting or consuming them. A name is just a name, and names can be forgotten or confused. It is like running into an acquaintance and forgetting their name—but still remembering the scent of their perfume. Names can aid our memory, but they do not tell us what a plant looks like, smells like, tastes like, or where it grows. To add to the complexity, botanists sometimes reclassify a plant's family based on new insights into its phytochemical composition.

As you go out and forage, you will begin to notice the diversity and uniqueness of each plant. I have seen hybrids and distinct variations depending on where and how the plant grows. Like people, plants can develop their own personality as they mature. This is what makes foraging so endlessly fascinating. So do not judge a book—or a plant—by its cover. Learn the names to help organize your knowledge, but truly get to *know* the plant before making assumptions.

When teaching about wild plants, I encourage my students to find creative ways to memorize plant names—through rhymes or melodies, such as "I am liking the lichen!" or "Sedum, you eat 'em!" Learning the historical and esoteric associations can also be helpful in this process. For instance, *Achillea millefolium* (yarrow) is named after the Greek hero Achilles, who used the plant to make himself invincible. The Latin name itself offers clues: *millefolium* means "a thousand leaves" (*mille* = thousand, *folium* = leaf). Take a close look at yarrow and you will see why.

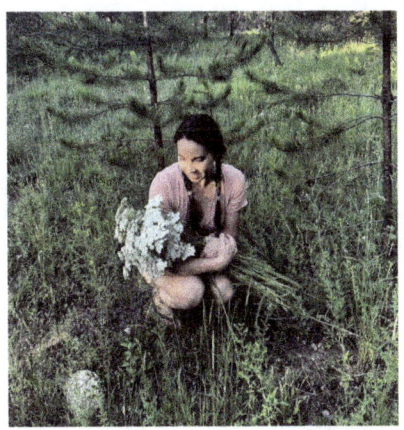

Acknowledgements

This book is the fruit of many seasons of learning, gathering, and growing—and it could not have been written alone. I am deeply grateful to all who have walked this path with me.

To my family: thank you for your patience and encouragement as I disappeared into the woods with baskets and books, and later into long hours of writing and editing. Your love anchors me.

To my dear forest students: your curiosity and joy have reignited my own wonder, again and again. Teaching you has been one of my life's greatest honors. You have inspired much of what blooms on these pages.

To the wise herbalists, elders, teachers, authors, and plant lovers whose works have informed and guided my understanding: thank you for lighting the way and reminding us of our ancient connection to the plants.

To the Freeborn Family Forest School and the wider foraging community: thank you for your friendship, support, and commitment to sharing this knowledge with respect and integrity.

To the ancestors: both of blood and spirit—who lived in close relationship with the land, who gathered wild food and medicine long before these teachings were written down—I honor your wisdom and give thanks.

And lastly, to the plants themselves—my teachers, companions, and healers. Thank you for your generosity, resilience, and quiet grace. You have changed my life.

May this book serve as a humble offering in return of the wild wisdom and gifts received.

ACKNOWLEDGEMENTS

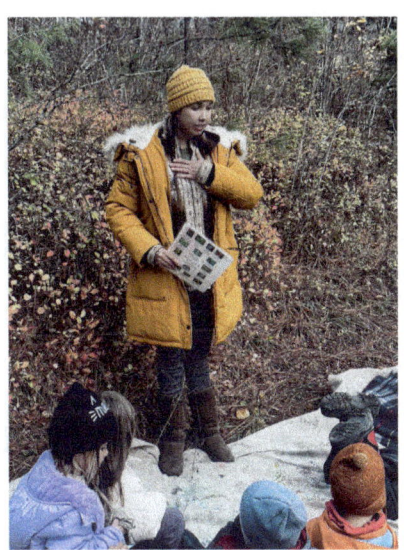

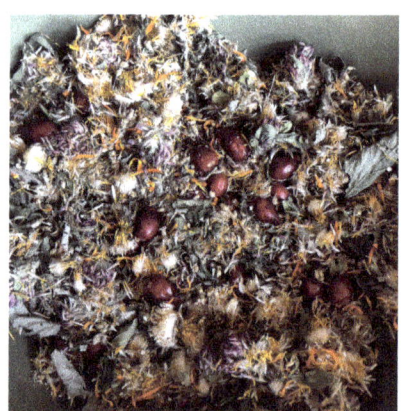

Dedication

This book is dedicated first and foremost to Almighty God, the Creator of all plant medicines—gifts of healing and nourishment provided for us in perfect wisdom. Everything we need to grow, to heal, and to thrive has been lovingly placed upon this earth. *"...herb for the service of man: that he may bring forth food out of the earth."* —Psalm 104

To my brilliant and beautiful boys, Jacob and Jared—thank you for teaching me so much through our shared explorations. I love you more deeply than words on these pages could ever express.

To all my forest students who have so richly blessed my life, I wish you abundant joy and discovery on your foraging journeys. May this guide serve you well as you blaze your own trails and come to know the healing plants that await. And remember—eat something wild every day.

To my husband and forever foraging partner, Jason—thank you for walking beside me on this path, for learning the plants with me, for teaching and inspiring me daily, and for keeping me safe as we wander mountains and unknown terrain. Much of the knowledge within these pages is grounded in your firsthand experience as a forest farmer and lover of wild places. It is no wonder you were born on Earth Day! This book would not exist without your steadfast support.

I would also like to dedicate this book to Craig Welsh, my stepfather, "Fajah," who raised me into the medicine woman I am today. He passed away as I was editing this book. Bittersweet that I was birthing this book as he was crossing the rainbow bridge. The Welsh Woods, Fajah Craig's 5-acre pine forest, was my first Idaho classroom, and Fajah cleared the trails to access the wild woods.

DEDICATION

To the miraculous plants featured in this book, I dedicate my love, time, and energy to the flora of the wild terrain. These are the plants I have known, harvested, and worked with through the seasons. They have kept me, my family, and our forest tribe strong, healthy, and resilient.

Lastly, this book is dedicated to the "step-over plants"—the ones dismissed as weeds, eradicated, and forgotten. Though trampled and sprayed, they endure as "people's plants." Once beloved and domesticated across cultures, many now grow quietly in the margins. May we never forget them. In reverence, I honor their resilience and their quiet, steadfast power.

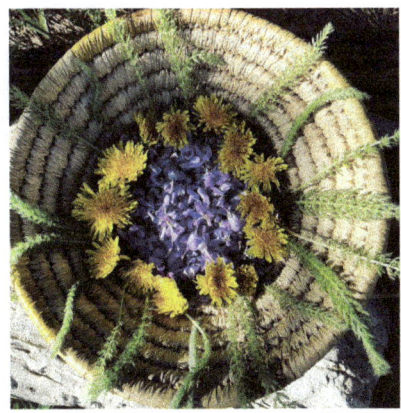

Reclaimer

May this book inspire you to wander into the wild, to question everything, and to become a steward of the healing plants that await you.

Instead of a disclaimer, I offer a Reclaimer—an invitation for you to reclaim your health, your intuition, and your deep relationship with the healing power of plants. This book is intended to awaken your divine right to understand and work with the plant medicine that surrounds you. It is intended to inspire you to research, explore, and deepen your connection with the plants that grow close to home.

The information shared here is for educational purposes only and is not intended to treat, diagnose, or cure any medical condition. These words reflect my personal journey, research, and experience. They are not to be copied or plagiarized. The responsibility for reclaiming your health lies with you, the reader. Trust your intuition. Honor your own healing path. The author is not liable for any injuries that may result from working with the plants described. I encourage you to approach this work with humility and reverence: take a moment to say a prayer, ask for guidance, and listen deeply. We all have access to ancient, collective wisdom. It is time to remember.

Plant medicine is original medicine. Healing is sacred. It happens through mindful, prayerful intention. Whether wildcrafting or cultivating your own medicine, do so with love and care.

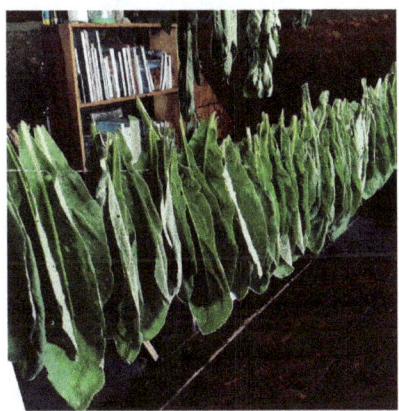

Collecting and Preserving

Collecting wild plants is my favorite part of the whole medicine-making gig. I suit up with my foraging belt, bag, gardening shears, and digging knife. Sometimes I bring a large basket, depending on the day's haul. After collecting, I rinse anything dirty and then begin the drying process.

Preserving your harvest is simple. We air-dry delicate herbs in bunches, often using drying racks in a well-ventilated space out of direct sunlight. For denser plant materials, we use a dehydrator or sometimes a low-heated oven (taking care not to burn them!). When dried properly, herbs can last for years; however, fading pigment is a good indication that they have lost potency.

Our medicine chest is a wall of mason jars filled with wildcrafted herbs, roots, tree medicine, and mushrooms. Miraculously, we always seem to have just enough to get us through the year, and we conveniently run low just in time for spring, when the wild garden calls again. It is a beautiful rhythm. Winter becomes a time of rest and regeneration for both land and gatherer.

In winter, we turn our stockpile into finished medicine: tinctures, infusions, extracts, oils, salves, ointments, incense cones, and more. Bringing the wilderness indoors with wild-harvested remedies is a powerful way to lift the winter blues. Boughs of cedar and evergreen brighten the darkest days, filling the home with life and scent.

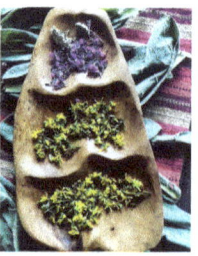

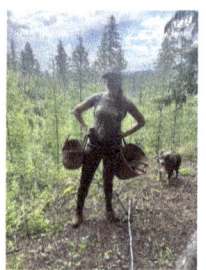

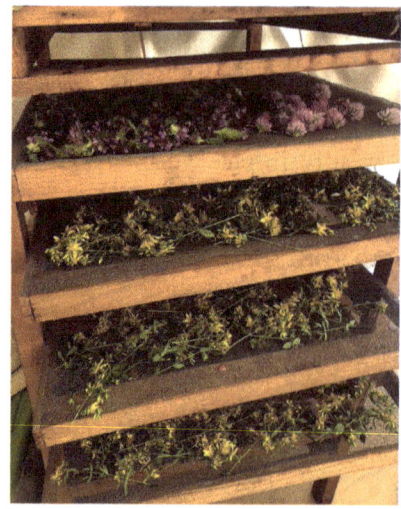

Wild Versus Domesticated

To Be Native or Invasive? That Is The Question...

Some of the plants discussed in this book may not be considered native to North America, depending on your definition of "native." Many traveled great distances to become naturalized here, either intentionally or accidentally, having been brought by people from around the world. Just like our human communities, these plants are a melting pot.

To me, "native" includes plants that have domesticated *themselves*, thriving in untamed forests and countrysides without cultivation. The plants I have chosen to include are those I have personally encountered during my foraging journey and believe are essential for healing and wellness. Many are often overlooked or dismissed as weeds and quickly eradicated.

However, this overlooks their value. We have strayed from the shared wisdom of our ancestors. Through this book, I hope to shine a light on the forgotten wild wisdom of plants and rekindle the forager within each of us. As I have explored, I have uncovered a treasure trove of folklore and mythology. These stories reconnect us to the natural world and the enduring medicine it holds.

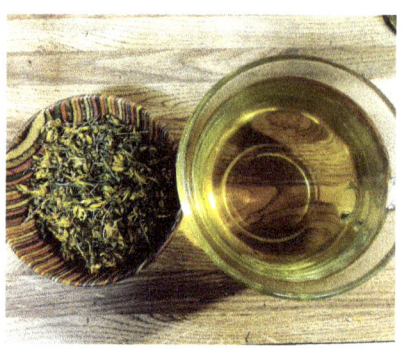

Dosages

One Size Does Not Fit All

Many people ask me about dosage and how to determine the right amount of herbs to use. I tell them to relax and trust their intuition. Start small and work with the plant in a traditional manner. I am a huge advocate of taking plant medicine as tea—hydrating, gentle, and easy to digest. Begin with a single herb to understand how it feels in your body, and from there, you can build confidence in formulating combinations tailored to your unique needs.

Part of my lesson plan with students includes sharing a tea ceremony that incorporates wild-harvested plants. I have even become known as the **tea-cher**.

Raw wild greens can sometimes contain alkaloids and oxalates, which may be harmful to the kidneys when consumed in excess. Cooking certain plants can help neutralize these compounds. Always taste a small sample first and see how it agrees with you. Some people may experience allergic reactions or sensitivities, such as a rash or digestive upset. For children and babies, a simple skin patch test is a great precaution: gently rub the plant on a tender area, such as the underside of the wrist, and wait 10 minutes to observe any reaction.

How to Properly Dose Children

Children are smaller than adults and therefore require smaller doses. I usually wait until a baby is over one year old before working with certain herbs, though very gentle herbs may be appropriate in smaller amounts. Here is a simple guideline based on an adult dosage of 1 cup (240 mL):

- **Under 1 year:** ½ to 1 teaspoon (3–5 mL)

DOSAGES

- **Ages 1–2:** 1 to 2 teaspoons (5–10 mL)
- **Ages 3–7:** 2 teaspoons to 2 tablespoons (10–30 mL)
- **Ages 8–12:** 2 to 4 tablespoons per day
- **Ages 13–18:** Full adult dose (¾ to 1 cup), depending on the herb

Always consider the strength of the herb and the child's constitution. When in doubt, go slow and observe.

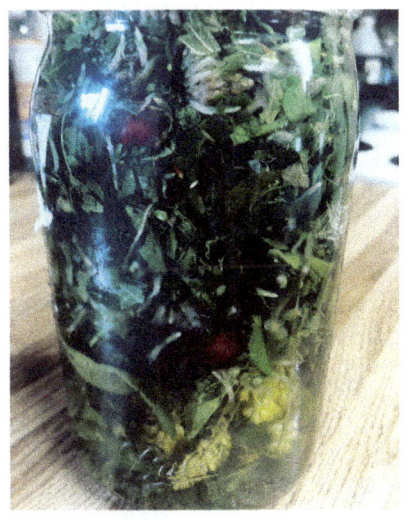

The Doctrine Of Signatures

The Other Language of Flowers

To make sense of the natural world, many ancient herbalists believed that plants were stamped with images of their healing properties by the Creator. The concept held that a plant's appearance, scent, environment, shape, and color could offer clues to its medicinal purpose and the bodily systems it supports.

This idea, known as the **Doctrine of Signatures**, is an ancient, metaphysical approach to herbalism. For instance, walnuts resemble the brain and are rich in Omega-3 fatty acids and B vitamins, both of which support brain function. Wild ginger has heart-shaped leaves—perhaps hinting at its ability to stimulate circulation and benefit the heart. Horsetail (Equisetum) resembles a horse's tail, suggesting its value for strengthening hair. Bright yellow roots, like those of Oregon grape or devil's club, point to their usefulness in clearing bile, a similarly yellow substance associated with liver function.

Though modern science tends to dismiss this doctrine, I find it useful as a way to remember and relate to plant medicine. It is an intuitive approach that blends observation, imagination, and deep listening. The Doctrine of Signatures is rooted in ancient teachings, dating back to Plato, who spoke of the **eidos**—the idea, essence, or archetype that underlies all forms.

"The Signatures likewise are taken notice of, they being as it were the book out of which the ancients first learned the vertues of herbes; Nature or rather the God of nature, having stamped on divers of them legible characters to discover their uses."— *William Coles, Adam in Eden (1657)*

Using this concept while foraging invites you to dance between the mystical and the practical sides of herbalism. Nineteenth-century American historian and novelist Edward Eggleston observed, *"The wild woods were full of creatures (flora and fauna) whose value was written on each of them in the language of signatures...considerately tagged at the creation"* (Eggleston, 1901, p. 55). I resonate deeply with this notion. When I am out foraging in the forest, I often notice subtle connections between a plant's form and its function—shapes, colors, and textures that seem to speak their purpose if we take the time to listen.□

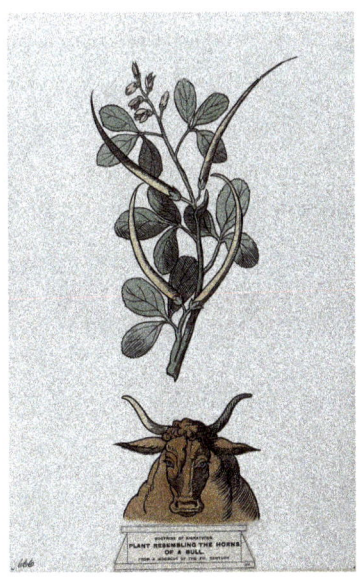

Fig. 1
Doctrine of signatures: a plant with seed-pods resembling the horns of a bull, above, and a bull's head, below
(coloured ink drawing, c. 1923). Wellcome Library, London; photo no. V0025791. CC BY 4.0.

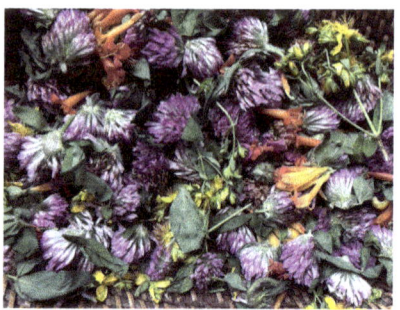

Herbs and Flowers

People's Plants

We begin with the sometimes delicate, yet potent and beautiful herbs and flowers of the wild garden. Simply looking upon their blooms can be therapeutic—a feast for the eyes and balm for the spirit.

These familiar friends often travel with us, thriving where people live and wander. Found on nearly every continent and easily planted in any cottage garden, they are what I like to call *people's plants*. Accessible, resilient, and generous, these wild weeds have walked beside us for generations.

Their healing gifts are profound. Rich in nutrients and potent in their medicine, these plants offer restoration not just for the body, but also for the heart and mind. To connect with them is to feel at home, no matter where your feet are planted.

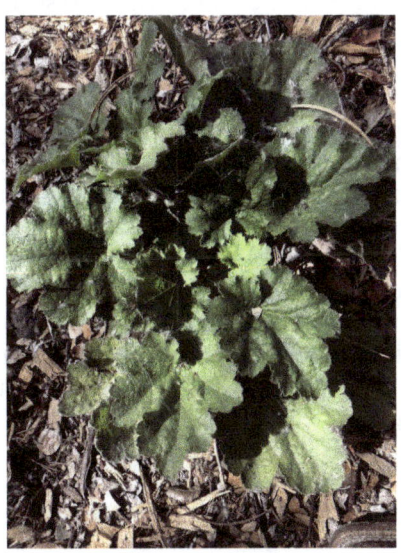

Alumroot

Heuchera parviflora

Saxifragaceae (Saxifrage) Family
Other common names: round leaf alumroot, little leaf alumroot, pink alumroot, coralbells, common alumroot, Heuchera
 Description: Alumroot is a low-growing, herbaceous perennial ground cover with bright green, heart-shaped leaves that are lobed and often form a dense mat. Its delicate flowers have a 5-lobed calyx and typically lack actual petals—the calyx itself is petal-like and serves as the showy part of the bloom. Flowers are usually yellowish-white with a greenish hue and grow in a spiked formation. Some varieties, such as the popular garden cultivar 'Coralbells', feature dainty pink flowers atop slender stalks that range from 2 inches to 1 foot tall. Below ground, the plant anchors itself with a stout, knotty, fibrous taproot.
 Where it grows: A widespread mountain plant, Alumroot thrives in subalpine forests, sunny meadows, disturbed soils, and along rocky slopes or ledges. Its adaptability makes it a common sight in the inland Northwest and throughout the West's mountain ranges.
 When and how to harvest: Harvest the rhizomes when the plant is dormant, typically in late fall or early spring, after the plant has rested

through winter. Fresh roots can be gathered year-round, provided they are gathered with care and reverence. Because harvesting roots means taking the life force of the plant, I harvest sparingly—only from colonies where other healthy Alumroot plants are nearby to ensure sustainability.

How to work with it/ Medicinal use: Alumroot gets its name from the powerful astringency in its root, similar to that of alum. This quality makes it especially beneficial in herbal first aid and digestive care. The root can be chewed to help with mouth sores, bleeding gums, sore throats, and even acid reflux or mild cases of food poisoning. It can also be rubbed directly on a teething baby's gums—just a tiny bit goes a long way. Externally, the mashed fresh root or an ointment made from it soothes minor burns, scrapes, cuts, and irritated skin. A sitz bath made from a decoction of the root can be beneficial for postpartum care and minor vaginal discomfort. Alumroot leaves, rich in tannins, are also a folk trick for pickling, helping keep vegetables crisp.

Healing constituents / Therapeutic actions: Alumroot contains flavonoids, ellagitannins, and gallotannins, giving it potent astringent and styptic actions. It is traditionally used to tone tissues and reduce inflammation.

Note of caution: Due to its high tannin content, Alumroot should be used in moderation and only for short periods. Overuse may irritate the kidneys. Occasional use is generally safe during pregnancy, but daily consumption should be avoided unless advised by a trusted herbalist or midwife.

Historical connection: The Blackfoot tribe and other Indigenous peoples used Alumroot roots as a gastrointestinal aid and topical medicine for wounds and burns. Early settlers, familiar with its strong astringency, used it to make homemade toothpaste by combining the powdered root with cream of tartar. Alumroot held a place in the U.S. Pharmacopoeia from 1820 to 1882 and was a respected remedy in the Eclectic medicine movement of the 19th century. The Eclectics adopted and refined many plant-based remedies through clinical observation, including Heuchera species, which were prized for their astringent, styptic, and tonic effects.

Jessica's notes: One of my favorite ways to help students connect with plants is through sensory exploration. At Forest School, I sometimes dare them to chew a small quantity of the root, to see what it feels like. The intense drying sensation caused by the tannins leaves no doubt about its astringency! It is a powerful teaching moment.

Cultivated forms of Alumroot, known as coral bells, are often grown in ornamental gardens, although they are hybrids of their wild cousins. When I think of *Heuchera*, I am reminded of this sweet folk tune, often sung in rounds around a campfire with girl scouts. It was first published in a Brownie Girl's Guide in 1975: *"White coralbells, upon a slender stalk, Lilies-of-the-valley deck my garden walk. Oh, don't you wish that you might hear them ring? That will happen only when the fairies sing."*

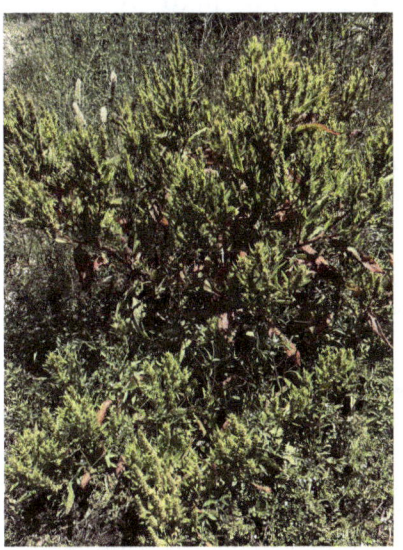

Amaranth

Amaranthus viridis

Amaranthaceae (Amaranth) Family
Other common names: Green Amaranth
Description: Amaranth is a vibrant, versatile plant that ranges in height from six inches to six feet. Its seeds cluster at the top of the plant, while the leaves, typically a bright lime green, are pointed and smooth-edged. Though Green Amaranth is most commonly this vivid green, other species in the Amaranth family may display red, bronze, or deep purple hues. A waxy, shimmering coating gives the entire plant a subtle luster under sunlight. The seeds also vary in color, from pale green to deep red and purple. There are over 70 recognized species in the *Amaranthus* genus, many of which are edible and have medicinal properties.
Where it grows: Green Amaranth is a prolific and adaptable plant, often found growing wild along roadsides, in gardens, hedgerows, and disturbed soils. Although it is technically an annual, in warmer climates it can behave like a short-lived perennial. It is drought-tolerant and thrives in full sun, often emerging in areas where other plants struggle to grow.
When and how to harvest: Harvest the young, tender leaves in spring and early summer, when they are at their most nutritious and palatable.

Seeds are best collected in late summer through early fall when the seed heads have fully matured and begin to dry. Allow the seeds to dry completely before winnowing and storing.

How to work with it / Medicinal use: The greens are mild, tender, and can be used much like spinach. They are excellent sautéed, steamed, added to soups, or eaten raw in salads. The seeds, similar to quinoa in texture and nutrition, can be cooked like a grain or ground into a gluten-free flour. Amaranth is considered a superfood due to its high nutritional value. Its combination of minerals and protein supports bone strength, recovery after illness, and overall vitality. Traditionally, the plant has also been used to promote healing from inflammation and support a healthy digestive system.

Healing constituents / Therapeutic actions: Green Amaranth is rich in dietary fiber, vitamins A and C, riboflavin, calcium, zinc, copper, and manganese. It is also a good source of lysine-rich protein and contains antioxidant compounds that help reduce inflammation and oxidative stress. The nutrients in both the leaves and seeds contribute to anti-inflammatory, alkalizing, and potentially anticancer effects. While many traditional uses have been passed down through generations, modern research continues to explore the full spectrum of its health benefits.

Historical connection: The name *Amaranthus* originates from the Greek "amarantos," meaning "unfading" or "immortal," which refers to the plant's long-lasting flowers and hardy nature. Amaranth was first cultivated in Central and South America around 6,000 to 8,000 years ago and was a sacred staple crop of the Aztecs. They incorporated the grain into religious rituals, even crafting statues of their gods from amaranth flour and honey—statues that were later ceremonially broken and eaten. This ritual use alarmed Spanish conquistadors, and in 1521, under Hernán Cortés, the use of amaranth was outlawed. Fields were burned, and those who cultivated the grain were punished. Although suppressed, amaranth survived in secret and was reintroduced to wider cultivation in the United States in the 1970s, though it likely persisted unnoticed for much longer.

Jessica's notes: Harvesting amaranth seeds is a meditative act. The process is slow and requires patience, but that is part of its beauty. These repetitive, grounding tasks have a way of bringing me back to the present moment. Sometimes, I use the time for quiet prayer; other times, I invite a friend to join in and we muse on life while we winnow the seeds. In today's fast-paced world, there is something profoundly healing about these old, rhythmic rituals of seed saving and hand-harvesting nourishment from the land.

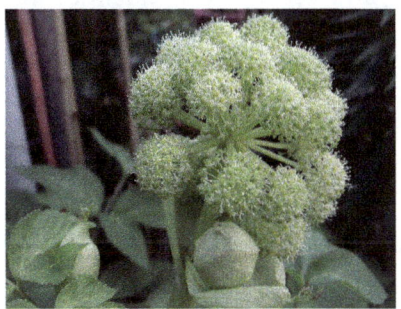

Angelica

Angelica archangelica

Apiaceae (Carrot) Family
Other common names: Wild Celery, Norwegian Angelica
Description: Angelica is a striking, upright herb that can reach heights of 3 to 9 feet. Its large, bipinnately compound leaves and prominent petiole sheaths at the base make it a standout in the wild. The delicate white flowers bloom in flat-topped umbels, a classic trait of the carrot family. Its stout taproot has a purplish tinge and grows deep and strong. Angelica is typically a biennial or short-lived perennial. Due to its close resemblance to poisonous lookalikes such as water hemlock, poison hemlock, and giant hogweed, accurate identification is crucial.

Where it grows: You will find Angelica near creeks and streambanks, where moisture is abundant. It thrives in swampy woodlands, floodplains, and river edges, often gracing these spaces with its tall, elegant stalks and delicate blooms.

When and how to harvest: Harvest the roots in early spring or late fall, ideally before the plant is older than two years. These younger roots are more potent and easier to work with. Seeds are ready for collection in late summer to early fall. As always, be mindful and respectful—harvest only what you need and be certain of your plant ID.

How to work with it / Medicinal use: Angelica is a powerful aromatic and warming herb, often described as a gift for digestive and respiratory complaints. It is beneficial for infants with colic or flatulence and can be made into a tincture from either fresh or dried roots. The seeds are aromatic and versatile, and can be infused into oils, honeys, glycerites, or alcohol-based tinctures. For infants or young children, the alcohol can be evaporated off through gentle heating.

Topically, Angelica is prized for massage oils, soaps, and bath preparations. Its warming and decongesting qualities stimulate the lymphatic system and ease conditions such as arthritis, rheumatism, fluid retention, and fatigue. As a nervine, it helps restore energy in states of burnout and tension. For respiratory conditions, its expectorant and decongestant actions make it helpful for chronic bronchial asthma, sinus congestion, or lingering chest colds. Use it in decoction, gently simmered in water, to extract its medicinal properties.

Angelica also has emmenagogue properties and may help bring on delayed menstruation or relieve cramping. It has been whispered through folklore that smoking the dried leaves could induce visions, though such practices are rare and should be approached with caution and reverence.

Healing constituents / Therapeutic actions: Angelica contains volatile oils, including α-pinene, limonene, and osthol, as well as furanocoumarins, flavonoids, and bitter principles. Its actions include: anti-spasmodic, antimicrobial, astringent, aromatic, anti-inflammatory, bitter, carminative, cholagogue, depurative, diaphoretic, digestive, diuretic, emmenagogue, expectorant, nervine, and stomachic.

Historical connections: The name *Angelica* is derived from the Greek *angelos*, meaning "messenger" or "archangel." The herb is steeped in folklore and legend. One tale recounts how an angel revealed the plant's healing powers to a monk during the 17th-century plague years. Angelica became known as "The Root of the Holy Ghost," believed to protect against contagion, evil spirits, and witchcraft.

John Gerard, in his famed *Herball or Historie of Plants* (1597), wrote of its power:

"If you doe take a piece of the roote and holde it in your mouth or chew the same between your teeth it doth most certainly drive away the pestilential aire, yea although the corrupt aire have possessed the hart, yet it driveth it out again."

This may be a poetic reference to its pungent aroma and digestive-relieving properties, particularly helpful in treating flatulence or the "bad airs" once believed to cause illness.

Caution: Angelica must be carefully identified before harvest. Its resemblance to toxic plants like poison hemlock and water hemlock makes foraging risky without proper knowledge. Key identifiers include its greenish or slightly purple stem (unspotted), the rounded shape of its umbels (in contrast to the flatter ones of hemlock), and its strong, sweet aroma (in contrast to hemlock's foul, mousey odor). Angelica contains furanocoumarins, which can cause photosensitivity. Avoid topical use followed by sun exposure unless precautions are taken.

Jessica's notes: Angelica is one of those ancient herbs that carries both mystery and practicality. When I work with its roots—digging, washing, chopping—I feel transported to another time. I imagine what it must have felt like centuries ago to reach for this plant in a time of sickness, placing hope in its angelic name and healing powers.

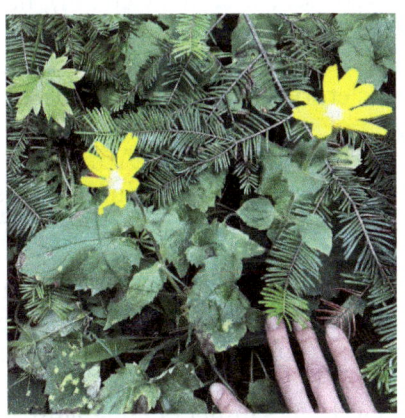

Arnica

Arnica cordifolia

Asteraceae (Daisy) Family

Description: This pubescent (covered with downy hair), short-lived, perennial has leaves that are heart-shaped and simple (not divided into leaflets), that bear radiate yellow, tubular disk flowers atop a two-foot stem.

Where it Grows: Heartleaf Arnica prefers subalpine fir forests and high mountain meadows. The mini yellow flowers brighten up the forest floor and fields in springtime. Simply looking at this bright yellow flower is a form of medicine.

When and how to harvest: Gather the flowering tops in late spring/early summer. It is a short-lived plant, so harvest it while it is in flower. Wear gloves while harvesting. Arnica contains a compound called Helanin, which can irritate the skin.

How to work with it/ Medicinal use: Arnica helps reduce pain through its anti-inflammatory properties, making it an excellent choice for poultices, salves, creams, ointments, massage oils, and liniments. Apply topically to promote healing on bruises, sprains, muscle aches, joint pain, inflammation from insect bites, and swelling from broken bones. Do not apply it to an open wound or abrasion. For internal use, it is best consumed diluted in a homeopathic application. In its homeopathic dilution, Arnica is used to treat trauma both internally and externally. It is toxic to ingest the plant in its raw form, but it is a powerful medicine when applied topically.

Healing Constituents/Therapeutic Actions: Key compounds include sesquiterpene lactones (notably helenalin), flavonoids, terpenoids, phenolic acids, essential oils, mucilage, and polysaccharides. These contribute to Arnica's antibacterial, antifungal, antiseptic, anti-inflammatory, antioxidant, and antisclerotic effects. It is considered a first-aid medicinal herb for trauma.

Historical Connection: Historically, Arnica was used as a cardiovascular stimulant. A small dose of arnica tincture was once used to treat acute heart weakness associated with aging, cardiovascular disease, or other episodes that result in heart weakness. This historical application may not be the most effective treatment for heart disease today, as we now understand the connection between cardiovascular disease and inflammation. Hawthorn may be a more suitable approach to alleviate heart conditions.

Arnica has been a staple of homeopathic medicine since its introduction in 1796 by German physician Samuel Hahnemann.

Jessica's Notes: Arnica has proven to be one of our most dependable first-aid allies. I always keep it in our herbal toolkit for treating bruises, sprains, and inflammation. I have watched Arnica ointment prevent bruising in toddlers and soothe sore muscles after forest school adventures. We also turn to it for recovery after childbirth or surgery. I have noticed that our wildcrafted Arnica ointments feel more potent and soothing than those purchased from stores. The forest's touch makes a difference.

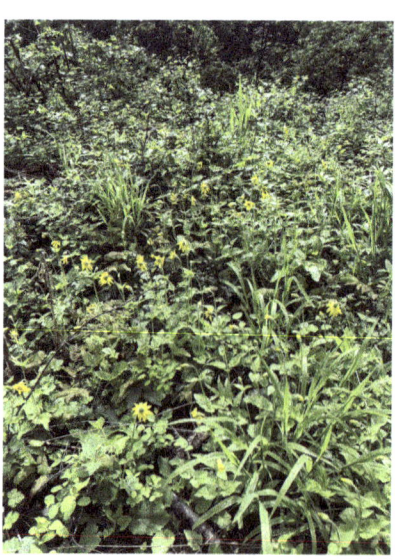

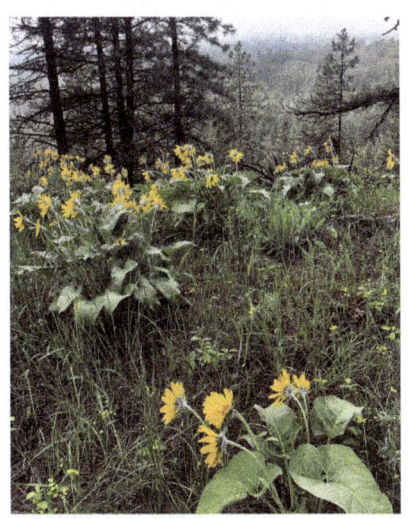

Arrowleaf Balsamroot

Balsamorhiza sagittata

Heliantheae (Sunflower) Family

Description: This perennial's long, basal, silvery-green, arrow-shaped leaves are a key giveaway of Arrowleaf Balsamroot. Its roots are legendary—able to survive forest fires and live for over forty years. In early spring, the plant produces radiant yellow, sunflower-like blooms that rise above the leaves on tall, slender stems. Underground, the roots can grow to the size of a human head, with some weighing up to thirty pounds. These roots are rich in resin and have a pungent, pine-like scent that speaks to their potency.

Where it grows: Arrowleaf Balsamroot thrives on open hillsides, prairies, and sun-drenched, south-facing slopes. It prefers dry, well-drained soils and is often found in large colonies in the inland Northwest.

When and how to harvest: The roots are bulbous and rugged, with a large central taproot and many side shoots. Harvest in late summer or early fall, when the plant is dormant. Use care and conservation—take only one root from each colony. These roots are enormous and powerful; one is often more than enough. I recommend using a Pulaski, strong hands, and plenty of patience to dig out this resinous treasure.

How to work with it/ Medicinal use: Arrowleaf Balsamroot is a powerful stimulant and expectorant. Its root is most effective when prepared as a tincture, particularly for acute to subacute bronchitis accompanied by thick mucus and phlegm. It also makes a potent honey-based syrup for dry or irritating coughs. Though not widely used by modern herbalists, I believe this plant deserves a revival.

A strong decoction or extract effectively captures its medicinal properties. The root can be shredded and used in a poultice for bites, blisters, sores, bruises, and wounds. A leaf poultice is an excellent treatment for burns. The root infusion has traditionally been used for fevers, headaches, whooping cough, tuberculosis, stomachaches, and even as a birthing aid. It can also serve as a coffee substitute!

Internally, the plant functions as an immune stimulant; externally, its antibacterial and antifungal properties make it useful in liniments or salves. For athlete's foot or fungal conditions, infuse the crushed root in rubbing alcohol. For skin healing, infuse in oil and use it as a base for an antibacterial balm.

I often use the tincture in a throat spray and sometimes add honey to create a pleasant and effective cough remedy.

Healing Constituents/ Therapeutic actions: Arrowleaf Balsamroot contains dihydroxy-cycloartenol, hydroxy-cycloartenol, cinnamic acid, eudesmols (alpha and beta), carnosol, beta-selinene, montarusin, and several other compounds that give it its antibacterial, antifungal, and immune-enhancing effects. These phytochemicals make it valuable for both internal and external applications.

Historical connection: Among the Great Basin tribes, Balsamroot was a prized medicinal herb for the lungs. It was traditionally used to treat whooping cough, bronchitis, and other respiratory ailments. The ash of the leaves was applied as a burn remedy. This plant has long held a significant place in Indigenous healing traditions across the Western United States.

Jessica's notes: Our first Balsamroot harvest was on my grandparents' land in Goldendale, Washington. When we unearthed the enormous, sap-heavy root, I briefly mistook it for a ponderosa pine. The preparation was memorable—shredding the resin-rich root into strips by hand was a lesson in respect for the plant's strength. There is no substitute for working with the plant yourself. You engage all your senses, and in doing so, you develop a deeper understanding of the plant's character and medicine.

ARROWLEAF BALSAMROOT

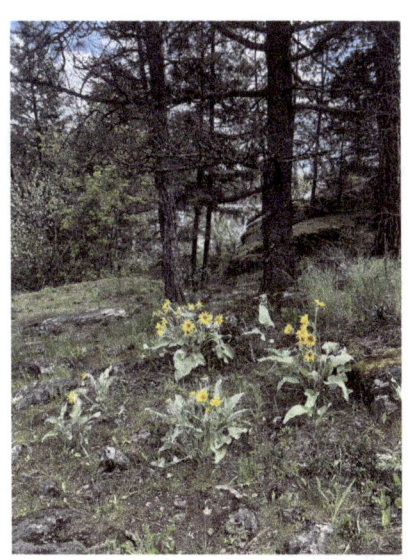

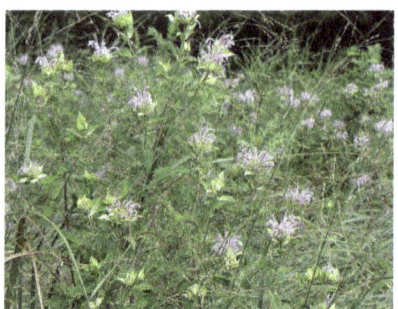

Bee Balm

Monarda fistulosa

Lamiaceae (Mint) Family

Other common names: wild bergamot, sweet leaf, horsemint, oregano de la Sierra

Description: Bee Balm is a member of the mint family, with the typical square stem, holding large, oval, green-gray leaves. The plants stand 2 to 3 feet tall. The pinkish to scarlet red tubular flowers in terminal whorls appear in summer and look like fireworks that attract butterflies, bees, and hummingbirds. This reminds me to go out looking for it around the 4th of July, as it blooms from June to September.

Where it grows: Bee balm prefers to grow at higher elevations in moist, well-drained soil. It is found in alpine meadows along running or dry creek beds, fields, and clearings. This aromatic perennial stands out when in full bloom, covering a vast area of wild meadows.

When and how to harvest: Harvest the leaves from late spring to summer. The flowers can be harvested when they are in full bloom, typically in mid-to-late summer.

How to work with it/ Medicinal use: Dry the leaves and flowers for tea. Use leaves in Mexican or Italian cooking as an oregano substitute, or infuse in butter to add a savory herbal note. Steam inhalation with Bee Balm eases sinus and lung congestion. Poultices made from the plant relieve burns, wounds, and rheumatic pain. Honey infusions serve as effective cough syrups. Tinctures may help with menstrual cramps and stomach discomfort. Bee Balm tea soothes gas and upset stomachs.

Monarda acts as a nervine tonic, calming the nervous system and easing anxiety in adults and children alike. Topical salves promote the healing of wounds and skin infections. Traditionally, Bee Balm has been used to treat colds, flu, sore throat, congestion, gas, diarrhea, and nausea.

Healing constituents/ Therapeutic actions: Bee Balm contains thymol, a potent antimicrobial and antiseptic. It exhibits aromatic, diaphoretic, antiseptic, antimicrobial, emmenagogue, antispasmodic, carminative, anti-inflammatory, diuretic, expectorant, bitter tonic, sedative, and local anesthetic properties.

Historical connections: Native to North America, Monarda has been used for thousands of years by many Native American tribes. It was used to treat fevers, coughs, congestion, infections, insect bites, and venomous bites, and served as a food preservative and flavoring agent for meats. Steam inhalation was also used in ceremonial sweat lodges. The red flowering bee balm, *M. didyma,* was an ingredient in the blend of native plants made into "Liberty Tea," which colonists drank in protest of the tea tax from England after the Boston Tea Party. The genus "Monarda" originates from the Spanish physician and botanist, Dr. Nicholas Monardes (1493-1588). He wrote the book "Joyful News: The Botany of the New World." Interestingly, he had never visited North America, but his people had sent him seeds for his gardens in Spain. John Bartram (March 23, 1699 - September 22, 1777), an American-born botanist, horticulturalist, and explorer who lived in Philadelphia, is said to have sent Monarda seeds to England in the mid-1700s, where the plant is known today as Bee Balm or Wild Bergamot, not Gold Melissa or Indian Nettle. Bartram made notable contributions to the collection, study, and international publicizing of North American flora and fauna, and was a frontiersman in importing and cultivating non-native plants. In the early 1730s, he established the Bartram Botanic Garden and Nursery near Philadelphia.

Jessica's notes: Bee Balm flowering tops and leaves are a staple in my winter medicine chest. I like to add Monarda to teas with other respiratory supportive herbs to help relieve coughing fits and the common cold. I also enjoy its perennial return in my healing garden, where the hummingbirds drink nectar from the hot pink flowers.

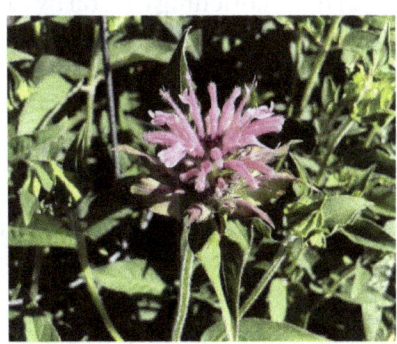

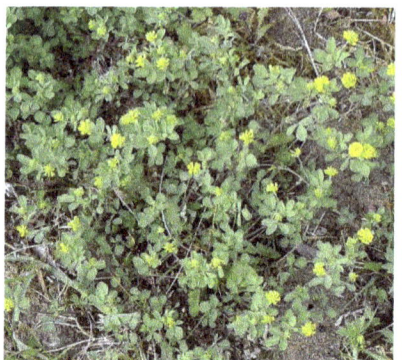

Black Medic

Medicago lupulina

Fabaceae (Legume) Family
Other common names: Hop Clover, Black Clover, Yellow Trefoil

Description: Black Medic is a low-growing, creeping annual legume with many-branched, slender, and slightly hairy stems. Its leaves are trifoliate—composed of three leaflets—arranged alternately along the stem. Small yellow flowers form tight, hop-like clusters that bloom in spring and summer, later turning into tiny, hard black seed pods that give the plant its name.

Where it grows: This common groundcover thrives in lawns, meadows, roadsides, disturbed areas, and fodder fields. Like its clover cousins, Black Medic is a nitrogen fixer, enriching the soil by capturing atmospheric nitrogen through symbiotic relationships with bacteria that reside in its roots.

When and how to harvest: Harvest the leaves and flowers in late spring through summer, ideally before they dry or go to seed. Select healthy-looking plants that are growing in clean, chemical-free environments.

How to work with it / Medicinal use: Use the tender leaves and flowers in soups, stir-fries, or dry them for herbal teas. Due to the plant's fibrous nature, it is best to lightly cook or steam the leaves before consuming. The fiber supports healthy digestion, and the plant has a mild laxative action, which may relieve occasional constipation. Because the leaves provide a sense of satiety, Black Medic may support healthy weight management.

Traditionally, it has also been used for its antibacterial properties, helping the body respond to minor bacterial infections and foodborne illnesses.

Its coagulant properties make it suitable for minor bleeding, although caution is advised for individuals taking blood pressure or anticoagulant medications due to its potential to induce clotting.

Healing constituents/ Therapeutic actions: Black Medic is a surprisingly protein-rich wild plant. Every 100 grams of leaves contains approximately 23 grams of protein and about 25 grams of fiber—impressive for a wild green. It is also rich in calcium, phosphorus, potassium, and magnesium. Therapeutic actions include coagulant, mild purgative (laxative), antibacterial, nutritive, and digestive supportive properties.

Historical connection: Native to Eurasia, Black Medic was introduced to North America by European settlers and spread rapidly during the 18th and 19th centuries. It was cultivated as a nutritious potherb and valued for its high protein content. In California, Indigenous groups collected and ground the black seeds into flour, utilizing the entire plant.

Its Latin species name, *lupulina*, is derived from the word lupus (meaning "wolf"). This is a nod to the flower's resemblance to hop blossoms (*Humulus lupulus*), also named after the wolf—an allusion to their vigorous, climbing nature and association with the "Willow Wolf tree" (*Lupus silicarius*) in German lore. The double "wolf" reference endures in the botanical name, linking this humble legume to ancient symbolism and storytelling.

Jessica's notes: Though small and unassuming, Black Medic has much to offer. I appreciate how it grows quietly among more dominant plants, improving the soil while offering subtle healing. It is one of those herbs you overlook until you need it, and then it proves itself in simple, nourishing ways. I like to remind my students that sometimes the medicine is growing right at their feet.

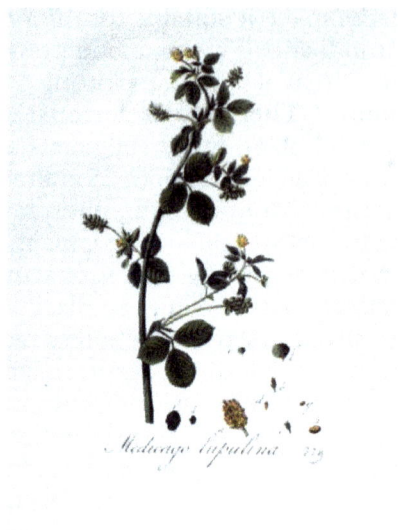

Permission granted to use under GFDL by Kurt Stueber, Source: www.biolib.de □

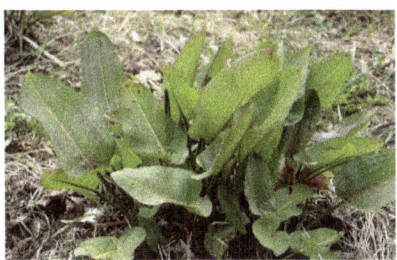

Broadleaf Dock

Rumex obtusifolius

Polygonaceae (Buckwheat) Family
Other common names: Bitter Dock, Broad-leaved Dock, Blunt Leaf Dock, Dock Leaf, Butter Dock

Description: Broadleaf Dock is a hardy, resilient perennial with large, broad, smooth leaves that can grow up to 12 inches long. The leaves are oval-shaped with blunt tips and a distinctive red central vein. As the plant matures, its seed clusters turn a reddish-brown color and persist through the winter, making it a year-round foraging option.

Where it grows: Broadleaf Dock thrives in moist soils and disturbed areas such as farmlands, ditches, riverbanks, and along creek beds. It is widespread near water sources and often found growing alongside stinging nettle. Though considered invasive across many temperate regions worldwide, its abundance speaks to its resilience and usefulness.

When and how to harvest: Harvest young, tender leaves in late spring to early summer before they become tough or overly bitter. The roots are best gathered in early spring or late fall, when the plant's energy is concentrated underground. Seeds can be harvested throughout the year—even in winter if needed—making them a reliable wild staple. Always forage responsibly, leaving enough for the plant to regenerate and for other creatures to share.

How to work with it / Medicinal use: Every part of Broadleaf Dock is edible and medicinal. The younger leaves can be cooked like spinach, bringing a tart, lemony flavor to soups or sautés. Seeds can be toasted or ground into flour, much like buckwheat, and serve as an excellent alternative to wild grains. The root is rich in medicinal compounds and can be made into a tea to aid digestion, support liver detoxification, and relieve coughs or jaundice. Its laxative effects are mild but effective.

Broadleaf Dock is also a trusted topical remedy. The leaves are famously soothing for skin irritations, especially when applied directly to nettle stings, burns, insect bites, blisters, or boils. At Forest School, we often use fresh Dock leaves to soothe Stinging Nettle stings—a perfect example of nature's balance.

Healing constituents / Therapeutic actions: Broadleaf Dock contains tannins, oxalic acid, phosphate, potassium, and magnesium. Its primary therapeutic actions include astringent, laxative, antipyretic (fever-reducing), antioxidant, and antimicrobial effects. The root also stimulates bile production, supporting healthy digestion and liver function.

Historical connection: In medieval European folklore, dock held magical significance. People carved the roots into the shape of a desired partner, carrying the root effigy in their pockets as a charm until their love appeared. Shopkeepers washed their store doors and doorknobs with dock root-infused water, believing it would invite prosperity and good fortune.

Broadleaf Dock was also a practical staple. In the 19th century, European farmers wrapped freshly churned butter in the broad, waxy leaves, giving rise to the name "Butter Dock." This traditional use not only protected the butter from spoilage but also infused it with a touch of the plant's earthy vitality.

Despite its current status as a "weed," dock was once a cornerstone plant in ancestral food and medicine traditions. Its widespread growth is an invitation—a reminder not to overlook the everyday plants beneath our feet. As the old saying goes, "The cure grows beside the cause," and dock's proximity to nettle seems to echo that truth.

Even the nursery rhyme "Hickory Dickory Dock" may hint at this plant's widespread cultural familiarity. While the rhyme's origin is uncertain, the use of the word "dock" might reference this once-essential plant.

Jessica's notes: Dock is a humble but powerful plant ally. It is one of the first I teach at Forest School, especially for its role in helping little ones soothe nettle stings. I have used the leaves as emergency wraps and have come to appreciate the fiber rich seeds for flour and an addition to granola. Eating wild edibles return us to the rhythms of the land—and remind us that weeds are often the most generous givers. One of my favorite forest school memories is feeding the little forest school students like baby birds wild salad greens garnished with dock seeds!

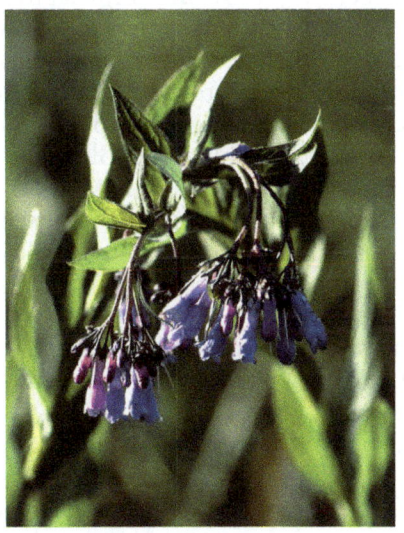

Bluebells

Mertensia paniculata, ciliata

Asparagaceae (Asparagus) Family
Other common names: Mountain Bluebells, Chiming Bluebells
  Description: Bluebells are delicate spring bloomers with ovate to lanceolate leaves that may be smooth or softly hairy. Their alternating leaf pattern climbs gracefully up the flowering stalk. The bell-shaped, tubular flowers hang in loose, nodding clusters, ranging in color from soft pink to royal purple. True to their name, these blossoms resemble tiny chimes, ringing in the arrival of spring.
  Where it grows: One of the first heralds of the season, Bluebells emerge with the spring rains and melting snow. They favor sunny mountain slopes, open meadows, and fields across the Mountain West. You will often find them scattered like soft notes of color, soaking up moisture from alpine terrain before the heat of summer.
  When and how to harvest: Harvest the flowers and leaves from early spring through late summer. Always forage with reverence—take only what you need, and never uproot the plant. Pinch off just a few flowers or leaves from each plant, allowing the plant to continue thriving and reseed for future seasons.

How to work with it / Medicinal use: Bluebells can be worked with in a similar manner to comfrey. How amazing that they look alike! They are soothing to the skin and excellent in healing face oils, salves, and liniments. Use poultices made from the fresh plant on sprains, bruises, or broken bones to ease inflammation and promote healing. Internally, a light tea or infusion may help soothe a cough, although it should only be used during an acute illness, not as a daily tonic. Bluebells contain low levels of alkaloids, so moderation is key.

Healing constituents / Therapeutic actions: Bluebells are known for their diuretic and styptic properties. These qualities make them useful both internally for short-term support during illness and externally for healing wounds or irritated skin.

Historical connections: Historically, Bluebells had more than just medicinal significance—they were also practical and artistic tools. Their sticky sap was once used to glue book pages and fletch arrows. In Elizabethan England, crushed bulbs were used to make starch for the elaborate ruffs that adorned collars and cuffs. Despite their versatility, their internal use in high doses was discouraged due to potential toxicity. Sir John Hill, an 18th-century English botanist, composer, and author, praised their medicinal strength but cautioned that doses should not exceed three grains. He noted their decisive diuretic action and warned of their potency.

Jessica's notes: Bluebells are a plant of joy for me. Their appearance signals the actual start of spring, and they seem to lift the spirits just by being there. There is something so comforting about that soft blue-violet glow on the mountainside after a long winter—like nature whispering, "We made it." I first discovered Bluebells on an early spring day while teaching a class on the medicinal plants of spring on a friend's property at the edge of Lake Coeur d'Alene. I didn't know what it was, but I kept it in my memory, noting that its flowers looked similar to comfrey's. Months later, I found the mystery spring flower in the foraging book I was reading at the time: *Mountain States Foraging* by Briana Wiles. Another powerful plant ally was discovered and remembered.

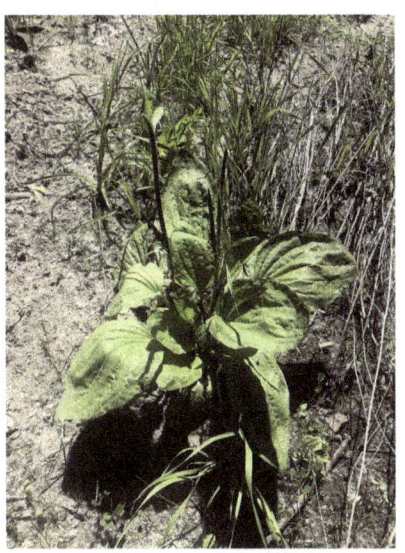

Broadleaf Plantain

Plantago major

Plantaginaceae (Plantain) Family

Description: Broadleaf Plantain is a hardy perennial that can also act as an annual or biennial, depending on its growing conditions. It forms a low-growing basal rosette of broad, dark green leaves connected to the base by strong fibrous threads. These leaves range in size from a modest inch to over a foot long. The flowers are small and inconspicuous, growing on tall, upright spikes. This unassuming plant is often overlooked, yet it carries powerful healing potential.

Where it grows: Plantain is one of the most widely distributed plants globally. It thrives in disturbed soils, along roadsides, in farmlands, beside creeks, and within forest understories. Though often dismissed as a weed, this plant is a gift found almost anywhere, from backyards to deep mountain valleys.

When and how to harvest: Harvest the vibrant green leaves from late spring through late summer, before they begin to yellow or dry out. Choose healthy, intact leaves and always leave enough behind to support the plant's continued growth.

How to work with it / Medicinal use: Broadleaf Plantain is one of my favorite herbs to share with children. It is an unassuming, accessible plant that introduces them to the power of plant medicine. Though now considered a weed, it may have been brought to North America from Eurasia as a food crop. Its leaves are edible both raw and cooked and have a mild flavor, reminiscent of Swiss chard.

We use bruised or chewed leaves topically for spider bites, splinters, and insect stings—its signature drawing action helps to pull out toxins and irritants. Dried leaves can be infused in oil to create soothing salves for the skin. Internally, plantain is healing to the digestive system and can help soothe inflammation. The seeds also have medicinal value and may help lower cholesterol levels, as noted by Tilford (1997). In survival situations, the plant's inner leaf fibers can even be used for thread or fishing line—another testament to its resourcefulness.

Healing Constituents / Therapeutic Actions: Broadleaf Plantain is rich in vitamins A, C, and K—nutrients also found in powerhouse greens like kale and chard. Its medicinal effects come from alkaloids, flavonoids, phenolic acid derivatives, and terpenoids. These contribute to its anti-inflammatory, astringent, drawing, and anti-tumor actions.

Historical connection: Plantain's healing legacy stretches back centuries. Carl Linnaeus named the species in 1753, though it had been used in folk medicine long before that. The name derives from the Old French *plantin*, related to the Latin *planta*, meaning "sole of the foot," a reference to its flat, footprint-like leaves. It was often used to soothe sore feet on long journeys—a fitting symbol for a plant that has walked alongside humanity for thousands of years.

Plantain is depicted in medieval manuscripts and artwork, including images of the Nativity. Shakespeare mentions it as a household remedy in *Romeo and Juliet* (1592), and Chaucer referenced it in *The Prologue to the Yeoman's Tale*. Puritans brought plantain to New England, where it rapidly spread across the colonies. Native Americans called it "white man's foot" because it seemed to grow wherever settlers traveled.

Even older evidence of its use comes from bog mummies in Northern Europe, dating back to the 3rd and 5th centuries A.D., showing that humans have valued this plant for a very long time.

Jessica's notes: The Broadleaf Plantain on the mountain grows to a magnificent size—one leaf was as big as my son's head! This plant has been a true staple in our foraging adventures. It is my go-to for bug bites, sore feet after barefoot hikes, and stomach upset. Whether stirred into soups, brewed into tea, or sautéed like spinach, plantain has supported our family's well-being again and again. It is a perfect example of how the so-called "weeds" are often the most powerful and generous healers. I have adopted my dear herbalist friend, Sandy's morning ritual of eating a small plantain leaf to stimulate the pituitary gland.

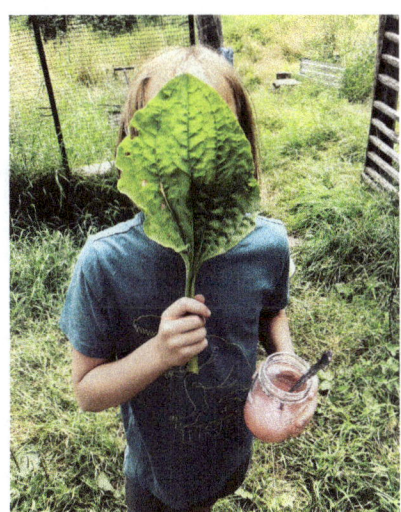

Plantain Mask!

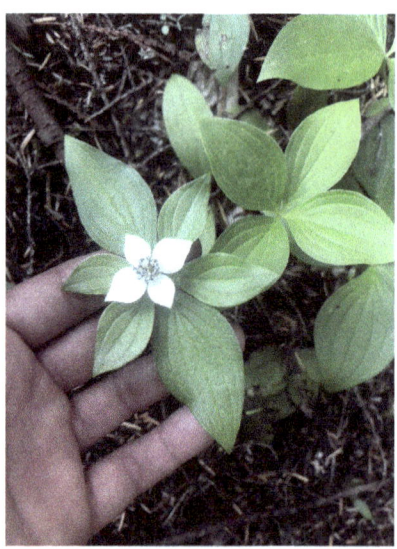

Bunchberry Dogwood

Cornus canadensis

Cornaceae (Dogwood) Family
Description: Bunchberry Dogwood is a charming, low-growing ground cover that typically grows to a height of 3 to 6 inches. It produces brilliant red, button-like berries that grow in clusters—hence the name *Bunchberry*. Its leaves are velvety, deep green, and arranged in whorls that give the plant a miniature dogwood appearance. The flowers are equally remarkable: when they bloom, the petals spring back and the stamens launch pollen at an astonishing acceleration of 24,000 m/s^2—about 800 times the force experienced by astronauts during launch (Stephenson, 2021). This catapult-like action sends pollen ten times higher than the flower itself—an event that would be mesmerizing to witness with a time-lapse camera.

Where it grows: Bunchberry thrives in cool, shady, and moist environments within coniferous, deciduous, and mixed forests. It is commonly found beneath the canopy of spruce and fir trees. The plant favors moist, organically rich, acidic humus in partial shade—think dappled forest floors or near-full shade.

When and how to harvest: Harvest the aerial parts—leaves, berries, and stems—in late summer to early fall, when the plant is lush and vibrant.

How to work with it / Medicinal use: The fruits and seeds are edible, either raw or cooked, though the berries are somewhat mealy and not very sweet. They pair well with other wild fruits in jams and preserves. The berries are rich in vitamin C, offering immune-boosting and antioxidant benefits. You can also use the boiled plant liquid to make pectin, which I am eager to try in our wild berry jams. In addition to its culinary uses, pectin can help lower cholesterol, ease inflammation, support digestion, and may even protect against heavy metal poisoning.

Medicinally, tea made from the leaves and berries is used to treat colds, flu, coughs, fevers, and stomach infections. Fresh leaves can be applied to open wounds to help stop bleeding. The mashed fruits and leaves work well as a poultice for mouth ulcers and sore throats. Interestingly, modern researchers are now exploring members of the Dogwood family, including Bunchberry, for their potential in natural cancer treatments.

Healing constituents / Therapeutic actions: Bunchberry contains vitamin C and pectin, as well as antibiotic, antiseptic, anti-inflammatory, analgesic, and febrifuge properties.

Historical connection: In Alaska, Bunchberry has long served as a vital food source—not only for humans, but also for moose, black-tailed deer, mule deer, and a diverse array of birds. Indigenous peoples traditionally used Bunchberry to help draw out toxins, which may have inspired modern scientific interest in its potential as a pharmaceutical.

Jessica's notes: Bunchberry's resilience and beauty always bring me joy when I find it carpeting the cool, shaded forest floors. I admire how such a small, unassuming plant holds so much hidden vitality and healing potential. One of my foraging goals is to experiment with making pectin from this sweet forest gem and to weave it into our wild berry preserves—another way to preserve the gifts of the wild.

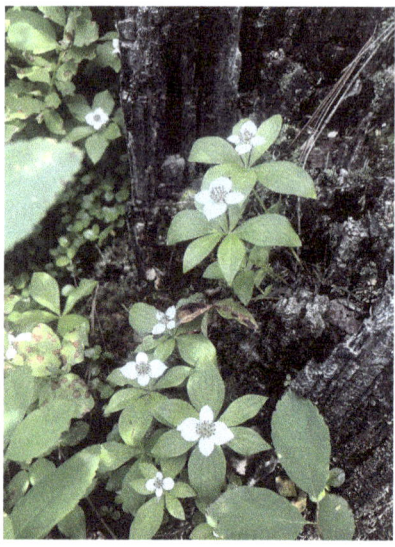

A bunch of Bunch Berry Dogwood

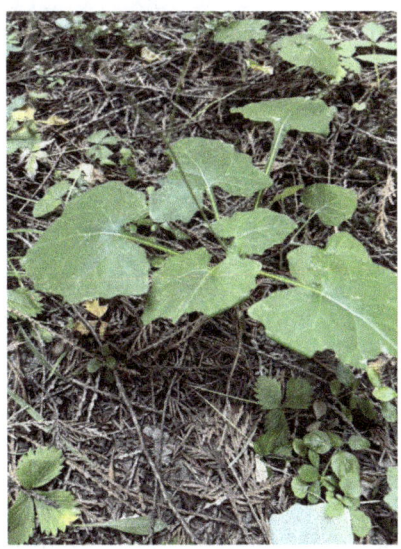

Burdock

Arctium lappa

Asteraceae (Daisy) Family
Other common names: Elephant Ear
Description: Burdock grows to an impressive 3 to 6 feet tall, with enormous leaves measuring up to 12 inches long and 8 inches wide. These coarse, hairy leaves resemble elephant ears—hence one of its common names. Its prickly seed heads, or burrs, are nature's Velcro and will cling stubbornly to clothing, animal fur, and anything passing by. Anyone who has walked a dog through a Burdock patch knows how challenging these burrs can be to remove! Burdock is a biennial plant that was introduced to North America by early European settlers.
When and how to harvest: Harvest the roots from summer through late fall, ideally before the burrs go to seed. At this stage, the root is full of stored energy and nutrients.
Where it grows: Burdock thrives in disturbed areas, preferring sunny, dry, open fields. You will often find it near roadsides, in pastures, and along fence lines.

How to work with it / Medicinal use: Nearly the entire plant is useful. The young leaves, stalks, and roots can all be cooked and eaten. The Japanese traditionally prepare the roots in a stir-fry dish known as gobo. In Russia, the roots have been used as a potato substitute. The root is especially valued for its medicinal properties. A tincture or decoction of Burdock root is a classic blood purifier and is used to support liver detoxification. It is highly effective for treating chronic skin conditions, including eczema, psoriasis, acne, and skin infections. Burdock can also help balance and soothe the digestive system, assisting the body in processing proteins and supporting hormonal regulation.

Topically, a poultice made from the leaves is excellent for cradle cap, eczema, boils, insect bites, and even minor skin cancers. Many herbalists also use Burdock to support the body's elimination of heavy metals and environmental toxins. In our household, we prefer to harvest and dry the roots before the burrs mature, storing them for use in teas, decoctions, and tinctures throughout the year.

Healing constituents / Therapeutic actions: Burdock root contains fatty acids, carbohydrates, starch, and is particularly rich in inulin polysaccharides (about 45%) (Schauenberg). It also provides vitamin C, calcium, magnesium, and iron. Its primary therapeutic actions include blood purification, liver support, digestive balancing, diuretic effects, and skin healing (Hobbs, Tilford).

Historical connection: Burdock has been valued medicinally since at least the Middle Ages. During the Industrial Revolution, the root was used to purify water and dispel industrial pollutants. As we now face modern environmental challenges, Burdock remains a reliable ally in detoxifying the body from heavy metals and contaminants.

Russian author Leo Tolstoy once reflected on the plant's resilience: *"Black from dust but still alive and red in the center. It reminded me of Hadji Murad. It makes me want to write. It asserts life to the end, and alone in the midst of the whole field, somehow or other had asserted it."* — Leo Tolstoy, journal entry (July 1896), upon observing a tiny Burdock shoot surviving in a ploughed field.

Jessica's notes: Burdock is one of those humble but mighty plants that I return to again and again. It may not dazzle like showier herbs, but its roots run deep—both literally and figuratively. I love the process of harvesting Burdock roots in late fall, knowing I am gathering a powerful ally to support my family's vitality through the winter months. In our home, it is a staple in our skin-supportive formulas and liver-cleansing teas.

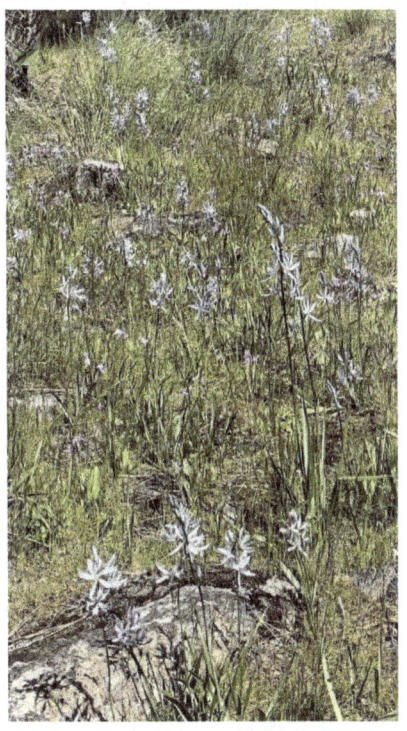

Camas

Camassia leichtlinii

Asparagaceae (Asparagus) Family
Other common names: Common Camas, Wild Hyacinth, Quamash, Prairie Camas, Leichtlin's Camas

Description: Common camas is a striking wildflower with star-shaped blossoms ranging from soft blue to deep indigo. It grows from a teardrop-shaped bulb and sends up tall flower stalks above slender, grass-like leaves. Its blooms are showy and elegant, with six delicate petals that spiral gently open, attracting bees and butterflies alike. From a distance, camas can appear like a shimmering sea of blue across a springtime meadow.

Where it Grows: Camas thrives in moist meadows, grassy flats, and forest openings, especially in the Pacific Northwest, the Sierra Nevada foothills, and areas of the Rocky Mountains. It favors well-drained soils that are seasonally wet in spring and dry out in summer.

When to Harvest: Harvest occurs after flowering—typically in late spring to early summer—when the blossoms have faded and the seed pods begin to form. This timing ensures the bulbs have reached their peak starch content and that the plant has had a chance to reproduce. Traditionally, camas was dug with specialized tools like fire-hardened sticks, and only mature bulbs were taken, leaving smaller ones to regrow.

Caution: Common camas looks alarmingly similar to *death camas* (*Toxicoscordion venenosum*), a highly toxic plant that grows in similar environments. Death camas has white to cream-colored flowers, and its bulbs are deadly even in small amounts. Because both plants may grow side by side, it is absolutely essential to positively identify camas before harvesting. If you are not 100% sure—do not eat the bulb.

How to Work With It / Medicinal use: The bulbs are the primary part used. They must be slow-roasted, pit-baked, or steamed for many hours—sometimes up to two days. This long cooking process converts the inulin in the bulbs (a complex carbohydrate) into sweet, digestible fructose. Once cooked, the bulbs are soft, sweet, and almost fig-like in taste. They can be eaten fresh, dried for winter storage, or ground into a flour. Medicinally, camas was used to support postpartum recovery, ease difficult labor, and occasionally to soothe persistent coughs when made into a tea.

Healing Constituents/ Therapeutic Actions: Camas bulbs are rich in inulin, a prebiotic fiber that feeds beneficial gut flora and provides a slow-release energy source without spiking blood sugar levels. This made camas a deeply nourishing food for sustaining energy through long winters. Therapeutically, its gentle action on the digestive system and blood sugar balance speaks more to its value as a food-medicine than a potent herbal remedy.

Historical Connections: Historically, camas prairies were actively tended and maintained by Native communities through controlled burns and careful digging practices. Common camas was one of the most important staple foods for many Indigenous peoples of the Western United States, including the Nez Perce, Coast Salish, and Klamath. Harvesting camas was a communal, ceremonial event, marked by seasonal migrations and intergenerational teachings. Women were often the primary stewards of camas meadows, passing down knowledge of how to tend, dig, and replant. Camas fields were not "wild" in the modern sense—they were carefully maintained food forests, shaped by fire and care over centuries. These meadows represent one of the oldest known examples of sustainable land management in North America.

Jessica's Notes: When I first discovered common camas, it was growing wild among Lomatium, a familiar herbal ally. Its historical reverence made me stare in awe and connected me to the people that once cared for this wild garden. We must be mindful when harvesting its bulbs—taking only what is needed, replanting as we go, and honoring the sacred relationship between people and place. In doing so, we bring back earth stewardship principles and help reawaken these forgotten fields where camas once thrived in abundance.

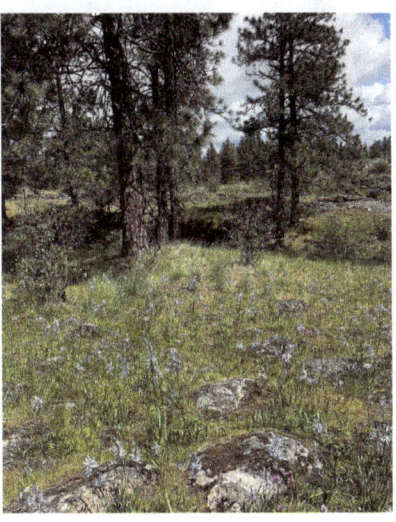

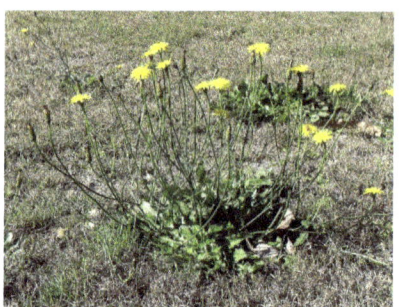

Cat's Ear

Hypochaeris radicata

Asteraceae (Daisy) Family

Other common names: Hairy cat's ear, flatweed, false dandelion, California dandelion, frogbit, gosmore, Australian Capeweed, Flatweed

Description: Cat's Ear is named for the fine fuzz that covers its leaves, giving them a soft, velvety texture reminiscent of a cat's ear. The toothy leaves resemble those of a dandelion and grow in a basal rosette close to the ground. From this rosette, a slender stem can rise to two feet tall, topped with bright yellow flowers. The blooms resemble dandelions, although they are more compact and exhibit a slightly more intricate, compound structure. When plucked, the stem exudes a milky white sap, another feature it shares with its dandelion cousin.

Where it grows: Cat's Ear favors open fields, pastures, and farmlands, often appearing in disturbed soil. It is a common sight in both rural and suburban settings.

When and how to harvest: Harvest the leaves and other plant parts from early spring through late summer. Keep in mind that as the season progresses, the leaves become more bitter; early harvest yields the tenderest greens.

How to work with it / Medicinal use: Every part of this plant is edible, and its culinary versatility is impressive. You can enjoy Cat's Ear raw in salads, or steam, sauté, marinate, and boil it for use in a variety of dishes. Its bitter profile makes it a superb digestive tonic, supporting bile production and aiding the function of the liver, kidneys, gallbladder, pancreas, and spleen. In short, it is a cleansing plant that gently stimulates and tones the body's major detoxification systems. The roots can also be harvested, roasted, and brewed as a coffee substitute—a testament to their versatility as a wild food.

Healing constituents / Therapeutic actions: Cat's Ear is rich in essential vitamins and minerals, including vitamins A, B, and C, copper, phosphorus, potassium, iron, calcium, and magnesium (Kallas, 2010). Its therapeutic actions include anti-inflammatory, bitter tonic, and mild laxative effects.

Historical connection: Cat's Ear is a quintessential "people's plant." It thrives where human activity occurs and can now be found on every continent except Antarctica. Originally a perennial weed from Eurasia, it has successfully traveled the world thanks to its tiny, windborne seeds, which parachute through the air to colonize new terrain. Its Latin name, *radicata*, meaning "with conspicuous roots," speaks to its strong and easily recognizable taproot. The Greek origins of *Hypochaeris* loosely translate to "under" and "young pig," a curious but fitting reference for a plant so common in the fields where livestock once grazed.

Jessica's notes: Cat's Ear is an excellent example of a humble plant with generous gifts. It is a frequent addition to my spring greens and digestive teas. Its sunny yellow flowers are a welcome sight in early spring, and its resilience reminds me that even the simplest plants can offer powerful support to our bodies.

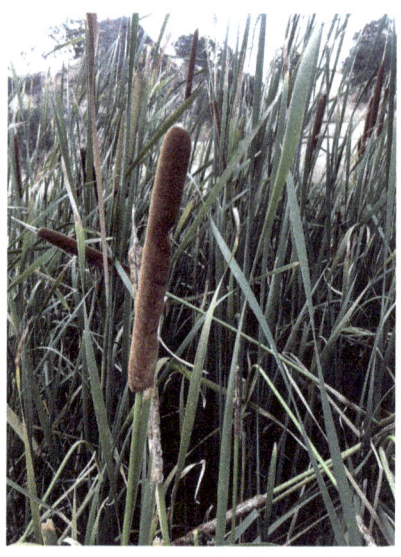

Cattail

Typha latifolia

Typhaceae (Bulrushes) Family

Description: Cattails are tall, slender plants that can reach heights of up to 8 feet. Their long leaves wrap gracefully around the central stalk. In late summer, mature cattails develop their distinctive brown, velvet-like flower spikes, which my children fondly call "hot dogs on a stick." These iconic features make cattails instantly recognizable in any wetland setting.

Where it grows: Cattails thrive in wetlands, marshes, and along the edges of ponds, lakes, and slow-moving streams. They are an integral part of healthy aquatic ecosystems, providing habitat and shelter for many birds, insects, and amphibians.

How to work with it / Medicinal use: Cattail is a remarkably versatile plant—almost every part is edible. In early spring, the young shoots, often referred to as "Cossack asparagus," can be eaten raw or cooked. The roots, rich in starch, can be dried and ground into flour for baking. The immature green flower spikes (those famous "hot dogs") can be boiled or steamed and eaten like corn on the cob. In summer, the pollen can be gathered and used as a flour extender, adding a nutritional boost to baked goods.

Medicinally, the gel-like sap that seeps from cut leaves is cooling and soothing to the skin, similar to Aloe Vera. It can be applied to burns, rashes, insect bites, and other minor skin irritations.

Healing constituents / Therapeutic actions: Cattails are a valuable energy source, rich in calories and carbohydrates. They also provide a good amount of vitamins A and C, as well as potassium and phosphorus. The plant exhibits antiseptic, styptic (stops bleeding), and anti-inflammatory properties.

Historical connections: Cattails have served as an essential staple for millennia. They are referenced multiple times in ancient texts, including the Bible. In the Old Testament (Exodus 2:3), the basket that carried the infant Moses was hidden among the "bulrushes"—likely cattails. In the New Testament, the reed mentioned during the Crucifixion of Christ (Mark 15:19) may also have been a species of cattail.

Beyond the Judeo-Christian tradition, cattails appear in mythologies worldwide. In Greek, Eurasian, and Asian lore, reeds such as cattails are often linked to dragons, water serpents, and primordial creation stories. Many indigenous cultures honor wetlands as sacred spaces, viewing them as portals between worlds. Cattails, with their roots in ancient waters, are frequently woven into these origin myths as symbols of life's emergence.

Jessica's notes: When harvesting cattails, always be mindful of where they grow. Because they thrive in water, they can easily absorb pollutants. Ensure the wetland is free of chemical runoff, sewage, or heavy metals. Check with local environmental agencies and avoid harvesting near roads or industrial areas. Wetlands are increasingly threatened by development, so I encourage you to forage consciously and consider cultivating cattails on your land if you have a suitable spot. These generous plants provide food, medicine, and habitat, and they deserve our care and stewardship.

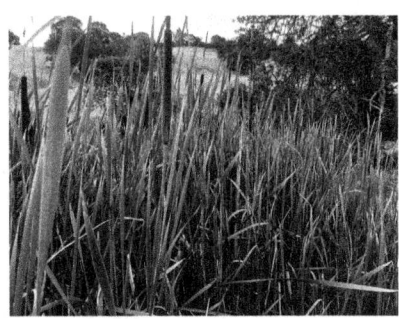

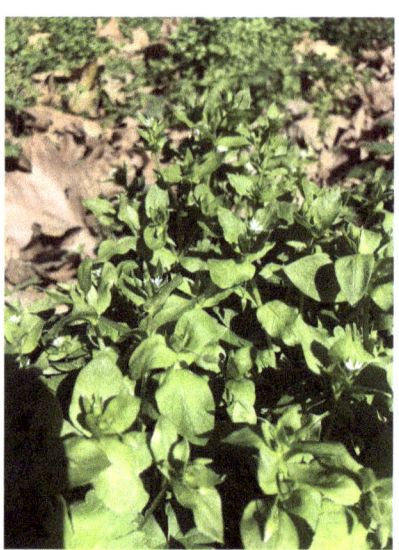

Chickweed

Stellaria media

Caryophyllaceae (Carnation) Family
Other common names: birdweed, chickenweed, common chickweed, starweed, starwort, winterwort, winterweed

Description: Common Chickweed is a charming winter annual that grows in a dense mat across the ground. It emerges in late spring, summer, or early fall, then lies dormant over the winter, setting seed in early spring. Its stems are covered with tiny hairs—an important identifying feature that sets it apart from potentially poisonous look-alikes such as *Euphorbia*. If you observe the stem closely, you will notice a distinct "Mohawk" line of hairs running up one side—this is Chickweed's signature trait.

Its dainty white flowers, shaped like stars, give rise to its botanical name, *Stellaria*. These tiny blossoms are tucked neatly into the upper leaf axils. The plant's tender, spatula- or egg-shaped leaves range from about 0.8 to 2.5 cm long and 0.6 to 1.2 cm wide. Chickweed itself is a low-growing plant, typically 5 to 50 cm tall, creating a lovely green carpet across fields and gardens.

Where it grows: Chickweed thrives in farm fields, pastures, meadows, and gardens—anywhere with partial to full sun and moist, fertile soil. It is often seen as a common "weed," but those of us who know it recognize its actual value!

When and how to harvest: Harvest the tender aerial parts of Chickweed from early spring through late summer. The leaves and stems are at their best when young and fresh.

How to work with it / Medicinal use: Chickweed is one of my favorite wild salad greens. Its mild, slightly sweet flavor makes it perfect for adding raw to salads, sandwiches, pestos, stir-fries, and soups.

Topically, Chickweed is an exceptional remedy for eczema, dry, inflamed, and itchy skin. I love adding it to my *Heals All Balm* because of its cooling, soothing qualities.

As a tincture, Chickweed is used to support urinary, kidney, and bladder health. Its gentle action makes it an excellent choice for many common inflammatory conditions.

Healing constituents / Therapeutic actions: For such a delicate little plant, Chickweed is impressively nutrient-dense. It contains vitamins A, D, B-complex, and C, along with rutin (a potent bioflavonoid), calcium, potassium, phosphorus, zinc, manganese, sodium, copper, iron, and silica. Believe it or not, Chickweed contains as much iron as spinach!

It is deeply soothing and cooling for inflamed, irritated, or itchy skin. Internally, it offers gentle laxative action, is demulcent (soothing to the digestive tract), refrigerant (cooling to the body), and anti-inflammatory. Its cool, moist nature makes it ideal for balancing hot, dry, or irritated conditions.

Historical connection: Native to Eurasia and North Africa, Chickweed made its way to the Americas with European settlers and quickly became beloved here as well. It has a long history of use for both people and animals. In fact, chickens are particularly fond of it—hence its common name. Chickweed is referenced in ancient Greek botanical texts and was regularly consumed in early Ireland, where it was valued both as a nutritious food and a gentle medicine.

Jessica's Notes: Chickweed has earned a permanent place in my apothecary. I especially love adding it to my skin balms—it has helped me personally. I once suffered from a stubborn skin rash that would not clear up with other treatments. After incorporating a Chickweed-infused balm, the rash healed beautifully, and I have trusted it ever since.

I also adore making pesto with Chickweed. Its mild flavor pairs so well with garlic, lemon, olive oil, and wild foraged pine nuts—sometimes I blend it with wild greens or garden herbs. It is the perfect way to celebrate spring and to nourish the body from the inside out.

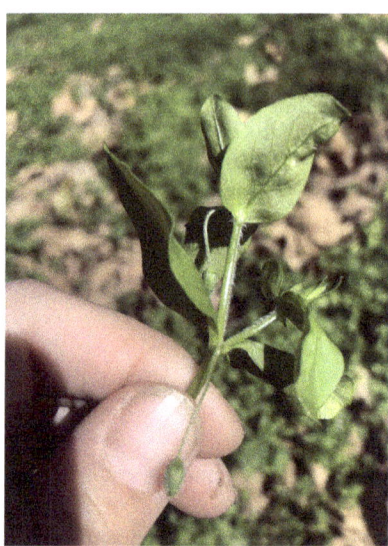

Mowhawk-line of hairs

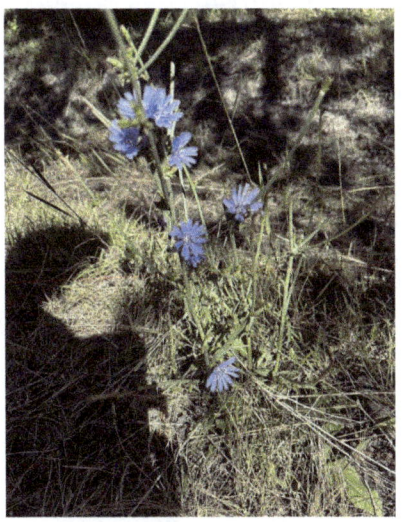

Chicory

Cichorium intybus

Asteraceae (Daisy) Family

Description: Chicory leaves grow in a basal rosette near the base of the plant, much like dandelions. The flowers have a striking periwinkle to purple hue, with daisy-like petals that feature serrated clefts at their tips. A hardy perennial, Chicory can grow from one to four feet tall. The flowers bloom spontaneously along the stem, creating a beautiful display against dry and rugged landscapes.

Where it grows: Chicory prefers dry soil and is commonly found in abandoned lots, open fields, and ditches. I first discovered a Chicory plant on a family foraging trip to Rose Lake. We had stopped to stretch our legs, and there it was—blooming right off the roadside. It felt like bumping into an old friend, a sign that we were on the right path. There is something special about seeing those vibrant purple flowers standing tall in an unexpected place.

When and how to harvest: Like dandelion greens, the older the leaves, the more bitter their flavor becomes. For the best taste, harvest greens in spring to early summer. The flowers can be gathered when in bloom—usually late summer—to brighten up salads or use as an edible garnish. Roots are best harvested in late summer to early fall.

How to work with it / Medicinal use: Every part of the Chicory plant is edible and offers valuable nutrients that support the liver and kidneys. The greens can be eaten raw or cooked. The roots can be roasted and ground as a decadent, earthy coffee substitute. The flowers, with their mild sweetness, can be sprinkled over salads or used to decorate cakes and savory dishes. Chicory's bitter qualities help stimulate digestion and promote detoxification.

Healing constituents / Therapeutic actions: Chicory leaves are a rich source of vitamins A, B, C, E, and K, as well as minerals such as potassium, calcium, phosphorus, copper, zinc, and magnesium. The bitter compounds found in the leaves and roots provide powerful support for the liver, kidneys, gallbladder, and pancreas, encouraging gentle detoxification and improved digestion.

Historical connection: Chicory's reputation as a coffee substitute dates back to the 18th century in Europe. In the Prussian Empire, Frederick the Great restricted coffee imports to limit consumption, which spurred interest in local coffee alternatives. Chicory quickly gained popularity due to its widespread availability and palatable flavor.

During the early 19th century, Napoleon's Continental Blockade similarly restricted coffee imports in France, leading to the widespread adoption of chicory as a substitute for coffee. Over time, this sparked an entire agricultural industry around Chicory, with France exporting as much as 60 million pounds of Chicory per year during the 19th century.

The tradition spread throughout Europe and later to the French colonies, including parts of Canada and the Caribbean. From there, it found its way to New Orleans, where Chicory coffee became a cultural staple, especially after the Civil War, when coffee imports were once again scarce. To this day, New Orleans is known for its signature Chicory coffee blends.

Jessica's Notes: As a lifelong coffee drinker, I have enjoyed researching the rich historical connection between chicory and coffee. It inspired me to start adding roasted chicory root powder to my morning brew. It feels good knowing that while I am sipping that familiar cup of Joe, I am also supporting my liver and kidneys thanks to the healing properties of Chicory. I love thinking about how our ancestors valued this plant, not only for its practical uses but for the comfort and nourishment it provided in lean times. I would call Chicory a "people's plant"—one that continues to serve us today.

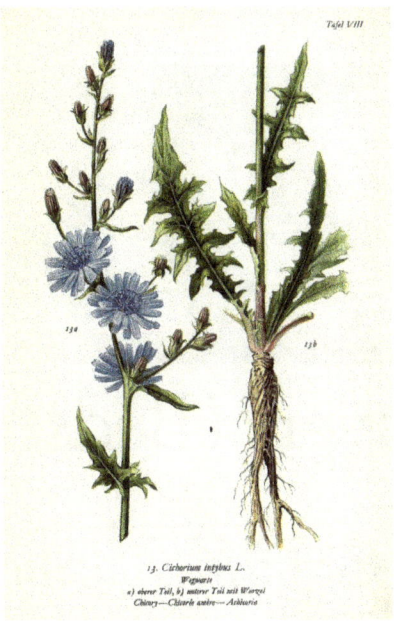

Common chicory, from an anonymous plate (Tafel VIII, 13) in the Apotekarsocieteten Museum, Sweden (public domain).

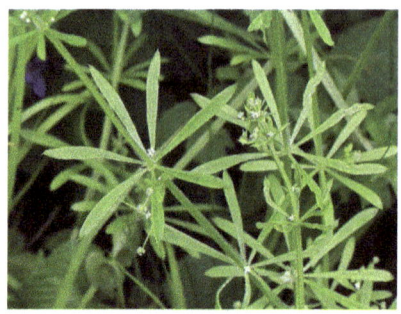

Cleavers (Bedstraw)

Galium aparine

Rubiaceae (Madder) Family
Other common names: Sticky Willy, Nature's Stickers
   Description: Cleavers are a long-lived annual that can grow from just a couple of inches to an impressive six feet tall. They lean and cling to neighboring plants, thanks to tiny hooked hairs on their stems and leaves that act like natural Velcro. These hairs allow Cleavers to sprawl and climb, attaching themselves to whatever they can find. The leaves grow in whorls of up to eight around the stem, and in spring and early summer, delicate, whitish-green, star-shaped flowers emerge in clusters of two or three from the leaf axils. As the plant matures, it produces tiny globular fruits covered in sticky hairs, perfect for hitching a ride on the fur of animals or human clothing—nature's clever seed dispersal system at work.
   Where it grows: Cleavers thrive in open fields and moist, fertile woodlands. They prefer soil rich in nutrients and are often found sprawling through meadow edges and under the dappled shade of trees.
   When and how to harvest: Spring is the time to gather Cleavers—before they flower and set seed. Once the plant has gone to seed, its medicinal strength fades. When harvesting, look for healthy, vibrant plants that emit a sweet honey-vanilla scent. Harvest the aerial parts of the plant, and as always, take only what you need with reverence.
   How to work with it / Medicinal use: Cleavers are one of my favorite spring "cleansing" herbs. The young leaves, stems, and seeds are edible. We prefer to cook the hairy leaves for about ten minutes to soften them. Fresh Cleavers are ideal for teas, tinctures, and infusions. They gently stimulate the lymphatic system, making them the perfect tonic for clearing out winter stagnation. The Doctrine of Signatures supports this seasonal

wisdom—Cleavers appear in spring, signaling the body's readiness for renewal and detoxification.

In Native American tradition, Cleavers are considered "Deer Medicine." This has two meanings: mama deer often bed their young in bedstraw to mask their scent from predators, and Cleavers' gentle, nurturing energy is particularly suited for deer-like personalities—artists, healers, and the soft-hearted among us.

Externally, an oil infusion of Cleavers makes a beautiful addition to lymphatic massage. Internally, Cleavers tea is known to aid in the elimination of kidney stones and promote urinary tract health. As a skin wash, it soothes psoriasis, eczema, freckles, and sunspots. The dried, powdered leaves can be used on wounds to stop bleeding. Modern studies have shown Cleavers' potential to inhibit cancer cell growth and act as an immunomodulator. (Ilina et al., 2019). According to the American Cancer Society, immunomodulators help regulate immune pathways, supporting treatments for various cancers.

Healing Constituents / Therapeutic Actions: Cleavers contain a powerhouse of healing constituents: quercetin, glycosides, saponins, flavonoids, organic acids, minerals, vitamin C, and essential oils. These components give Cleavers their antioxidant, cytotoxic, antimicrobial, protective, endocrine-supportive, and lymphatic-cleansing properties.

Historical connection: The name *Galium* comes from the Greek word for "milk," as species like *Galium verum* were traditionally used to curdle milk in cheese-making. "Cleavers" and "Bedstraw" refer to the plant's historical use as stuffing for mattresses. The sticky leaves would adhere to fabric, creating soft, plump bedding. There is even a folk belief that Mary lined Jesus's cradle with Cleavers—a lovely image that captures this plant's nurturing energy.

Jessica's Notes: Nature's stickers! My forest school students and I have a great deal of fun with Cleavers—wearing them proudly on our shirts as foraging badges. Cleavers is one of the ingredients of my Muscle Massage Balm that we use to soothe sore muscles, aches, and pains. One of my favorite camping hacks is to gather Cleavers and stuff them into a pillowcase (or even a shirt) for a surprisingly soft and fragrant cushion. I adore the sweet scent of Bedstraw—it brings peaceful dreams and adds an uplifting note to my solar-infused herbal teas.

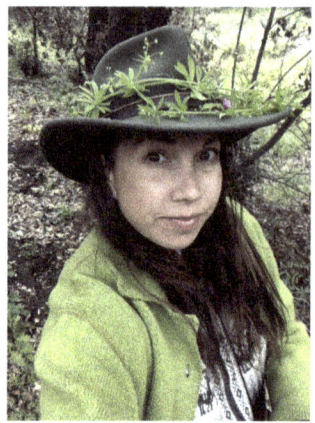

Cleavers are nature's stickers!

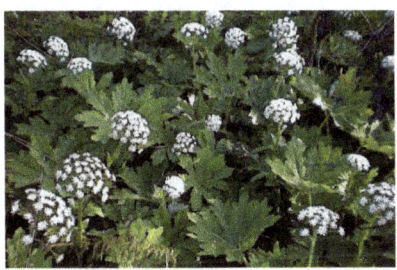

Coltsfoot

Petasites frigidus (sweet coltsfoot)
Petasites frigidus var. sagittatus (arrow-leafed coltsfoot)

Asteraceae (Daisy) family

Other common names: Arctic sweet coltsfoot, sweet coltsfoot, western coltsfoot, arrow-leafed coltsfoot, cough-wort, palmate-leaved coltsfoot, Arctic butterbur

Description: Coltsfoot is a perennial herb characterized by its milky sap. In early spring, the flowers emerge before the leaves, producing clusters of small, white blossoms that brighten the moist meadows. The seeds carry feathery bristles, parachuting on the wind to new growing spots. Stems grow between 10 and 50 centimeters tall, while dark green, toothed leaves form at the base. These leaves, measuring 2 to 18 centimeters long, are soft with fuzzy undersides. The shape of the leaves varies by subspecies—*Petasites frigidus* tends toward heart-shaped leaves, while *Petasites frigidus var. sagittatus* has elegant arrow-shaped foliage.

Where it grows: Coltsfoot prefers damp places, making its home in moist meadows, lakeshores, and forested areas. You will often spot it where water lingers.

When and how to harvest: Leaves are best harvested from mid to late summer. The roots and stalks are gathered in late fall or early spring, either before new growth begins or after the plant has stored its energy in the roots and stalks for the winter.

How to work with it / Medicinal use: Dried coltsfoot leaves create a soothing tea or cough syrup, used traditionally to calm coughs and ease upper respiratory troubles. Coltsfoot is particularly valued for relieving chest discomfort from persistent coughing. Herbalists reach for it in cases of chronic asthma, bronchitis, whooping cough, dry hacking cough, laryngitis, lung cancer symptoms, sore throat, and wheezing. Its sedative and antispasmodic properties relax the lungs and calm the nerve impulses that trigger coughing. As an expectorant, it helps move phlegm from the lungs. Applied externally, poultices made from the leaves and flowers are used to soothe eczema, insect bites, and inflamed skin. The leaves are sometimes included in herbal smoking blends to help open the lungs and ease coughing fits.

Healing constituents / Therapeutic actions: Coltsfoot contains soothing mucilage, along with anti-catarrhal, antispasmodic, demulcent, diaphoretic, diuretic, emollient, expectorant, pectoral, sedative, and tonic properties.

Historical connections: In the seventeenth century, physician and astrologer Nicholas Culpepper wrote, "The plant is under Venus; the fresh leaves or juice, or syrup thereof is good for a hot dry cough, or wheezing and shortness of breath." John Gerard's *The Herball* (1597) also included coltsfoot as a valued herb, noting its uses for treating ulcers and inflammation. Decoctions of the leaves and roots were used to alleviate coughs, and smoke from the dried leaves was believed to aid those struggling with breathlessness. In northern Indigenous traditions, such as among the Inuit, the ash of coltsfoot served as a substitute for salt. Green leaves were rolled into balls, dried, and burned on fire-heated stones, with the resulting black ash collected for use as a seasoning in cooking.

Jessica's Notes: I have yet to fully work with Coltsfoot, but it is high on my list to add to my wild medicine chest. I find it fascinating how this plant has been used for lung support through so many generations and cultures. In my wanderings, I have spotted it growing along cool, damp forest edges, and each time I take it as a gentle nudge from nature: "learn me!" It feels wise to have a plant like Coltsfoot in your herbal toolkit, especially for those lingering winter coughs or upper respiratory challenges. I look forward to building a relationship with this plant and discovering firsthand what it has to teach me.

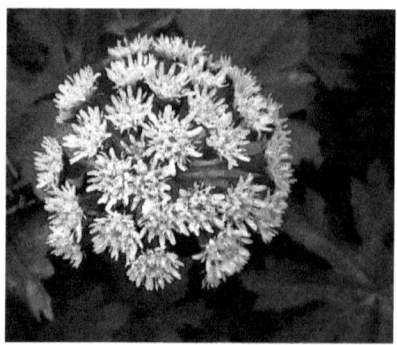

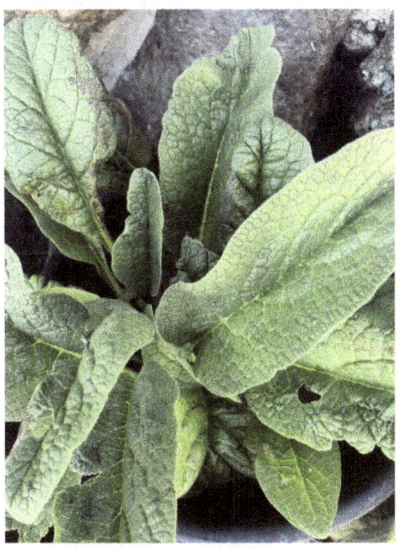

Comfrey

Symphytum officinale

Boraginaceae (Borage) Family

Other common names: True comfrey, common comfrey, boneset, knitbone

Description: Comfrey is a striking perennial with a thick, hairy stem and dark green leaves. The lower leaves can reach lengths of up to 12 inches and are ovate, while the entire plant can grow anywhere from 2 to 5 feet tall. The bristly hairs along the stem and leaves can cause skin irritation for some, so it is wise to handle them with care. Comfrey's flowers grow densely in clusters, arranged in a graceful scorpoid curve that resembles a scorpion's tail, gradually arching from fully opened blossoms to tiny, undeveloped buds at the tip. The flowers vary in hue, ranging from pink to purple, white, or dull blue. The bell-shaped corollas and five-parted calyx add to the plant's distinctive beauty.

Where it grows: This hardy perennial thrives in wet grasslands, ditches, and along riverbanks. I have also come across it growing in wild cottage gardens and around the edges of old abandoned homesteads—places where the land remembers the hands that once tended it.

When and how to harvest: Harvest the leaves when they are mature, ideally before the plant goes into full bloom. We gather comfrey leaves throughout the summer and into early fall, ensuring that the plant has had time to soak up the season's vitality.

How to work with it / Medicinal use: Comfrey has long been revered for its remarkable ability to knit and repair broken bones, torn ligaments, and damaged tissue. It is one of the finest plants for soothing arthritic conditions, sports injuries, and sprains, thanks to its anti-inflammatory and analgesic properties. I prepare poultices, compresses, and fresh applications of crushed leaf or root for injuries, allowing comfrey's medicine to do its deep-healing work. Internally, comfrey is now approached with caution due to its pyrrolizidine alkaloids, which can be toxic to the liver if consumed in large amounts or over extended periods. For this reason, comfrey is no longer sold for internal use in the United States; however, the homeopathic preparation known as Symphytum can still be found on the market. The external applications, however, remain time-honored and highly effective.

Healing constituents / Therapeutic actions: Comfrey leaf and root contain allantoin (a key tissue regenerative compound), mucilage polysaccharides, phenolic acids such as rosmarinic acid, chlorogenic acid, oleanolic acid, lithospermic acid, and caffeic acid, along with glycopeptides, amino acids, and triterpene saponins. These constituents synergistically promote deep tissue repair, reduce inflammation, alleviate pain, and accelerate the healing of wounds and musculoskeletal injuries. It is, quite literally, a plant that helps knit the body back together—living up to its common name, *knitbone*.

Historical connections: The Latin name *Symphytum* originates from the Greek word symphyo, meaning "to unite," which is an apparent reference to its reputation for bone mending. Comfrey was revered by our European ancestors for both its medicinal virtues and its value in the garden as an organic fertilizer and companion plant. The radical 17th-century English herbalist Nicholas Culpepper sang its praises in his *Complete Herbal*, recommending it for a wide range of ailments, from gout and internal bleeding to wound healing. An article from *The Chemist and Druggist* in 1921 reflected the longstanding trust in this plant among country folk: "Allantoin is a fresh instance of the good judgment of our rustics, especially of old times, about the virtues of plants. The great Comfrey or consound...was held almost infallible as a remedy for both external and internal wounds, bruises, and ulcers."

Jessica's Notes: I have personally witnessed and experienced the miraculous healing powers of Comfrey. When my knee flares up, I love to gather fresh young leaves, bruise them, and apply the crushed leaves directly to my inflamed knee. The relief is nearly immediate, and I am always left in awe of this plant's gift. Comfrey has earned a permanent place in my wild medicine chest and my heart. Thank you, God, for providing such a healing ally for our bodies.

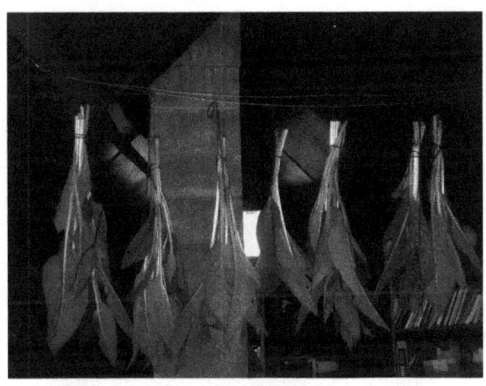

Comfrey drying in the cabin loft

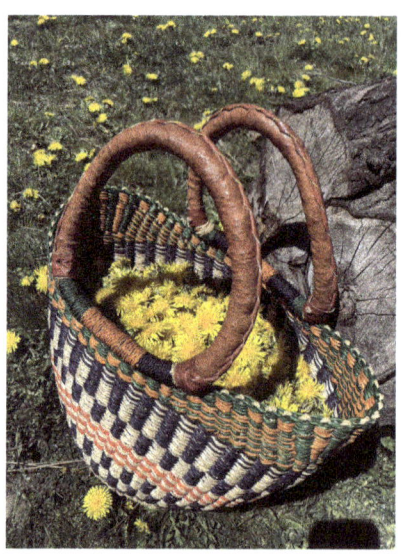

Dandelion

Taraxacum officinale

Asteraceae (Daisy) Family

Description: This herbaceous and hearty perennial is wonderfully easy to identify. Its deeply veined, toothy leaves grow in a rosette, funneling rain down into the nourishing roots below. Atop each hollow stem blooms a cheerful cluster of bright yellow flowers. Interestingly, each petal of what we call a dandelion "flower" is a tiny individual flower, complete with its stamen and pistil. A single flower head can contain between 60 and 100 seeds! The hollow stems, by the way, make fun biodegradable straws for children.

Where it grows: It always amazes me that people complain about dandelions in their lawns, going to great lengths to spray them away, when this humble plant is such a gift! Dandelions love to grow among grasses and thrive in disturbed soils, along garden edges, meadows, roadsides, and just about anywhere you venture. They are a true companion plant of the l and.

When and how to harvest: Harvest the greens when they are young and tender, as their bitterness increases with age. The flowers can be gathered from early spring to late summer, while they are in bloom. For the roots, the ideal time to harvest is in early spring, before the plant flowers.

How to work with it / Medicinal use: Dandelion is sometimes affectionately called "Poor Man's Ginseng," because the root carries many of the same healing virtues as ginseng—especially for building vitality and balancing the body's systems. This hardworking plant benefits not only us but also the earth beneath our feet. Its long taproot helps to break up compacted soil and draw nutrients up toward the surface, nourishing neighboring plants. Similarly, when consumed, the root helps to break up stagnation within the liver, supporting detoxification and nutrient absorption.

I love adding dandelion flowers to my wintertime teas for both their sunny flavor and nourishing qualities. They also make their way into my *Glow-up Face Oil*. The leaves are wonderful in smoothies or tossed into a spring salad. If their bitterness is too strong for your palate, sautéing them gently tempers their flavor. Moreover, of course, roasted dandelion roots make an excellent coffee substitute—delicious and fortifying.

Healing Constituents / Therapeutic Actions: Dandelion blossoms are rich in vitamin D, the "sunshine vitamin." The roots and leaves offer a treasure trove of bioavailable minerals, including calcium, iron, copper, magnesium, manganese, phosphorus, potassium, selenium, silicon, and zinc. They also contain generous amounts of vitamins A, B-complex, C, and D. Dandelion is abundant in carotenoids, fatty acids, flavonoids, and phytosterols. The leaves in particular are strongly diuretic, helping the body release excess fluids and cleanse the system.

Historical Connection: Dandelions originated in Asia and Europe. Though they were not native to North America when Europeans first arrived, they quickly made their way here, following people as one of their beloved plant companions. Their feathery, wind-borne seeds have allowed them to spread across every continent on Earth. Ancient texts reference dandelions, and they were used medicinally by Arabic physicians as far back as the tenth and eleventh centuries.

The name *Taraxacum* stems from the Latin *Dens Leonis*, meaning "lion's tooth," which in French became *Dent de Lion*, a reference to the toothed leaves and the flower's golden mane. The English later adopted this as "Dandelion." One folk name for this plant is *pis en lit*—meaning "piss in the night"—a playful warning about its diuretic nature. (Best not to drink dandelion tea before bedtime!)

Jessica's Notes: When dandelion flowers are blooming in abundance, and we have fired up the grill for a summer barbecue, I love to toss the fresh flowers in an herbal marinade and grill them. They taste surprisingly like tender, buttery artichoke hearts! It is such a joyful way to celebrate this humble, nourishing plant that grows so freely all around us.

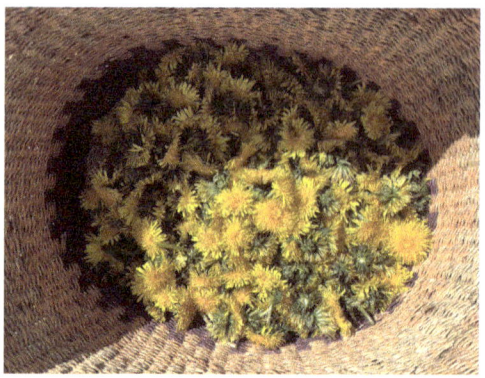

A basketful of springtime dandelion flowers

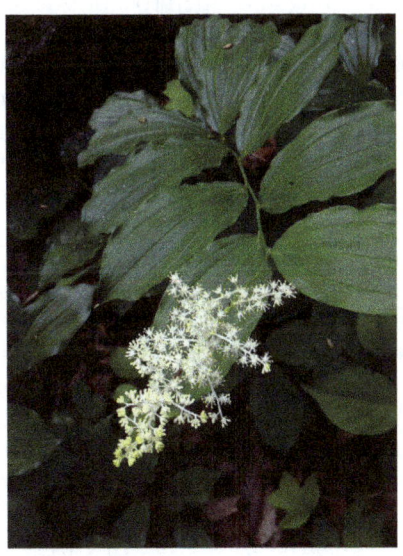

False Solomon's Seal

Maianthemum racemosum subsp. amplexicaule, Maianthemum stellatum

Liliaceae (Lily) Family

Other common names: False Spikenard, Solomon's Plume

Description: False Solomon's Seal brings an elegant touch of spring to the forest floor with its gracefully arching stalks and fragrant white flower clusters. This perennial plant grows to a height of 1 to 3 feet, with its unbranched stalks arching outward and adorned with 5 to 12 alternately arranged leaves. These leaves, oblong-elliptical to egg-shaped, range from 3 to 8 inches long and are smooth-edged, with parallel veins. The leaves are stalkless and often taper where they meet the stem. In mid-spring, creamy-white flowers bloom in pyramidal clusters at the tips of the stalks, their fragrance beckoning both pollinators and passing foragers alike. Each flower displays six distinct tepals—structures that are not clearly differentiated into petals and sepals.

As summer progresses, the plant produces berries that start light green with golden-brown mottling and ripen to a bright red. These berries contain one to two seeds each. The roots of star-flowered false Solomon's seal (*Maianthemum stellatum*) are smaller than those of *Maianthemum racemosum*; *stellatum* also bears fewer flowers and darker berries. False Solomon's Seal spreads by branching rhizomes, often forming thick mats across the forest floor. Its name arises from its similarity in growth habit, leaves, and habitat to true Solomon's Seal (*Polygonatum biflorum*).

Where it grows: You will find False Solomon's Seal thriving in the shaded understory of forests. It favors dense woodland ground cover beneath shrubs and trees, preferring nutrient-rich soil to create a lush, graceful carpet of green.

When and how to harvest: The rhizomes and roots are best harvested in autumn, once the plant's above-ground parts have died back. It is important to harvest with care—take only a few plants from each healthy colony. After gathering roots, you can encourage future growth by replanting a 3-inch section of the bud-bearing rhizome. The bright berries, tart and sweet like cranberries, can be harvested in late summer to early fall. If saving seed, sow it soon after the berries ripen.

How to work with it / Medicinal uses: This beautiful plant nourishes the body's inner waters and lends flexibility to stiff joints and tissues. Its flowing, graceful form offers a visual signature of its gifts: promoting ease and suppleness. Tea or tincture made from the roots helps hydrate the connective tissues of joints, making them less prone to injury. Because the roots contain steroidal saponins, a tincture may also help regulate the menstrual cycle and balance mood swings related to hormonal fluctuations.

The soothing, moistening qualities of False Solomon's Seal also make it an excellent remedy for sore throats. Taken as a tea or gargled, it helps ease coughs and inflammation. In the field, bruised leaves can be applied as a poultice for scrapes, rashes, insect bites, and minor cuts, providing quick, gentle relief.

Healing constituents / Therapeutic actions: The roots are sweet, bitter, astringent, and rich in saponins. These properties help hydrate connective tissue, regulate hormones, soothe sore throats, and support tissue healing.

Historical connections: Though not as widely chronicled as its close relative, authentic Solomon's Seal, this North American plant has long been used for similar healing purposes. In his classic text *The Herbal*, John Gerard wrote of Solomon's Seal: "The root stamped and applied in manner of a poultice and laid upon members that have been out of joint, and newly restored to their places, driveth away the pain, and knitteth the joint very firmly, and taketh away the inflammation, if there chance to be any." These same healing virtues are found in False Solomon's Seal, though its story has long remained somewhat hidden in plain sight, ready now to be rediscovered.

Jessica's notes: I have always felt a pang of discomfort when referring to this plant as "false." There is nothing false about it! It is a profoundly healing and virtuous ally of the forest. During my herb walks and tea talks, I make a point of explaining this to my students, referring to it by its common name while acknowledging its true gifts. I hope that, with more awareness, this plant will gain the full respect it so richly deserves.

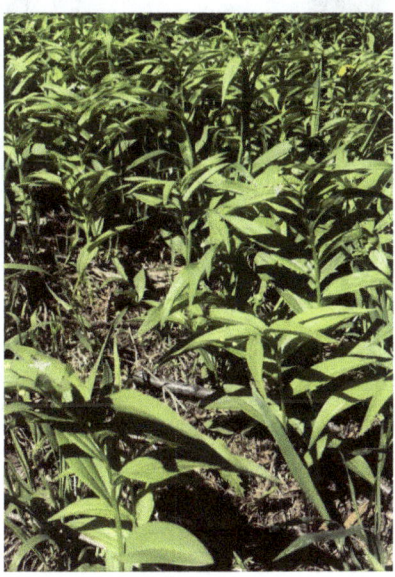

Mainthemum stellatum

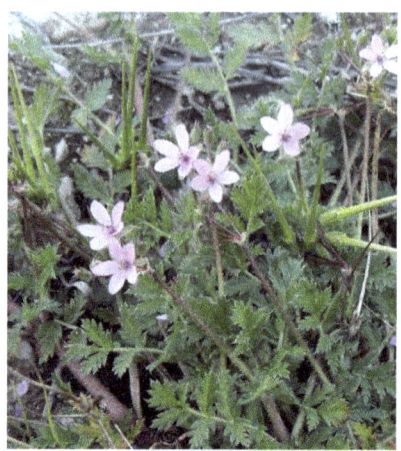

Filaree

Erodium cicutarium

Geraniaceae (Geranium) Family
Other common names: storksbill, cranesbill
   Description: Filaree is a low-growing perennial, with its dainty pink five-petalled flowers appearing in small clusters. The plant earns the common name "storksbill" from its long, beak-like fruits, which resemble the bill of a stork. The stems, often tinged red, emerge from a basal rosette. Its feathery, dark green leaves are finely divided into delicate segments. When the seed heads dry, they curl tightly and are cleverly adapted for seed dispersal—easily catching in socks, animal fur, or anything passing by.
   Where it grows: Originally introduced to North America from Europe and Asia as a foraged crop, Filaree is now a familiar lawn and garden "weed." It thrives in disturbed areas—gardens, meadows, lawns, pastures, and roadsides—and is found throughout much of the world. Wherever people settle, Filaree often follows.
   When and how to harvest: Harvest the young greens in the spring and early summer, when the leaves are at their tenderest and most flavorful.
   How to work with it / Medicinal uses: Filaree leaves are edible and versatile. They can be eaten raw or cooked, with a sharp, parsley-like flavor that adds brightness to green salads or serves as a flavorful garnish for soups and stews. In traditional Chinese medicine, tea made from Filaree leaves has been used as a kidney tonic and to treat urinary tract bleeding. The

herb's mild diuretic and astringent actions make it a gentle support for urinary health and inflammation.

Healing constituents / Therapeutic actions: Filaree offers subtle but beneficial healing properties. It is considered astringent, diuretic, and anti-inflammatory, supportive for urinary tract health, and helpful in reducing minor inflammation.

Historical connections: Filaree's relationship with humans stretches back millennia. In Mexico, it has been used for centuries to help prevent postpartum hemorrhage and infections following childbirth. With more than 10,000 years of association with people and livestock, Cranesbill is truly a "people's plant," thriving wherever humans travel and settle.

Jessica's notes: When I was a child, one of my favorite recess pastimes was gathering Cranesbill seed stalks and turning them into miniature scissors. I have always been enchanted by tiny objects and loved creating miniature fairy villages with them. At the time, I had no idea Filaree was edible—no one taught me that! Years later, on a forest school outing, I spotted a patch of Storksbill growing as a ground cover near a landscaped trailhead. I pointed it out to my students, though we did not harvest it—there was a chance the area had been sprayed. A few weeks later, we returned to the spot, only to find that the Parks and Rec landscapers had removed the "weed." Moments like this remind me of the importance of preserving and honoring the plants we often overlook. Furthermore, if you wish to abolish these abundant weeds, try nibbling on some of the tender greens to receive the earth's medicine.

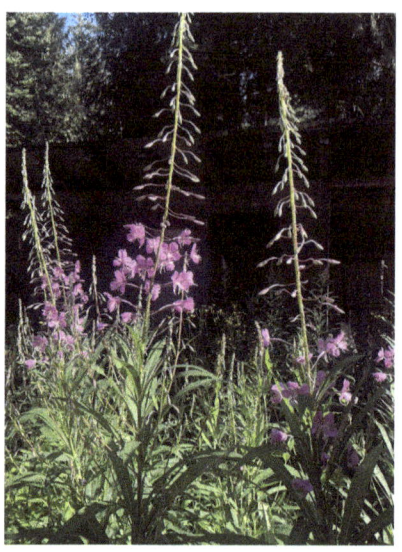

Fireweed

Chamaenerion angustifolium

Onagraceae (Evening Primrose) Family
Other names: *spukWu'say* (Twana), willow herb, *Epilobium angustifolium*

Description: Fireweed is a tall and striking wildflower with brilliant magenta-pink blooms that catch the eye of both humans and pollinators alike. The reddish stems rise above the forest floor, adorned with dark green, alternately arranged lanceolate leaves that spiral upward. The flowers, each 2 to 3 centimeters in diameter, open from the bottom of the stalk to the top, creating an elegant, tapered spire. After flowering, Fireweed produces slender seed capsules, each containing 300 to 400 tiny brown seeds—nearly 80,000 seeds per plant! These seeds are attached to silky hairs that allow them to drift on the wind like tiny parachutes, helping Fireweed swiftly colonize disturbed landscapes. Once established, its robust underground root system forms a dense and resilient perennial patch.

Where it grows: A true pioneer species, Fireweed thrives in disturbed soil and is often one of the first plants to reclaim land after a wildfire, which is how it earned its evocative name. It flourishes in open fields, meadows, pastures, and recently burned areas, favoring locations with ample sunlight. Its vibrant pink floral spikes bring beauty and life to stark or recovering landscapes, where it rarely grows alone but instead forms vast colonies of color and resilience.

When and how to harvest: In early spring, harvest the tender young shoots when they are still succulent and mild. Throughout summer and into early fall, gather the leaves and flowers at their peak.

How to work with it / Medicinal use: Both Fireweed's flowers and leaves are delicious and nourishing additions to tea, soups, and stews. The young shoots can be eaten raw, sautéed, or pickled—Yukon tradition includes making a fragrant jam from its flowers. Fireweed honey is especially prized for its light, floral flavor. The flowers can also be added to bathwater to soothe inflamed skin conditions, such as eczema. In Russia, a traditional fermented tea called *Ivan Chai* is made by rolling and drying Fireweed leaves, which is enjoyed as a flavorful and healthful substitute for black tea. Medicinally, a strong decoction of Fireweed is an effective remedy for fungal and yeast infections, both internally and topically. It supports gut healing and restores balance to the digestive microbiome. In this way, Fireweed mirrors its role in nature—just as it rehabilitates the land after fire or devastation, so too can it help regenerate the human body after imbalance and illness.

Healing constituents / Therapeutic actions: Fireweed contains quercetin and oenothein, compounds known for their natural antihistamine effects, which are excellent for treating seasonal allergies and fungal skin infections. It is considered a superfood, rich in vitamins A and C, as well as bioflavonoids that support overall wellness. The young shoots are exceptionally high in mucilage, a soothing agent for the intestinal tract and digestive system.

Historical connections: For centuries, Fireweed has been an important food and medicine for Indigenous peoples of the Pacific Northwest and Alaska. The stem pith was used to thicken soups, gravies, and puddings, while the fibrous seed fluff was woven into mountain goat wool for soft, insulating blankets. Early pioneers, fur traders, and trappers also embraced Fireweed as a staple. The Eclectic Physicians of the 19th and early 20th centuries documented Fireweed's usefulness as a gentle astringent and tonic for chronic diarrhea, recovery from food poisoning, prostate inflammation, sore mouths, and swollen gums. Remarkably, Fireweed was among the first plants to return after the 1980 eruption of Mt. St. Helens, once again demonstrating its role as a healer of the land.

Jessica's notes: Fireweed holds a special place in my heart and our family's foraging traditions. Each spring, we joyfully pickle the tender shoots—they taste much like pickled asparagus and are enhanced with healing herbs in the brine. Throughout the growing season, we gather leaves and some flowers, always mindful to leave plenty for pollinators, and store them for fall and winter teas. Just as Fireweed brings beauty and resilience to recovering landscapes, it brings healing and harmony to the body.

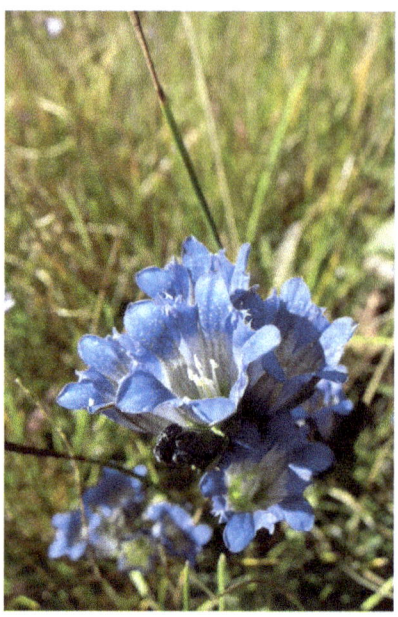

Gentian

Gentiana affinis Griseb.

Gentianaceae (Gentian) Family
Other common names: Explorer's gentian, Mountain bog gentian, *Gentiana parryi* Engelm.

Description: The three species of Gentian described here are herbaceous perennials with opposite leaves and a low-growing habit, reaching heights of approximately 1 to 1 ½ feet. Their deep violet to blue tubular flowers stand out amongst other ground-hugging forest herbs. *Gentiana affinis* sprouts from a well-developed root crown, with lance-shaped to ovate leaves measuring ½–1 inch in length. The bluish-purple, funnel-shaped flowers develop at the upper leaf axils. *Gentiana calycosa* features ovate leaves of similar size, with dark blue to violet flowers that are often solitary. *G. parryi* is a multi-stemmed herbaceous plant with lanceolate to ovate leaves. The flowers appear in groups of up to six, arranged in terminal or subterminal whorls, and display vibrant violet petals accented by green bands. In all species, the elongated seed capsules are approximately ½ inch long and contain brown seeds.

Where it grows: Gentian commonly inhabits moist mountain meadows, fields, and pine forests, often blooming alongside wildflowers such as yarrow and St. John's wort.

When and how to harvest: Gather Gentian's taproot in late summer and early fall. Its simple taproot is easily forked out of the earth. The herbage can also be used if it is sufficiently bitter—taste it to be sure.

How to work with it/ Medicinal uses: Gentian is known as the "champion bitter tonic" of Western herbal medicine. While it is not the most pungent bitter, it is considered the purest (Kane, 2017). Gentian stimulates digestion and bile production. A tea or tincture taken before meals supports the breakdown of food and encourages optimal nutrient absorption. It stimulates the secretion of pepsin, hydrochloric acid, and mucus, making it particularly useful for gastric deficiency and chronic dry mouth resulting from reduced saliva production.

Gentian is often combined with aromatic herbs, such as Monarda and mountain mint, to create an aromatic, bitter blend. This blend is generally superior to using Gentian alone. However, in cases of acid reflux or gastritis, it may be better to pair Gentian with gentler herbs, like mugwort.

One of Gentian's lesser-known yet valuable uses is in helping to restore digestive function after interruptions caused by conditions such as anorexia nervosa, orthorexia, temporary feeding tubes, or chronic gastrointestinal injuries. In such cases, taking Gentian 5–10 minutes before meals can be highly effective in rebuilding appetite and digestive strength.

Though not as strong as milk thistle or turmeric, Gentian does exhibit hepatoprotective (liver-supportive) actions. It stimulates the upper digestive tract, which, in turn, promotes liver and kidney function, helping to reduce liver inflammation.

Gentian also has a mild blood-sugar-lowering effect and can aid circulation in those with type 2 diabetes or hyperglycemia. For best results, it should be combined with a healthy diet, regular exercise, and other supportive herbs.

Topically, Gentian ointment or salve is an effective antibacterial and antifungal dressing, particularly for minor wounds prone to infection. Gentian is an ingredient in Angostura bitters, a popular tonic used in spirits and cocktails.

Healing constituents/ Therapeutic actions: Gentian contains a suite of bitter and stimulating compounds, including anthocyanins, flavones, iridoids, secoiridoid glycosides, sterols, and triterpenoids. It is valued for its stomachic (digestive-stimulating), hepatoprotective (liver-supporting), and tonic actions.

Historical connections: Gentian has been used for centuries. The flowers of *Gentiana pneumonanthe* were once used to create blue dye. The genus name *Gentiana* derives from King Gentius of Illyria (181–168 BC), who, according to Greek historians, was the first to recognize its medicinal value.

Gentian has also served as a substitute for hops in brewing beer, and gentian-infused liqueurs and wines have been popular in Europe for centuries. In the 18th century, gentian wine was a common stomachic, taken before meals to aid digestion.

Nicholas Culpepper, in *The Complete Herbal,* wrote that Gentian was "under the dominion of Mars" and a remedy for putrefaction, poison, pestilence, weak stomachs, fainting, and venomous bites. He advocated for the use of English Gentian for English bodies—a sentiment that resonates with today's emphasis on bioregional herbalism.

Jessica's notes: Although Gentian is not a plant I gather often due to its relatively small populations in certain areas, I hold great respect for its powerful medicinal properties. I was first surprised to find Gentian growing at *The Welsh Wood*—my parents' land in North Idaho—where I began learning about many of the wild plants that now fill this book. Amongst the yarrow and St. John's wort, those striking blue flowers caught my eye and stayed with me. Now, whenever I encounter Gentian on my foraging walks, it brings back memories of those early plant studies at The Welsh Wood. I look forward to one day crafting a local bitters blend with our native Gentian, wild Monarda, and perhaps fireweed—a true digestive bitter blend.

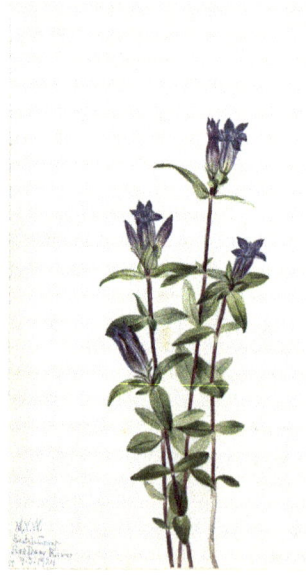

Riverbank gentian painted by Mary Vaux Walcott, 1924. Public domain image courtesy of the Smithsonian American Art Museum.

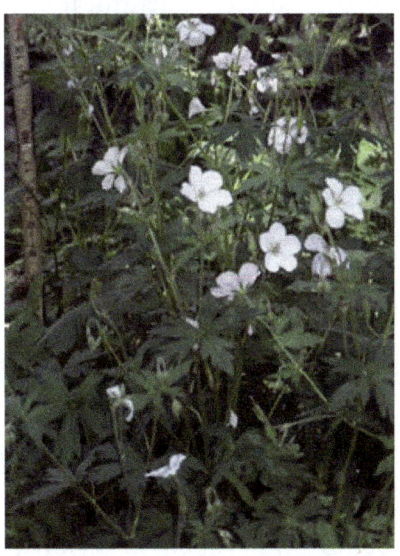

Geranium

Geranium caespitosum, Geranium richardsonii

Geraniaceae (Geranium) Family
Other common names: Pineywoods geranium, Wild geranium, White geranium, Richardson's geranium

Description: Both species are small, herbaceous, subshrub perennials that grow no more than 3 feet tall and 3 feet wide. The leaves are dark green, palmate, and deeply cut or lobed. The five-petaled flowers develop from the leaf axils on long stalks. *Geranium caespitosum* flowers are purple to pink and are composed of five disk-shaped petals. The leaves are five-parted, with each part divided into three lobes. *Geranium richardsonii's* flowers are white to pale pink. When examined closely, there are striking purple veins from the base of each petal that radiate toward the tip. The leaves are 2 to 5 inches wide and distinctly lobed.

Where it grows: *G. richardsonii* is more commonly found in mixed conifer/aspen forests, while *G. caespitosum* is more frequent in Ponderosa pine forests. Both species prefer woodland margins and forest openings over dense, shady forests.

When and how to harvest: Harvest the narrow taproots in late summer and early fall. Be sure to verify identification, as basal leaf growth resembles that of Aconite and Larkspur, which are toxic when ingested.

How to work with it / Medicinal uses: Geranium root is similar to tannin-rich Alumroot and can be used in the same astringent manner. Gargle an infusion of the root for bleeding gums and short-term relief of a sore throat. A nasal wash can help alleviate chronic sinusitis, particularly when there is significant mucus buildup. Geranium is an intestinal binder, like other tannin-rich plants; drinking Geranium root tea can help alleviate diarrhea. If there are accompanying spasms, add Monarda and Mint. With its intestinal binding actions, Geranium can help the bowels form a complete stool before it leaves the body. The root tea or tincture may help with nausea and gastritis. Start with a small amount and increase the dosage if there is improvement. A room-temperature sitz bath is soothing for vaginal irritations and hemorrhage and can be used as a postpartum toner. As a field poultice, Geranium comes in handy for insect bites, cuts, and stings. The powdered root can be applied to wounds due to its antibacterial and anti-inflammatory properties, which aid in healing.

Healing constituents / Therapeutic actions: Geranium is rich in phenolic acids, including quinic acid, shikimic acid, neochlorogenic acid, chlorogenic acid, ellagic acid, galloylglucoses, ellagitannins, and flavonoids such as quercetin, myricetin, kaempferol, and malvidin. Therapeutic actions include anti-inflammatory, antibacterial, and astringent.

Historical connections: Wild Geranium has been used for centuries by Native Americans. It is still used today to treat inflammation of the mouth and bowels.

Jessica's notes: The smell of Geranium always brings me back to carefree childhood afternoons spent playing make-believe in my grandparents' backyard. Their garden was filled with cultivated varieties of Geranium, a common landscaping plant, but the scent and feel of the leaves created an indelible imprint in my memory. Now, when I encounter wild Geranium in the forest, it reminds me how the cultivated and the wild are connected—how many of the plants we see in gardens today were once wild herbs, valued for their beauty and healing properties. The wild Geranium helps me bridge those worlds, honoring both the wisdom of the wild and the legacy of the cultivated.

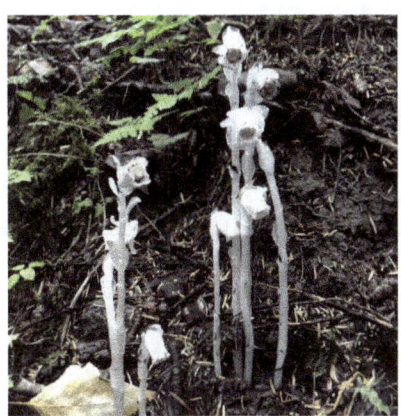

Ghost Pipe

Monotropa uniflora

Monotropaceae (Monotropa) Family
Other common names: Indian Pipe

Description: A parasitic perennial of the forest. Not quite a plant or a fungus, it is considered a saprophyte that garnishes nutrients from decaying organic material. Translucent ghost-white stalks bear scales and grow 4 to 8 inches long. Each stalk supports a single, nodding flower resembling those of blueberries — in fact, Ghost Pipe was once classified in the same family as blueberries and huckleberries. It often emerges in eerie clusters, peeking out of the forest loam. It requires no photosynthesis to grow; hence its translucent, pale-white appearance.

Where it grows: Found in old-growth forests amongst decaying organic material and fungi. It haunts the deep shadows of the forest floor, standing aloof and ghostlike, its life intertwined with the unseen mycorrhizal networks below.

When and how to harvest: Harvest with great care in mid-summer to early fall, when the plant is above ground but before it oxidizes and turns black. Tragically, this plant has been over-harvested and is now endangered in many states. Only gather where there is true abundance, and take only what you need. Cut at the base of the stalk—never uproot it—as this will impede future growth. Ghost Pipe is very delicate and oxidizes quickly, so fresh plant material must be transferred into alcohol shortly after harvesting.

How to work with it/ Medicinal use: Ghost Pipe tincture is a profound pain reliever, addressing both physical and emotional pain as well as intense nerve pain. It offers gentle support for highly sensitive individuals and those on the autism spectrum. Just a few drops of tincture can help ease suffering. Once the fresh stalk is placed in alcohol, the extract transforms into a stunning violet-purple hue through oxidation. Traditionally, Ghost Pipe tonic has been used for convulsions in children, epilepsy, chorea, spasmodic affections, febrile diseases, restlessness, nervous irritability, acute anxiety, and even psychotic episodes. When paired with rose water, Ghost Pipe juice can also be used topically to treat ulcers, bladder inflammation, ophthalmic inflammation, and other conditions.

Healing constituents/ Therapeutic actions: The plant contains salicylic acid (the same pain-relieving compound found in aspirin) and acts as a tonic, nervine, diaphoretic, and sedative.

Historical connection: An old Cherokee tale teaches that when selfishness first entered the world, people began to quarrel. The chieftains gathered to smoke a peace pipe but argued for seven days and nights. As punishment for using the peace pipe before true peace was achieved, the Great Spirit transformed the chieftains into gray, ghostly flowers that would grow where families and friends quarreled—a haunting reminder of the dangers of selfishness.

Interestingly, nineteenth-century American poet Emily Dickinson's favorite flower was the Ghost Pipe. After her death, her friend Mabel Loomis Todd and her publisher selected Ghost Pipe to adorn the cover of Dickinson's first published collection of poems in 1879. Dickinson referred to Ghost Pipe as her "preferred flower of life," believing that "being a flower is a huge responsibility." She had gathered Ghost Pipe in her youth and pressed it into her teenage herbarium, enchanted by its "almost supernatural" appearance.

Here is her poem in full:

'Tis whiter than an Indian Pipe
Emily Dickinson, ca. 1879

'Tis whiter than an Indian Pipe —'Tis dimmer than a Lace —No stature has it, like a Fog When you approach the place —

Not any voice imply it here —Or intimate it there —A spirit — how doth it accost —What function hath the Air?

This limitless Hyperbole Each one of us shall be —'Tis Drama — if Hypothesis —It be not Tragedy —

Jessica's notes: I first discovered this mysterious plant when I moved to Idaho and was exploring the old-growth forest near my new home. The moment I saw it, standing luminous and otherworldly amongst the duff, I knew it was something unusual. Serendipitously, that very week, I listened to a podcast that happened to cover the medicinal qualities of Ghost Pipe — and I realized they were describing the exact plant I had found. I returned soon after, carrying a mason jar of vodka just as the herbalist had recommended, and harvested a small amount with reverence and bare hands. That night, I had a vivid and lucid dream: I was in a distant, ancient time, seated around a fire preparing herbs. Suddenly, Ghost Pipe emerged from the earth and flowered above my head, speaking to me: *"We are sacred medicine, and we choose you to work with us."* I awoke in a sweat, deeply moved by the experience. Since then, Ghost Pipe has been one of my most trusted allies, especially after my knee dislocation and surgery, when pharmaceuticals upset my stomach, Ghost Pipe tincture brought gentle relief and allowed me to rest.

I must also emphasize that this plant is endangered in many places. If you come across it, please do not harvest unless the colony is abundant and thriving. Let it haunt the forest floor as it is meant to — a living reminder of humility, reverence, and restraint. May we remember the Cherokee wisdom: selfishness will lead to our ruin—Harvest Ghost Pipe only with the utmost respect and mindfulness.

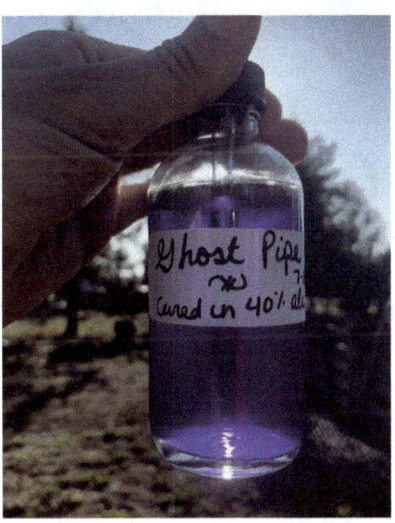

My first wild crafted ghost pipe tincture

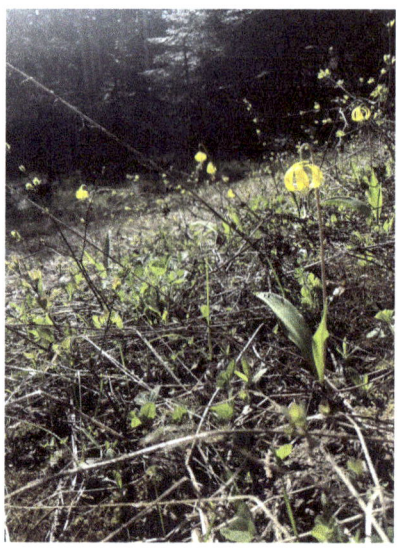

Glacier Lily

Erythronium grandiflorum

Liliaceae (Lily) Family

Other common names: Fawn Lily, Trout Lily, Adder's Tongue, Dogtooth Violet

Description: One of the first showy wildflowers of early spring, Glacier Lily appears at the margins of melting snowfields. This perennial bulb begins as a pair of basal leaves. The beautiful, bright yellow flowers rise on leafless central flower stalks (peduncles). Each flower, about 3 inches in diameter, has six lance-shaped petals and six stamens, with a distinctive white-yellow band at the base of the flower.

Where it grows: Glacier Lily favors moist woods and meadows, from an elevation of around 2,500 feet to above the timberline. It often carpets subalpine meadows in early spring, following the retreat of the snow.

When and how to harvest: Harvest the leaves and flowers from April through June. The delicate flowers can be picked for culinary use, but they should be harvested sparingly, as they are a vital early food source for pollinators. The seed pods and leaves are edible but should be consumed in small amounts due to their laxative effect. The bulbs, although edible, are small and should be reserved as a last resort in a survival situation. The life of this beautiful plant does not justify aggressive harvesting — take only a few flowers here and there, leaving the majority to nourish the land and its creatures.

How to work with it/ Medicinal uses: Glacier Lily flowers make a cheerful addition to springtime salads, pasta dishes, and soups. Leaves and seed pods can also be eaten, but should be consumed in moderation. The leaf infusion, though seldom used in modern herbalism, exhibits antibacterial properties and is effective against a broad range of bacteria when used topically. Emerging research suggests that some of the plant's compounds may have tumor-reducing properties, though further study is needed.

Healing constituents/ Therapeutic actions: Leaf infusions exhibit antibacterial properties and show promise in laboratory studies for their potential to inhibit tumor growth. Historically, the plant was used to reduce fever, swelling, and infection.

Historical connections: First Nations lore tells of observing grizzly bears digging up Glacier Lily bulbs in springtime, then leaving them to wilt in the sun for a few days to sweeten and make them more digestible. This ancient wisdom was adopted by early peoples, who learned to dry and prepare the bulbs in the same manner. The Shoshone consumed the corms fresh or in soups and traded the dried bulbs among tribes. Various Native American nations used Glacier Lily to help ease fever, swelling, infection, and the risk of miscarriage.

Meriwether Lewis recorded Glacier Lily during the famed Lewis and Clark Expedition; Lewis mentioned it frequently in his diary. Some historians believe he used the Dogtooth Violet, an old familiar name for this plant, as a kind of "botanical calendar" to track the arrival of spring.

Jessica's notes: Whenever I see these gorgeous golden lilies blooming on the mountain, I cannot help but think of Easter and the resurrection of Christ, of life renewed after winter's cold and darkness. Their ephemeral return brings hope and the promise of new life — a fitting symbol of salvation and rebirth.

As naturalist and author Rick Bass so beautifully wrote in *The Wild Marsh: Four Seasons at Home in Montana*:

"The snow is melting. The grizzly bears that have been sleeping beneath the snow, suspended like seeds, will prowl the warm fields just beneath the snow, grazing on the delicious emerging lilies. Sometimes the yellow pollen gets caught on the fur and snouts of the great golden bears as they grub and push through the lily fields, pollinating other lilies in this manner. In this crude fashion, they are farmers of a kind, nurturing and expanding one of the crops that first meets them yearly. The lilies follow the snow, and the snow pulls back to reveal the bears, and the bears follow the lilies. The script of life begins moving with enthusiasm once again."

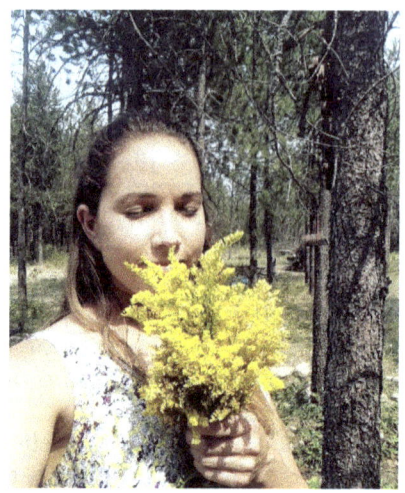

Goldenrod

Solidago canadensis

Asteraceae (Daisy) Family
Other common names: Golden woundwort
  Description: The name is perfectly descriptive of this radiant plant. A pubescent, short-lived perennial, Goldenrod sends up golden flower stalks that sway in the wind by mid-summer. The plant's toothed leaves alternate along the stem, and the flower cluster grows at the top of the stalk in both disk and ray flowers. Mature plants typically reach two to four feet tall.
  Where it grows: Goldenrod thrives in drier soils, open grasslands, meadows, old farm fields, and forest openings. It often flourishes where other plants might struggle, bringing color and vitality to the land.
  When and how to harvest: Harvest flowers and aerial tops early to mid-summer, before the plant goes to seed. If you wait too long, the dried flower clusters will turn into puffy seed clouds. Roots can be harvested in early spring or autumn.
  How to work with it/ Medicinal use: Goldenrod is both a tasty tea herb and a culinary delight. The flowers are edible and can be fried in batter for a seasonal treat. Young, tender leaves can be cooked like spinach and added to soups, stews, or stir-fries. The tincture is a valuable remedy to have on hand for seasonal allergies, colds, and flu, while a honey infusion soothes sore throats. Goldenrod tea supports the urinary tract and helps

nourish and restore kidney function. Chew the roots for toothaches and irritated gums. The flowers and leaves can also be infused in oil to create a salve with excellent wound-healing properties. The tea or tincture can help alleviate sore throats with its antiseptic and antimicrobial properties. As an expectorant, it helps clear mucus from the lungs. Goldenrod's diaphoretic action encourages sweating during a fever. Its antifungal properties make it helpful in combating candida overgrowth.

Beyond internal use, Goldenrod has numerous topical applications: the hydrosol is anti-inflammatory and antispasmodic, helpful for sore muscles, stiff necks, and repetitive strain injuries. A hair rinse made from Goldenrod flowers can naturally highlight golden-blonde tones.

Caution: Avoid use if you have known allergies to plants in the Asteraceae family.

Healing constituents/ Therapeutic actions: Goldenrod contains saponins with antifungal properties. Its astringent and antiseptic properties help tone and tighten the urinary tract and bladder, supporting healing in cases of bladder infection. It also contains rutin, a powerful antioxidant that supports overall well-being and can ease seasonal allergies.

Historical connections: Goldenrod's genus name, *Solidago*, is derived from the Latin words *solidare* ("to make strong and healthy") and *ago* ("to make whole"). The plant has been considered a symbol of good luck in many cultures. In Britain, Goldenrod was believed to mark hidden springs and treasure. During Queen Elizabeth's reign, the herb was highly prized for its healing properties, and powdered Goldenrod was imported and sold for nearly half a crown per pound.

Both Native American and Chinese healers worked with Goldenrod to treat arthritis, emphysema, nephritis, and periodontal disease. Native Americans also used *Solidago virgaurea L.* to create a lotion for wounds and ulcers. Ancient Germans gathered Goldenrod as a wound remedy before heading into battle. To this day in Germany, it is called "golden woundwort" and commonly referred to as "fastening herb."

After the Boston Tea Party, American colonists used Goldenrod as an ingredient in "Liberty Tea," brewing it alone or with other native herbs as an alternative to British-imported black tea. During World War II, Thomas Edison experimented with *Solidago leavenworthii* as an emergency rubber source. In parts of the East Coast, Goldenrod became known as Blue Mountain Tea and was often blended with wild mint.

Hildegard Von Bingen (1098–1179), the medieval herbalist and healer, included Goldenrod in her text *Physica*, advising that it not be used for sword wounds (as it heals the surface too quickly), but rather for blemishes, blisters, and animal sores.

Jessica's notes: Goldenrod has truly rescued my son and me during allergy season. We love to drink it as tea, combined with wild mint and sweetened with honey. It is considered a "singer's herb," and as a songbird myself, I turn to Goldenrod tea before performances or when my vocal cords need support. I can feel it loosening mucus in my throat and clearing my sinuses almost immediately. I am continually fascinated by this proud perennial and its wide-reaching history across the globe.

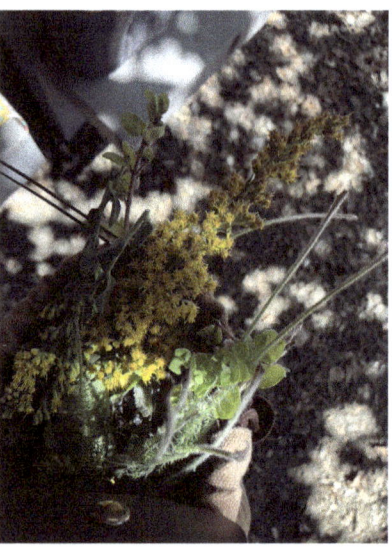

A full foraging bag of goldenrod, yerba buena and yarrow! This will become forest school tea.

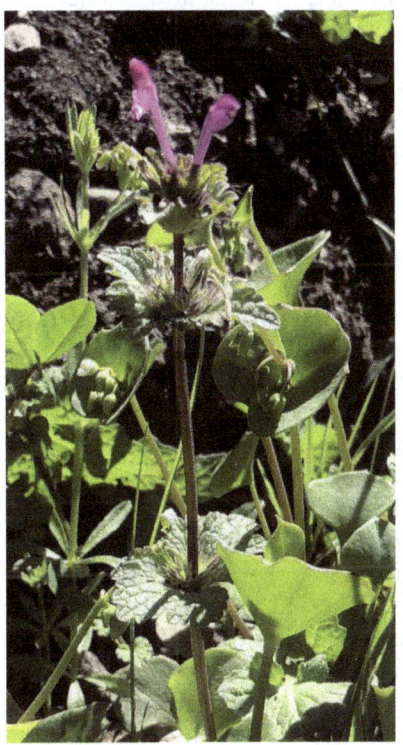

Henbit

Lamium amplexicaule

Lamiaceae (Mint) Family
Other common names: Common Henbit
Description: Henbit is a small, weedy annual introduced from Europe. Like other members of the mint family, it has square stems and leaves that are arranged oppositely. The leaves are rounded with deeply toothed edges and clasp the stem, giving the species the name *amplexicaule*, meaning "stem-clasping." The small, tubular flowers are a vibrant pinkish-purple, emerging intermittently from the upper leaf axils. Each flower has lobed petals and a fuzzy upper lip, resembling a tiny orchid. Henbit is a miniature herb that grows nestled among ground cover or just above it, rarely exceeding 6 to 12 inches in height.

Where it grows: Henbit is a common sight in disturbed areas, including lawns, fields, roadsides, gardens, and ditches. It thrives in cool-season conditions and is often one of the first green plants to appear in late winter or early spring.

When and how to harvest: Harvest the aerial parts—leaves, flowers, and stems—in early spring through summer. It is best gathered before flowering for tender greens or during full bloom for use in teas and poultices.

How to work with it/ Medicinal use: The entire Henbit plant is edible and can be eaten raw or cooked. It adds a delightful peppery flavor to salads, pizza toppings, pestos, and green smoothies. It is tender and mild when young, becoming slightly more fibrous as it matures. Henbit leaves and flowers can be brewed into a tea that soothes digestive discomfort and helps relieve diarrhea. Traditionally, a poultice of the fresh plant was applied to minor burns, insect bites, and wounds to promote healing. The tea is also known to help stop minor internal or external bleeding. Due to its gentle action, Henbit can be a nice addition to spring tonics or as a cooling herb for mild inflammation.

Healing constituents/ Therapeutic actions: Henbit contains anthocyanins, potent antioxidants that protect cells from oxidative stress. It is a source of vitamins A, C, and K, as well as iron and other trace minerals. The plant exhibits astringent, vulnerary (wound-healing), anti-inflammatory, and mild emmenagogue actions.

Historical connections: The common name "Henbit" comes from its popularity as a natural feed for chickens, who happily forage on it in the early spring. It likely arrived in North America with European settlers and quickly naturalized in gardens, fields, and along paths. In traditional folk practices, Henbit was valued both as a food and as a gentle medicinal herb, particularly in early spring after a long winter when fresh greens were scarce. Though not as widely written about in herbal texts, Henbit has long been appreciated in folk herbalism for its nutritive and healing properties.

Jessica's notes: Henbit is one of those humble little spring herbs that often gets overlooked, but I see it as a true gift of the season. I love to gather the delicate flowering tops to sprinkle into spring salads or to make a bright green pesto when the first greens are emerging. I have used Henbit tea to soothe a mild upset stomach and appreciate having this gentle, nourishing herb in my wild pantry. It is also a favorite plant for introducing young foragers and students to edible weeds—accessible, abundant, and friendly to harvest!

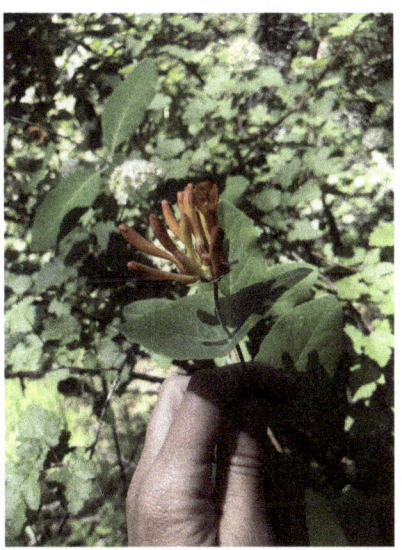

Honeysuckle

Lonicera ciliosa

Caprifoliaceae (Honeysuckle) Family
Other common names: Trumpet Honeysuckle, Orange Honeysuckle, Northwest Honeysuckle

Description: Honeysuckle is an eager, twining vine that can climb to the tops of towering pines in the forest. Young leaves are slightly hairy, while mature leaves are smooth, oval, and arranged in opposite pairs. Terminal flower clusters emerge from a disk-shaped fusion of leaves. The bright orange, trumpet-shaped flowers flare gracefully into five lobes at the tips, making them irresistible to hummingbirds and pollinators. After flowering, the vine produces clusters of translucent red-orange berries. The vines themselves are hollow and turn straw-yellow when dormant in winter.

Where it grows: This proud perennial thrives in open woodlands and along forest edges. It is commonly found trailing along shrubs and trees on forest trails. If you spot one vine, follow it upward as it weaves its way toward the light.

When and how to harvest: Harvest leaves and flowers in mid-to-late summer. The berries ripen from late summer to early fall and can also be harvested at this time.

How to work with it/ Medicinal use: Honeysuckle has a naturally cooling effect on the body. Honeysuckle tea can be used to soothe hot flashes, fevers, sunstroke, and overheated states. The sweet nectar can be sipped directly from the flowers—nature's candy and a refreshing trail-side treat. Prepare a glycerite infusion of the flowers for sore throats and persistent coughs. A poultice made from chewed leaves may be applied to bruises to help reduce inflammation. Traditionally, decoctions of the leaves have been used to treat tuberculosis and respiratory infections. Honeysuckle is also employed to ease inflammatory conditions, including arthritis and rheumatism, as well as certain bacterial or viral infections that contribute to sore throats, colds, and flu.

Healing constituents/ Therapeutic actions: While modern research on this particular species (*Lonicera ciliosa*) remains limited, the flowers are known to contain calcium, magnesium, and potassium. Based on traditional knowledge and related species (*Lonicera japonica* in Chinese medicine), Honeysuckle is considered antiviral, antibacterial, astringent, immune-modulating, blood sugar-regulating, and anti-inflammatory. It may also gently support digestion and urinary health.

Historical connections: Many Pacific Northwest tribes, including the Chehalis, Klallam, Lummi, and Nlaka'pamux, highly valued honeysuckle. An infusion of crushed leaves was used as a hair wash to encourage hair growth. Chewed leaf juice and bark decoctions were traditionally used for treating colds, sore throats, and tuberculosis. Vine segments were placed under pillows to promote restful sleep. The flexible stems were also used to make twine, thread, and black dye, as well as lightweight building materials. Honeysuckle was one of the flora collected and recorded by the Lewis and Clark expedition during their historic journey through the American West.

Jessica's notes: Our forest school students absolutely love Honeysuckle—especially sipping the nectar straight from the bright orange flowers. It is a joyful foraging moment when the children scramble up branches or reach through shrubs to collect their prized "nature's candy." Watching their delight reminds me that wild plants nourish not just our bodies, but also our spirits. Honeysuckle is one of those plants that invites us to engage playfully with the forest.

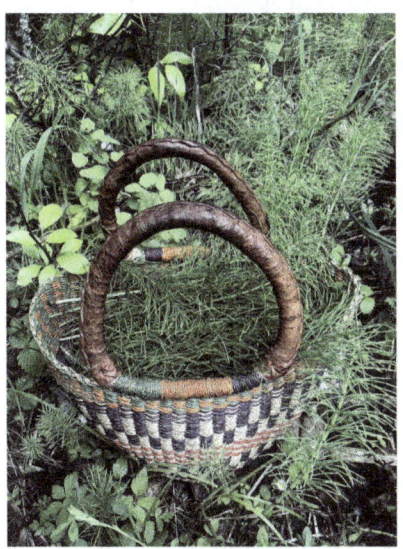

Horsetail

Equisetum arvense

Equisetaceae (Horsetail) Family
Description: An archaic perennial plant related to ferns, Horsetail spreads freely by rhizomes, which produce asparagus-like tubers in its first growth cycle. It is an ancient survivor, descended from massive tree-like plants that thrived 400 million years ago during the Paleozoic era. Today's Horsetail fans out in feathery green "tails" that can grow from one to four feet tall. Its rhizomes can extend as deep as six feet, drawing silica from the soil. Horsetail does not reproduce through pollen but instead through spores. The plant's structure speaks to its prehistoric origins, connecting us to Earth's ancient past.

Where it grows: Horsetail favors rich, moist soils and thrives along wetlands, riverbanks, creeks, springs, and streams. It grows in temperate zones of the Northern Hemisphere, including Asia, North America, and E urope.

When and how to harvest: Harvest the aerial "feathery tails" in early summer. Examine the plant closely—if you see crystals of calcium oxalates on the outer stems, avoid consuming them, as they can be hard on the kidneys. These crystalline Horsetails, however, are still helpful in scouring camp pots, brushing teeth, making foot soaks, and for external washes of hair, skin, and nails. The best specimens for medicinal use are those whose branches point straight upward—these indicate peak quality.

How to work with it/ Medicinal uses: Horsetail is remarkably high in silica, which helps the body build collagen, an essential protein found in connective tissues, skin, bones, cartilage, and ligaments. Because of this, Horsetail can support the healing of broken bones, strengthen hair, skin, and nails, and help prevent or mend osteoporosis. When prepared as a tea, it acts as a diuretic, promoting urination and aiding in the treatment of bladder and urinary tract infections. It can also soothe stomach ulcers and support the removal of kidney stones. A warm poultice may be applied to wounds to stop bleeding or ease pain from fractures and sprains. A cool wash is helpful for burns, bug bites, and skin eruptions. Horsetail is commonly included in natural shampoos, as its mineral-rich content, particularly silica, is known to stimulate hair growth. After shampooing, a simple Horsetail rinse works wonders for hair and scalp health. The Van Tat Gwich'in people of the Boreal North use the leaves to make a healing tea and prepare dried stems for foot soaks and hair rinses.

Healing constituents/ Therapeutic actions: Horsetail is rich in silica, organic acids, ascorbic acid, calcium, carotene, iron, magnesium, niacin, phosphorus, resins, riboflavin, starch, sterols, tannins, and thiamine. Its therapeutic actions include astringent, diuretic, styptic, and vulnerary properties.

Caution: Long-term internal use of Horsetail can deplete vitamin B1 (thiamine). If consuming it regularly, consider supplementing with a B-complex vitamin. Do not use Horsetail if you suffer from edema, gout, heart conditions, or kidney inflammation. Additionally, *Equisetum palustre* (Marsh Horsetail) is toxic to horses and is not recommended for human consumption. Proper identification is essential.

Historical connections: Horsetail is like a living fossil, connecting us to the days when dinosaurs roamed the Earth. Ancient Greeks and Romans used it to stop bleeding and promote the healing of ulcers and wounds. Across cultures, Horsetail has long been valued for its ability to strengthen the body from within and without. Early American pioneers used dried horsetail stems to score pots and pons. It earned the nickname "Pewter Wort" in the American colonies as it was commonly used to clean pewter and wooden kitchen utensils. In Europe, horsetail was employed by cabinet makers and carpenters for polishing metal and wood.

Jessica's notes: Whenever my nails begin to feel brittle, I turn to Horsetail, adding it to my mineral-supporting herbal teas. I am always amazed at how quickly my nails grow strong and resilient after incorporating this ancient plant. It is a humbling reminder that sometimes the simplest remedies are rooted in the deepest layers of time.

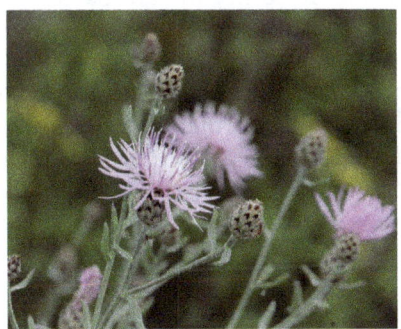

Knapweed

Centaurea stoebe

Asteraceae (Daisy) Family

Other names: Spotted Knapweed

Description: Knapweed is an invasive biennial or short-lived perennial with a stout taproot and pubescent stems when young. The leaves are deeply lobed and covered with fine, short hairs. In its first year, the plant forms a basal rosette, with alternate leaves that can reach up to 6 inches in length, divided into deep lobes. In its second year, it sends up a flowering stem, which can reach up to four feet in height. The upper stem leaves become progressively smaller and less lobed. From July to September, vibrant pink to lavender disk flowers bloom, protruding from distinctive black-tipped bracts. Each corolla has five narrow lobes. After flowering, the plant produces small, bristly achenes that spread through wind dispersal or tumbleweed-like rolling across the landscape.

Where it grows: Knapweed is most often found in disturbed areas: vacant fields, sand prairies, roadsides, streambanks, and pond shorelines. It thrives in dry, well-drained soils and easily outcompetes native vegetation.

When and how to harvest: Harvest flowers from mid-summer to early fall. Roots may be harvested in the fall or early spring. If harvesting for ecological reasons, it is best to uproot the entire plant to help prevent further spread.

How to work with it/ Medicinal uses: The hot root poultice can be used for abscesses, sores, wounds, jaundice, eye disorders, venomous bites, and nosebleeds. A decoction of the flowers may be used for fever, indigestion, and sore throat, or as a gargle for bleeding gums. An ointment prepared from the flowers is said to aid in the healing of bruises and wounds. Although not commonly used by modern herbalists, Knapweed's bitterness lends it stimulant, tonic, and antibacterial properties. Given its abundance in many regions, this invasive plant offers an opportunity for experimentation and the revival of traditional uses.

Healing constituents/ Therapeutic actions: Due to its bitter compounds, Knapweed acts as a stimulant, styptic, tonic, and antibacterial agent. Though modern phytochemical research on *Centaurea stoebe* is still limited, related species in the *Centaurea* genus contain sesquiterpene lactones, flavonoids, polyacetylenes, and tannins, which contribute to these therapeutic effects.

Historical connections: Nicholas Culpepper wrote in *The Complete Herbal* (1653), "It (Knapweed) is singularly good in all running sores, cancerous and fistulous, drying up the moisture, and healing them up so gently without sharpness. It doth the like to running sores or scabs of the head or other parts. It is of special use for the soreness of the throat, swelling of the uvula and jaws, and excellently good to stop bleeding, and heals all green wounds."

Spotted Knapweed likely arrived in North America from Eurasia in the late 1800s, probably as a contaminant in alfalfa seed. The first documented US sighting was in Bingen, Klickitat County, Washington. Since then, it has spread across 45 states and much of Canada. Unfortunately, when Knapweed replaces native grasses, it contributes to soil erosion and disrupts local ecosystems. However, it is an excellent nectar source for pollinators, and beekeepers prize Knapweed honey for its delicate flavor.

An old folk custom suggests that young women once tucked Knapweed beneath their bodices to attract a suitor—a charming example of this plant's role in human folklore.

Jessica's notes: Since Knapweed is so aggressively invasive, I think it makes sense to manage it by utilizing it as a medicinal resource rather than fighting it with harsh chemicals. It would be fun to organize foraging parties to harvest it collectively. Sometimes, the most aggressive "weeds" are simply the forgotten medicines of both people and animals. I have yet to try it, but I suspect a Knapweed ointment would also help treat abscesses on pets—another future project!

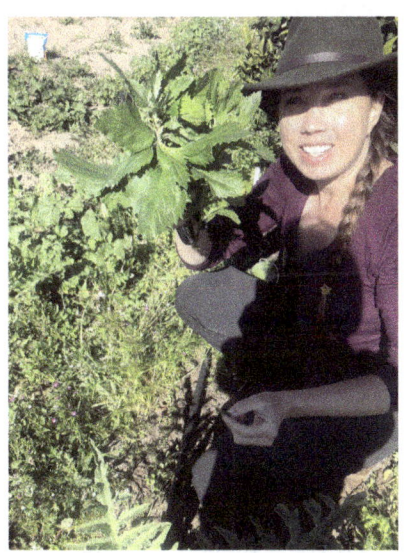

Lamb's Quarters

Chenopodium album

Amaranthaceae (Amaranth) Family
Other common names: Goosefoot, Pig's weed
  Description: Lamb's quarters is an annual weedy plant with dusty-looking leaves, covered in fine, fuzzy hairs. It typically grows up to 2 feet tall, although it occasionally reaches heights of up to 3 feet. The leaves are goosefoot- or diamond-shaped, slightly toothed, light green on top with a whitish-green underside. They can reach lengths of up to 10 cm. The small green flowers bloom in dense, granular clusters along the upper stem in late summer. The plant is highly prolific—one plant can produce up to 75,000 seeds!
  Where it grows: Lamb's quarters thrives in disturbed soils, meadows, gardens, and roadsides. It is found worldwide and is one of the most widespread edible "weeds."
  When and how to harvest: Harvest tender greens in the spring and summer. Seeds can be harvested from late summer to early fall.
  How to work with it/ Medicinal uses: Lamb's quarters is a highly nutritious plant. I like to call it "Nature's Spinach." Enjoy the fresh greens in salads or smoothies. Cooking the greens removes oxalates, making them

suitable for pesto, soups, stews, stir-fries, or any dish that requires greens. The greens can also be blanched and frozen for winter use or dried for when wild greens are scarce. Juicing the young goosefoot leaves in early spring can help the body flush toxins from the bloodstream. The whitish mineral dust on the leaves is highly nutritious and can be dried and powdered to create a seasoning salt. The seeds, harvested in fall, can be ground into flour for bread recipes or sprouted for an easily digestible source of vitamins and minerals. A poultice of chewed or crushed leaves can soothe bug bites, skin irritations, and arthritic joints. The saponin-rich roots can be brewed into a cleansing body wash or used in tea to support waste elimination.

Healing constituents/ Therapeutic actions: *Chenopodium album* is packed with vitamins and minerals. One cup of raw Lamb's quarters contains approximately 73% of the daily recommended intake of vitamin A and 96% of vitamin C (USDA). It is also an excellent source of B vitamins (thiamine, riboflavin, and niacin), as well as iron, calcium, magnesium, phosphorus, selenium, and zinc. Therapeutic actions include anti-inflammatory, anti-diarrheal, astringent, and detoxifying.

Historical connections: The genus name *Chenopodium* originates from the Greek words chen (meaning "goose") and podium (meaning "foot"), referring to the shape of the leaves. The species name *album* means "white," referencing the powdery undersides of the leaves. While *Chenopodium album* is commonly thought to have been introduced from Europe or Asia, archaeological evidence suggests North American tribes, such as the Blackfeet, were using native *Chenopodium* species prior to European contact. Prehistoric peoples worldwide likely relied on Lamb's quarters as a staple wild food. The common name "Lamb's Quarters" is associated with the ancient pagan festival of Lammas (Loaf Mass), the first harvest festival of the year, which is traditionally held on August 1st. This plant has long been gathered and celebrated as part of late-summer harvest traditions.

Jessica's notes: I feel so empowered knowing that I can freely forage for a bounty of easily digestible vitamins and minerals! Lamb's quarters provides everything my body needs to thrive. I always feel stronger and more vibrant when I consume the wild foods that grow naturally around me. Moreover, I do not need to eat much to feel the benefits—just a little goes a long way in nourishing my body and spirit.

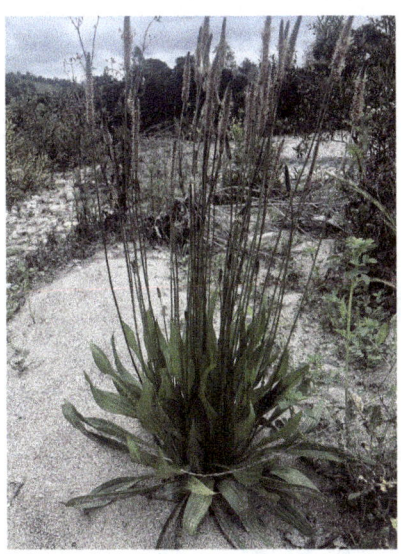

Lanceleaf Plantain

Plantago lanceolata

Plantaginaceae (Plantain) Family
Other common names: Ribwort, Narrow Leaf Plantain, English Plantain

Description: This common perennial plant has dark-green lanceolate leaves (hence its name) that form in rosettes. It produces leafless, silky, and hairy flower stems that range from 4 to 16 inches tall. The basal lanceolate leaves are spread or erect, with three to five parallel veins that narrow to a short petiole. The flower stem is square in profile, terminating in an ovoid inflorescence composed of multiple small flowers, each with a tapered bract. Each inflorescence can produce up to two hundred seeds.

Where it grows: It is found throughout the Americas and Australia, thriving in disturbed soil, garden beds, meadows, roadsides, and pastures. You can find it almost everywhere!

When and how to harvest: Harvest the leaves from early spring to late summer.

How to work with it/ Medicinal uses: Plantain is a versatile addition to the medicine chest, healing and soothing a multitude of external inflammatory conditions. Apply the fresh bruised leaves to spider bites, insect bites, stinging nettle stings, and splinters. The leaves can also be used to make tea as a cough remedy. The roots were traditionally used to treat rattlesnake bites.

Healing constituents/ Therapeutic actions: Plantain's major healing constituents are mucilage, iridoid glycosides (specifically aucubin), and tannins. Lanceleaf plantain offers therapeutic actions that include antihistamine, antifungal, antioxidant, analgesic, and even mild antibiotic properties.

Historical connections: In Celtic folklore, a young man and woman in love could predict their future happiness by collecting two kemps (the flowering spike of the ribwort plantain) and placing them under a rock. Two spikes—one to represent the lad, the other the lass—were plucked when in full bloom. After carefully removing all other blossoms, the kemps were wrapped in a dock leaf and laid beneath a stone. If the spikes had blossomed again when checked the following day, it was believed that there would forever be "Aye love between the twae."

Jessica's notes: The versatility of this so-called "weed" has always struck me as the mark of a universal healing ally. This was one of the first herbs I ever learned and added to my natural healing arsenal. My first memory of using plantain was while working at New Frontiers Natural Marketplace. One afternoon, my mother-in-law, who was also my manager at the time, took me outside to the landscaped beds surrounding the store. There, growing quietly along the lawn's edge, we found Lanceleaf Plantain in abundance. We would often take customers outside and show them how easy it is to identify this powerful plant right beneath their feet. Teaching them how to use it for splinters, insect bites, and skin irritations was such a joy. Tami taught me to listen deeply to the customers and offer practical, accessible herbal wisdom. Lanceleaf plantain will always remind me that some of the best remedies are the simplest—and are often growing right where we walk every day.

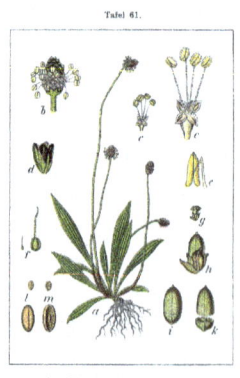

Spitz-Wegerich, Plantago lanceolata.

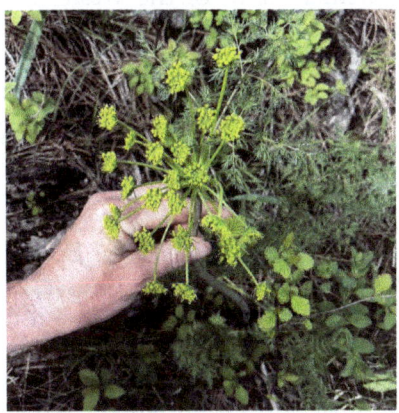

Lomatium

Lomatium dissectum, Lomatium triternatum

Other common names: Fernleaf biscuitroot

Apiaceae (carrot) family

Description: A perennial herb reaching 30–120 cm tall, with finely dissected, fern-like basal leaves and compound umbels of yellow flowers from late spring through early summer. It's flashy, bright yellow umbels remind me of fireworks, and it is a welcome presence in the spring and early summer. When crushed, the ½ long oblong to oval fruit are aromatic.

Where It Grows: Native to western North America, from coastal bluffs to dry foothills and rocky slopes, in habitats ranging from near sea level to 2,500 m elevation. Prefers sunny slopes and hillsides.

When to harvest: Harvest the thick taproot in spring or fall, once the foliage has died back. Take note of the plant in summer when it is in bloom, so when it has died back, you will know with certainty that you are harvesting the right root. Mid size roots are easier to harvest. The larger the basal crown, the larger the root.

How to work with it/ Medicinal uses: Prepare via decoction, tincture, poultice, smoke, or immersion (Neti pot use noted for sinus cleansing). Lomatium is an excellent bronchial stimulant and powerful aromatic-resinous medicine. It has a long history of use by Indigenous people in treating influenza, tuberculosis, and winter-time bronchitis. According to Charles Kane in Medicinal Plants of the Western Mountain States, Lomatium is a suitable remedy for individuals with dry skin conditions and an elevated temperature. With its skin-dilating and warming properties, Lomatium can also relieve pelvic congestion in menstruating women.

Topically, powdered Lomatium root has antimicrobial healing properties and can be applied to infected cuts, scrapes, burns, and boils. An oil infusion and salve can serve as a poultice and is the preferred method for topical applications.

For long-term auto-immune disease such as Epstein-Barr virus (chronic fatigue syndrome), HIV, and chronic Lyme disease, Lomatium may be able to strengthen the afflicted. It's worth a try, and if it makes you feel better, stick with it.

Caution: Some individuals may experience a rash from Lomatium, appearing like a hive breakout. Using refined extracts that remove these resins can mitigate this side effect.

Healing constituents/ Therapeutic actions: Lomatium contains Coumarins (furanocoumarins & pyranocoumarins), columbianin, nodakenetin isomer, luvangetin-like compound, and Coumarin glycosides. It also contains significant antioxidants, such as flavonoids and phenolics, as well as anti-inflammatory and immune-stimulating compounds, including saponins, terpenoids, and essential oils. Tetronic acids contribute to Lomatium's antimicrobial properties. Therapeutic actions include antiviral, antibacterial, expectorant, anti-inflammatory, antioxidant, and immune-supporting properties.

Historical Connection: Traditionally used by Native Plateau tribes for respiratory illness, including colds, flu, bronchitis, pneumonia, sinus infections, and asthma, as well as skin sores and joint discomfort. The Nez Perce, Salish, Ute, Navajo, Blackfeet, Paiute, Okanagan, and other tribes used Lomatium for respiratory and ceremonial purposes. It gained prominence during the 1917–18 influenza pandemic, credited with easing flu symptoms. Dr. Ernest T. Krebs observed that the Washoe people of Western Nevada and Eastern California who used Lomatium during the Spanish Flu had lower mortality rates than those who did not consume Lomatium. Dr. Krebs went on to formulate a Lomatium-based patent remedy called Balsamea.

Jessica's Notes: I am prone to chronic sinus infections. When I was learning about natural remedies working at the health food store, I was drawn to a Lomatium tincture. From the first taste, its earthy warmth and essence felt so familiar—it's been an herbal ally ever since. Discovering it growing wild was like bumping into an old friend!

LOMATIUM

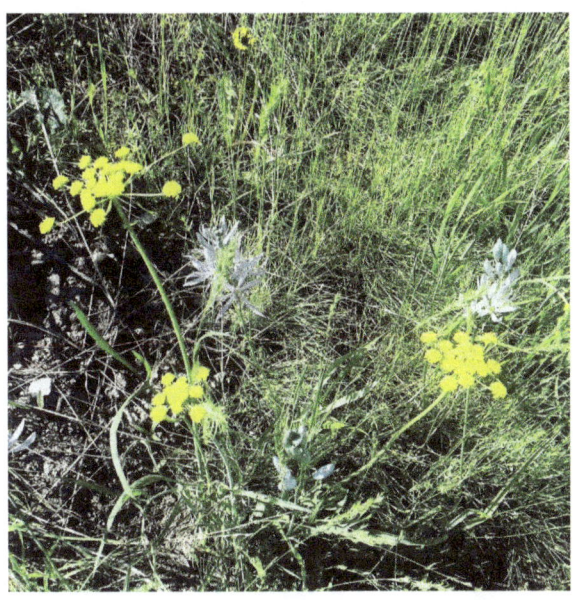

Wild Camas and Lomatium

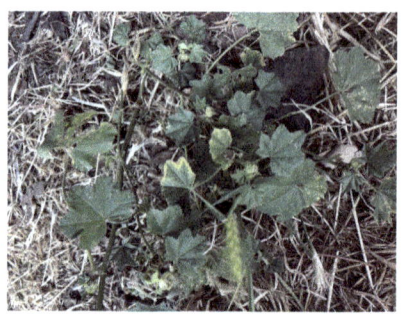

Mallow

Malva parviflora L.

Malvaceae (Mallow) Family
Other common names: Malva, Cheese Weed, Common Mallow
   Description: Common mallow is a low-growing, herbaceous perennial with an upright, branched stem that can reach up to 3 feet in length. The stems are covered with fine soft hairs, sometimes with a slightly bulbous base. The leaves are alternate, with a petiole up to 20 cm long, palmate and simple, measuring up to 7 cm long by 10 cm wide. They feature stellate hairs (i.e., several strands radiating from a common center) and notable veins on the underside. The flowers have five petals and five sepals and can be white, pink, or lavender. The fruits are shaped like a cheese wheel and have a round, flat appearance.
   Where it grows: Mallow is a common weed found in disturbed soil, meadows, garden beds, and prairies. I often find it growing in gravel and around people.
   When and how to harvest: Harvest the green leaves from spring to fall. Harvest fruits or seed pods in late summer.
   How to work with it / Medicinal use: The leaves, seeds, stems, and flowers can be eaten raw, steamed, boiled, or sautéed. Mallow is soothing to the digestive tract and can ease sore throats and irritated tissue. Topically, you can create a compress or poultice with the leaves to treat inflammatory conditions, such as mastitis. The plant's mucilage soothes irritated skin and can be added to creams and salves for added relief.
   Medicinal properties / Healing constituents: Mallow is mucilaginous and is related to okra. It is high in vitamins A and C and rich in minerals: copper, calcium, and iron. Therapeutic actions include antimicrobial, hepatoprotective, anti-inflammatory, and antioxidant properties.

Historical connections: Mallow is native to Northern Africa, Asia, and Europe, and has naturalized throughout the Americas. *Malva* is from the Greek word *malache*, meaning soft. The ancient Greeks would mix the cheese weed seeds into the filling of stuffed vegetables called *Dolmas*. Mallow became an important food source during Israel's War of Independence, from 1948 to 1949. During the siege of Jerusalem, when convoys of food could not enter the city, Jerusalemites foraged in the fields to gather mallow leaves, which they added to various dishes. In the Bible, Job describes "the juice of hallamut" (mallow) as insipid, so that even in his distress, "my soul refuses to touch them: they are as the sickness of my flesh." (Job 6:6). Sounds like Job had an extreme distaste for mallow! Horace Quintus Horatius Flaccus (65 BCE—8 BCE), the Roman poet, said his modest diet mainly consisted of olives, endives, and mallow. The Ancient Romans boiled the leaves like spinach. They served them as a vegetable, according to Marcus Gavius Apicius, the first-century author of *De Re Coquinaria* (On Cookery), during the reign of Tiberius. Roman author and naturalist, Pliny the Elder (23 CE–79 CE), mentioned *Malva* in his book *Natural History* XX.222–227: "...whoever swallows daily half a cyathus (cyathus is 45 ml) of the juice of any one of them will be immune to all diseases... The root of a single-stem plant stabs around an aching tooth until the pain ceases... The root boiled in milk and taken as a broth relieves a cough in five days."

Jessica's notes: Mallow has been part of my family's life since my children were babies. We first learned to eat the little "cheese wheels" from Teacher Tracy, founder of Acorn Village Forest School. The children loved picking them and popping them into their mouths. Now, mallow has become a staple green in my kitchen. It is one of those plants that seems to greet me wherever I go—abundant, generous, and nourishing. I love incorporating it into all kinds of dishes to support my family's health. The familiarity of it reminds me how simple and sustaining wild food can be.

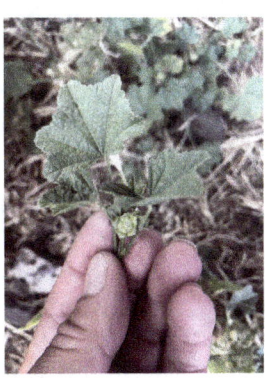

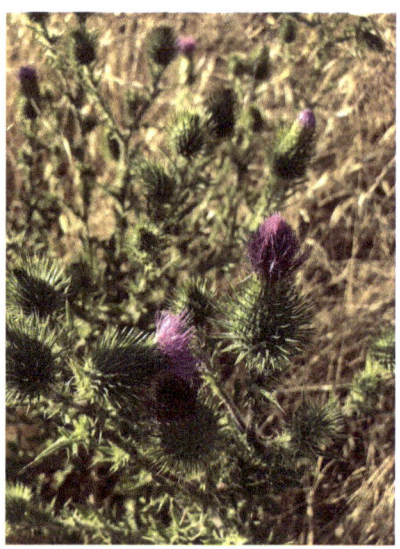

Milk Thistle

Silybum marianum

Asteraceae (Daisy) Family

Description: The main stem of Milk Thistle is hollow, stout, rigid, and branching. The plant can range in height from 2 to 6 feet. Its spiky, dark green leaves are marbled with distinctive white veins. The broad leaves are deeply lobed, and basal leaves can reach up to 20 inches long and 10 inches wide. The flowers are striking, ranging from hot pink to reddish-purple, measuring 4 to 12 centimeters in length and width. They bloom from June through August. Hairless bracts with triangular, spine-edged appendages surround each flower head.

Where it grows: Milk Thistle favors sunny hillsides, fields, farmlands, roadsides, and ditches.

When and how to harvest: Harvest the greens and stems from early to late summer. Roots can be gathered year-round, although they become more fibrous as the plant matures. Late fall or early spring is ideal for harvesting roots. Seeds ripen in late summer. Harvest flower buds before they open. Be sure to wear gloves to protect your hands from the plant's sharp spikes, and carefully remove all prickles before consuming the plant.

How to work with it / Medicinal use: The entire plant is edible once the prickles have been removed. The bitter leaves stimulate digestion and bile production. The stems taste much like cucumber, and the flower buds can be prepared and eaten like artichokes. Roasted seeds can serve as a substitute for coffee. The seeds of Milk Thistle have been used for centuries to support poor liver function. Modern clinical studies now confirm that Milk Thistle is a powerful liver protector. The seeds and leaves can help restore the liver and gallbladder from conditions such as cirrhosis, hepatitis, jaundice, liver infections, and damage from alcohol, drug use, or toxic substances such as painkillers and aspirin. Milk Thistle stimulates liver repair by enhancing protein synthesis and can even counteract poisoning from deadly substances, such as the Death Cap mushroom, if administered within 48 hours. The herb is also used to increase milk flow in lactating mothers and ease afterbirth cramps. Clinical trials suggest that Milk Thistle may complement chemotherapy by providing liver protection and supporting specific cancer treatments.

Healing constituents / Therapeutic actions: Milk Thistle seeds contain a complex of flavonolignans collectively known as Silymarin. Silymarin prevents toxins from entering liver cells and scavenges harmful free radicals. Its active compounds include silibinin A & B, isosilybinin A & B, silychristin, and silydianin (Anthony & Saleh, 2013). Together, these compounds promote liver detoxification and support the body's overall antioxidant action.

Historical connections: Milk Thistle has a history of use for over 2,000 years, primarily for treating liver dysfunction. The Greek physician Dioscorides (A.D. 40–90) documented its use as a cure for serpent bites. Pliny the Elder (A.D. 23–79) recommended that the juice of Milk Thistle mixed with honey be used to "carry off bile." During the Middle Ages, it was revered as an antidote for liver toxins. The 17th-century British herbalist Nicholas Culpepper wrote that Milk Thistle "opens obstructions of the liver and spleen and thereby is good against jaundice." In 1898, eclectic physicians Felter and Lloyd recommended it for congestion of the liver, spleen, and kidneys. Alaskan Native peoples and many American Indian tribes also used Milk Thistle for treating boils and skin diseases.

Jessica's notes: Milk Thistle is one of those remarkable herbs that connects herbalists and medicine people across time and cultures. I am fascinated by how ancient scholars already knew this plant was a liver cure—wisdom that modern science has now validated. It is such a powerful and protective plant, yet so often misunderstood or viewed as a nuisance weed. If more people realized its virtues, they might see its prickly nature as an armor of resilience—a fitting symbol for its liver-protective medicine.

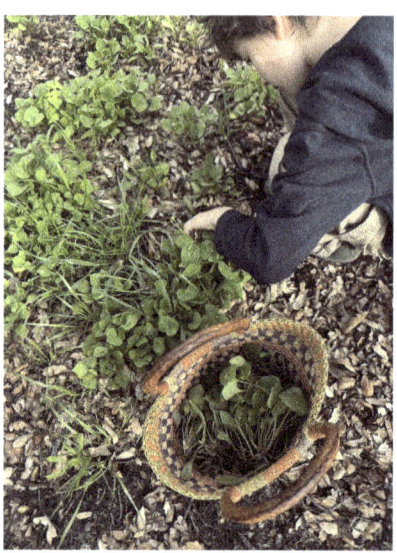

Miner's Lettuce

Claytonia perfoliata

Montiaceae (Miner's Lettuce) Family
Other common names: Winter purslane, Indian lettuce
Description: Miner's lettuce is a small, herbaceous annual plant that graces our presence in early spring. Its slightly succulent, bright green leaves may sometimes appear streaked with white or red from frostbite. The leaves occur in three types: the first growth leaves are basal, narrowly oblanceolate, and taper to a short petiole. The later growth leaves are oval to triangular and held aloft on long petioles. The two cauline leaves lack petioles and are fused at their base, forming a circular collar around the stem. Tiny white flowers emerge from the center of these fused leaves, either singly or in clusters. Each flower has five rounded (or occasionally notched) white petals, two sepals, five stamens, and one pistil with three elongated stigmas. The green, egg-shaped fruit capsule is nestled between the sepals, and when ripe, the small black seeds are explosively ejected from the capsule.

Where it grows: Miner's lettuce thrives in moist soils and is often found among grasses in fields, hillsides, meadows, and near creeks, springs, and streams. It frequently appears after spring rains, with the best leaves often growing in the shade of trees. Look for it on sunny south-facing slopes.

When and how to harvest: Harvest tender greens, stems, and flowers from early spring through summer, and sometimes into early fall. For the tastiest greens, pick before the flower stalk elongates.

How to work with it / Medicinal use: Miner's lettuce makes an excellent trail snack—refreshing, crisp, and hydrating. Enjoy it raw in salads or straight from the jar, or cook it as you would spinach: steam, sauté, or stir into soups and stews. It is a wonderful wild green for both nourishment and gentle cleansing.

Healing constituents / Therapeutic actions: Miner's lettuce is high in vitamin C, protein, and calcium. It is a mild laxative and a useful spring tonic to awaken the body after a long winter. It gently supports detoxification and helps refresh the system.

Historical connections: Native American tribes traditionally ate Miner's lettuce as a spring tonic. One delightful piece of regional lore from Placer County recounts how Native Americans would place leaves near red ant nests, allowing the ants to run over them and impart formic acid—a natural, vinegary dressing (naturescollective.org). The common name "Miner's lettuce" dates to the Gold Rush era, when miners consumed the abundant green to stave off scurvy.

Jessica's notes: This is a perfect foraging green for children and beginner foragers alike—easy to identify, highly nutritious, and delightfully palatable. I always caution that Miner's lettuce, like spinach, rhubarb, nuts, and chocolate, contains oxalates, so those with sensitivity should enjoy it in moderation. Still, it is one of the most refreshing and joyful wild foods of spring. There is something so satisfying about spotting its bright green leaves after a rain, and its presence always signals to me that the foraging season is truly underway.

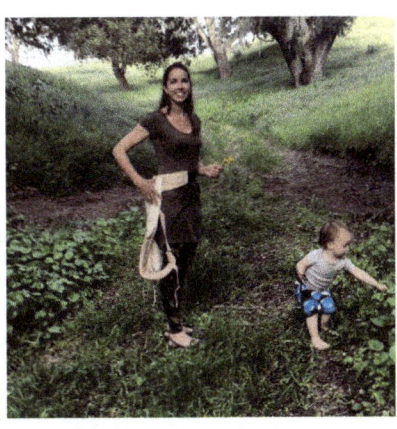

Little Miner's Lettuce Muncher: one of the first foraged feast for my babies!

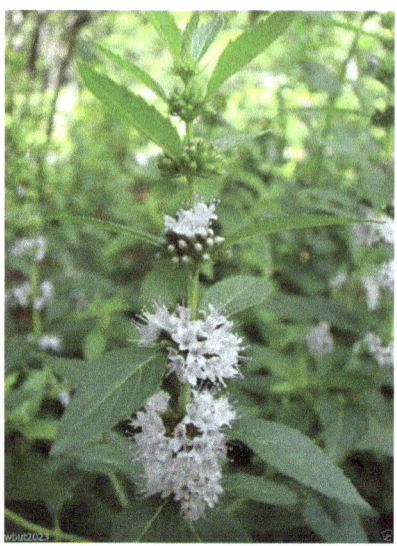

Mountain Mint

Mentha arvensis

Lamiaceae (Mint) Family
Other common names: Field mint
Description: Mountain mint grows up to 20 inches tall, though it more commonly reaches around 12 inches. Like all members of the mint family, it has a distinctive four-sided, square stem and opposite leaves. The plant blooms in whorls at the upper leaf axils and emits a delicious, minty, peppermint-like aroma. Its fresh scent is a hallmark of the moist places it grows—mountain mint typically flowers from July to August.
Where it grows: Mountain mint prefers moist soil and thrives along creeks, streams, brooks, and springs. It thrives in the cool, damp microclimates and grows vigorously when water is plentiful.
When and how to harvest: Harvest mints throughout spring and summer. For the most aromatic and potent leaves, gather them before the plant flowers or during the early bloom stage. Leaves can be used fresh or dried for year-round use.
How to work with it / Medicinal use: Mountain mint is a versatile herbal ally. The fresh or dried leaves make an excellent addition to medicinal tea blends. The tea soothes an upset stomach, alleviates gas pains,

calms colic in babies, and promotes a healthy digestive system. Due to its antibacterial properties, Mountain mint can freshen breath; an infused alcohol tincture can serve as a natural mouthwash. The aromatic plant can also be used as an insect repellent or placed around the home to deter rodents, such as rats and mice. Mint tea has a drying effect and can reduce milk supply in lactating mothers who are preparing to wean their babies.

Healing constituents / Therapeutic actions: The primary active constituent in Mountain mint is menthol, which acts as a carminative and a digestive antispasmodic. Other compounds found in mountain mint include menthone, isomenthone, neomenthol, limonene, methyl acetate, piperitone, tannins, flavonoids, and many other compounds, all of which contribute to its healing actions.

Historical connections: Wild mint has a long history of both culinary and medicinal use. Native American tribes prepared cold infusions of the mint plant to create cooling lotions for relieving fever and flu symptoms. Fresh mint leaves were used to preserve dried meats, layered between them for their antibacterial and fragrant qualities. Poultices of mint were applied to the chest to ease pneumonia. Mint was also used to season pemmican, a traditional and long-lasting food rich in fat and protein, essentially the original energy bar. The Ojibwa tribe regarded Mountain mint as a "blood purifier" and employed it to reduce fever. The Aztecs used mint to induce sweating and to treat insomnia. The name *Mentha* traces back to an ancient Greek myth: Persephone, the jealous wife of Hades, transformed a beautiful nymph named Minthe into the plant we know as mint, thereby preventing Hades from seducing her. Unable to undo the spell, Hades ensured that the plant would at least possess a sweet and pleasing fragrance.

Jessica's notes: Mountain mint is one of my favorite herbs to gather on hot summer days. Just rubbing a few leaves between your fingers fills the air with their refreshing scent—it is like inhaling a breath of cool, forest air. I love adding mountain mint to my wild tea blends, especially in the evenings when I want to relax my digestion after a big meal. It is also one of my go-to herbs to combine with Fireweed and wild ginger for a soothing tea. The plant's resilience and versatility remind me of how nature provides us with simple, accessible remedies that work beautifully with our bodies.

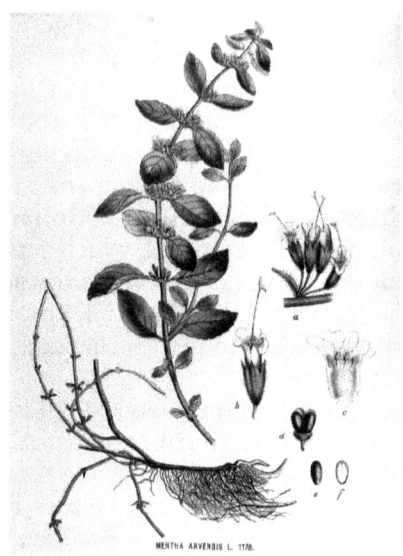

Corn mint (Mentha arvensis). Coloured engraving after James Sowerby, 1810. Wellcome Collection. Used under CC BY 4.0.

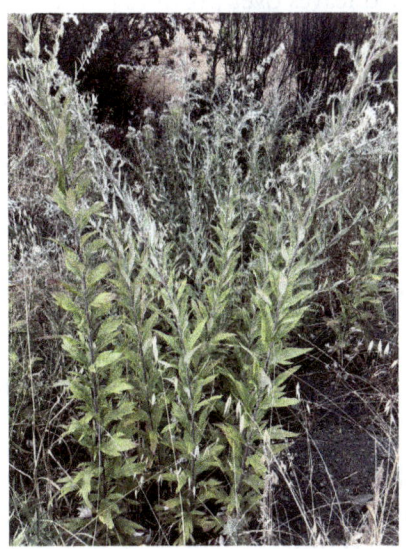

Mugwort

Artemisia vulgaris

Asteraceae (Daisy) Family

Description: Mugwort is an herbaceous perennial plant that grows 3 to 6 feet tall, with an extensive rhizome system. The leaves are 2-8 inches long, dark to light green, pinnate, and sessile, with white hairs on the underside. The erect stems are grooved and can have a red-purplish tinge. The flowers are small, yellowish or brown, rayless, radially symmetrical, and arranged in racemose panicles. Flowering from midsummer to early fall.

Where it grows: Found along creeks, springs, rivers, and streams. It likes to get its feet wet.

When and how to harvest: Harvest the leaves and flowers from early to late summer, and harvest the roots in autumn.

How to work with it/ Medicinal use: The aromatic and slightly bitter leaves can be eaten raw or cooked, supporting digestion, circulation, and respiratory health. Best picked before it flowers in July to September. Its bitter flavoring can be added to season fat, meat, and fish. Mugwort salve can be applied topically to bruises, itching sores, poison oak or ivy rash, and eczema. The tincture or extract can be taken orally to help alleviate fevers, stomachaches, liver complications, coughs, and colds. Artemisia essential oil can support blood pressure regulation, the menstrual cycle, and tumor growth. Burning dried leaves over pressure points on the body, known as Moxibustion, can support detoxification and the release of stagnant energy. Burn the leaves to purify the air and ward off negative energy. The essential oil diluted is an all-purpose insecticide for the garden.

Healing constituents/ Therapeutic actions: Various compounds in Mugwort oil exhibit antifungal, antioxidant, and antimicrobial properties. Its main constituents include camphor, cineole, α and β-thujone, artemisia ketone (CAS: 546-49-6), borneol, and bornyl acetate, as well as other phenols, terpenes, and aliphatic compounds.

Historical connections: Mugwort has traditionally been a people's plant worldwide. Ancient Roman soldiers would place Mugwort in their sandals to prevent their feet from becoming tired and sore. In the European Middle Ages, Mugwort was revered as a magical and protective plant. Mugwort was planted in the garden to repel insects, particularly moths. During ancient times, *Artemisia* was used to remedy fatigue and protect travelers against evil spirits and wild animals. Mugwort is one of the nine herbs invoked in the pagan Anglo-Saxon *Nine Herbs Charm*, documented in the *Lacnunga* (10th century).

Grieve's *Modern Herbal* (1931) states:

"In the Middles Ages, the plant (Mugwort) was known as cingulum Sancti Johannis; it is believed that John the Baptist wore a girdle of it in the wilderness... a crown made from its sprays was worn on St. John's Eve to gain security from evil possession, and in Holland and Germany, one of its names is 'St. John's plant, because of the belief that—if gathered on St. John's Eve—it gave protection against diseases and misfortunes."

On the Isle of Man, near the British Isles, Mugwort is known as *bollan bane* and is still worn on the lapel at Tynwald Day celebrations. Tynwald Day is usually held on July 5th and has a strong association with St. John.

In one of his poems, the famous Chinese poet Su Shi mentioned Mugwort in the 11th century. In Traditional Chinese Medicine, Mugwort is used in a pulverized and aged form, known as moxa, to perform moxibustion. This involves burning mugwort on specific acupuncture points on the patient's body to achieve therapeutic effects.

In Germany, Mugwort is traditionally used to season the roast goose eaten for Christmas. In India, the Mugwort plant is used in Ayurveda to treat cardiac complaints and alleviate feelings of unease and general malaise. In some regions of Japan, there is an ancient custom of hanging *yomogi* (Mugwort) and iris leaves together outside homes to ward off evil spirits, as these plants are believed to repel them due to their unpleasant smell.

North American Indigenous peoples used Mugwort as a medicinal herb to treat colds and fevers. Mugwort was also used in washes and salves to treat bruises, itching, poison oak, ivy, eczema, and underarm or foot odor. Some tribes called Mugwort *women's sage* because the leaf was taken to correct menstrual imbalances and also used to ease the delivery of babies.

Jessica's notes: Mugwort always lifts my spirits when I find it. As someone who loves water, discovering Mugwort along streams and springs feels like reuniting with an old friend who shares my affection for these places. Its intoxicating, fragrant aroma instantly brightens my mood. I love to burn Mugwort to purify the air after illness has visited our home or to clear out lingering negative energy. I also treasure Mugwort for its ability to enhance lucid dreams. I often tuck fresh Mugwort into my pillowcase to invite sweet, vivid dreams. There is something ancient about this plant—when I work with it, I feel a connection to my ancestors.

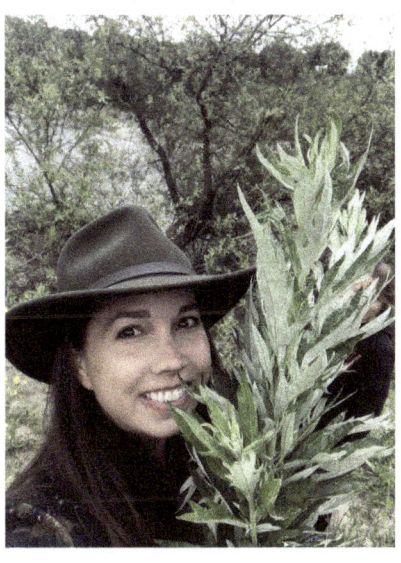

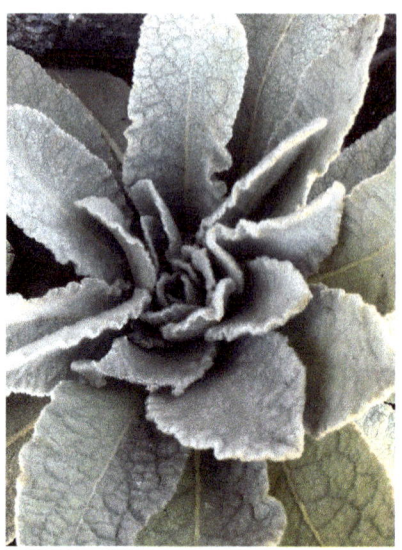

Mullein

Verbascum thapsus

Scrophulariaceae (Snapdragon) Family

Description: A fuzzy, greenish-gray, herbaceous biennial that can grow up to 10 feet tall. The early growth forms a rosette of leaves. The flower grows on tall spikes and blooms from May to September. The yellow flowers are tubular with five petal lobes, tightly packed in a terminal cluster. In the second year, the flower stalk rises, blooms, and sets seed before the plant dies. The basal leaves persist throughout the winter, being oblong and attached to petioles up to 1 foot long. The leaves are covered in soft, fuzzy hairs resembling rabbit's ears.

Where it grows: This common fuzzy herb is often found along roadsides, ditches, meadows, and gardens.

When and how to harvest: Harvest the leaves in their first growth cycle from spring through summer. Once the plant forms a stalk, the medicine is in the flowers. Harvest the flowers in late summer and into fall. The roots can be harvested in the fall and early spring.

How to work with it/ Medicinal use: Mullein leaf makes a healing infusion for colds and flu. The tincture can be used for asthma and chronic bronchitis. Topically, an ointment can be applied to burns and wounds.

The only human trial of mullein ointment was conducted on women who had an episiotomy during childbirth. In the study, the women participants applied mullein ointment to their episiotomy twice daily for 10 days. The mullein ointment helped expedite the healing of the episiotomy wound. (Taleb, Saeedi, 2021).

Mullein flowers can be added to oil to help soothe ear infections and reduce inflammation in the ear canal. Herbalist Matthew Wood has inspired me to try mullein for spinal damage and the nervous system. Mullein's doctrine of signature—an erect, sharp, spine-like stalk—indicates that it can strengthen the spine and nervous system.

Mullein contains saponins and pain-relieving active compounds that can help the body heal from injury and trauma.

A traditional way to use the mullein stalk is to turn into a candlestick. Simply dip the dried stalk with the flower and leaves removed into beeswax.

Healing constituents/ Therapeutic actions: Mullein contains flavonoids, saponins, and other active compounds that have been individually proven to be anti-inflammatory, anti-cancer, antihypertensive (lowering blood pressure), antiseptic, antimicrobial, astringent, diuretic, pain-relieving, emollient, expectorant, and spasmolytic (relieving muscle spasms and promoting wound healing).

Historical connections: Mullein has been used as a folk remedy for centuries throughout Europe, Asia, and the Americas. Roman soldiers were said to dip mullein stalks in tallow and use them as torches. In the Middle Ages, mullein was planted in gardens to ward off evil spirits. Native American tribes used mullein leaves as a poultice for wounds and inflammation, and smoked the dried leaves as a treatment for respiratory ailments. Its common nickname, "cowboy's toilet paper," comes from the soft texture of the leaves, which were used by pioneers and outdoorsmen as a natural alternative when no paper was available.

Jessica's notes: " Mulling over mullein," as Yarrow Willard (Herbal Jedi) would say. I developed a sensitive ear after getting a severe sinus infection. I created a soothing, wild-foraged ear oil using mullein flowers, St. John's wort flowers, usnea lichen, and garlic. This combination alleviated the pain and inflammation. I keep this oil on hand for any ear complaints as a tried-and-true formula. I string up the leaves we pick throughout the spring and summer to dry and keep them in the medicine chest for use during winter colds and flu. Sometimes we will add the leaves to our healing bone broths and soups. I like to refer to myself and Jason as the modern-day Johnny Appleseed, planting and spreading medicinal seeds wherever we go. Mullein has a brilliant seed dispersal ability, and it tends to grow wherever we go!

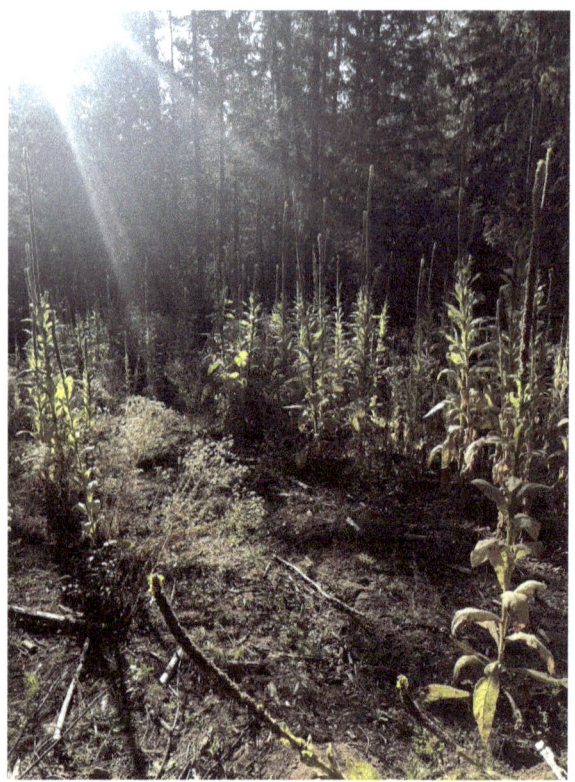

A field of mountain mullein

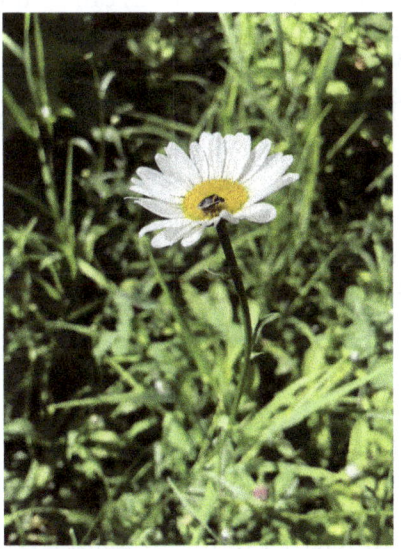

Oxeye Daisy

Leucanthemum vulgare

Asteraceae (Daisy) Family

Description: An herbaceous perennial that grows 1 to 2 feet tall. It has a creeping rhizome that spreads underground. The lower part of the stem is hairy, and the dark green leaves have up to 15 teeth or lobes on the edges. The larger leaves at the base of the plant are approximately 15 cm long and 2 cm wide, with a petiole, and decrease in size as they move up the stem. The upper leaves are deeply toothed and lack a petiole. The plant bears up to three flowers that look like daisies. Each flower head has fifteen to forty white petals, accompanied by 1–2 glabrous green bracts, ¼–3/8 inches long, edged in brown. Oxeye daisies flower throughout summer and into early fall.

Where it grows: Find wild daisies in fields, meadows, prairies, and roadside ditches.

When and how to harvest: Harvest the young shoots and buds in spring and early summer. Gather the flowers and aerial parts throughout the summer and into the fall when they are in bloom.

How to work with it/ Medicinal use: The plant can be added to salads, soups, and stews. Because the plant is bitter, add it sparingly to salads and other dishes. The young shoots and buds can be lightly steamed and eaten as a vegetable. The flower heads can be used to decorate cakes, salads, casseroles, and other dishes. Dry the flowers and add them to a wild tea blend. Medicinally, Oxeye Daisy supports the treatment of whooping cough, asthma, and nervous excitability. As a tonic, it is similar to chamomile and can help alleviate night sweats. Externally, it can be formulated into a lotion to aid in the healing of wounds, bruises, and ulcers.

Caution: Do not consume large quantities of fresh flowers, as they may cause an upset stomach.

Healing constituents/ Therapeutic actions: Oxeye daisy is rich in vitamins A and C, beta-carotene, riboflavin, niacin, and potassium. Therapeutic actions include anti-inflammatory, antispasmodic, diuretic, and tonic.

Historical connections: The ancient Greeks dedicated the Oxeye Daisy to Artemis, the goddess of women, considering it helpful in alleviating women's complaints. During the Christian era, it was transferred to St. Mary Magdalen and was called *Maudelyn* or *Maudlin Daisy*. English herbalist John Gerard referred to it as *Maudlin Wort*. Another English name for Oxeye Daisy was *bruise wort* because bruised leaves were applied to mend bruises.

John Gerard (16th century) writes: *"Dioscorides saith that the flowers of Oxeye made up in a seare cloth doe asswage and washe away cold hard swellings, and it is reported that if they be drunke by and by after bathing, they make them short in a short time well-colored that have been troubled with the yellow jaundice."*

Nicholas Culpepper (17th century) tells us that *"it is a wound herb of good respect, often used in those drinks and salves that are for wounds, either inward or outward"*... and that it is *"very fitting to be kept both in oils, ointments, plasters, and syrups."* He also notes that the bruised leaves reduce swelling and that *"a decoction thereof, with wall-wort and agrimony, and places fomented or bathed therewith warm, giveth great ease in palsy, sciatica, or gout. An ointment made thereof heals all wounds that have inflammation about them."*

Oxeye Daisy was a country folk remedy formerly used as a decoction of the fresh herb in ale to treat jaundice.

Jessica's notes: Seeing wild daisies brings me so much joy. It is a migratory plant brought to America by European settlers, where it domesticated itself and made a home in the untamed wilderness. Oxeye daisies remind me to grow and flourish wherever I land.

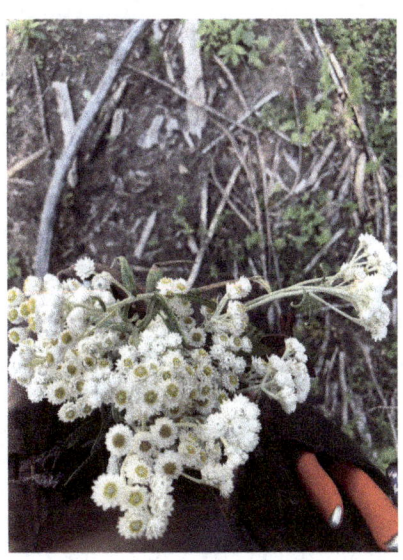

Pearly Everlasting

Anaphalis margaritacea

Asteraceae/ Compositae (Daisy) Family
Other common names: Everlasting, Life Everlasting

Description: Pearly Everlasting is an herbaceous perennial that grows erect up to 3 feet tall, with dark green alternate leaves. The underside of the leaves is covered with tiny fuzzy hairs. The flowers are white, sometimes with a hint of yellow, and measure approximately ¼ inch long. They form a corymb inflorescence. The most striking part of the plant is the pearly white bracts that surround the disc florets. Its pearly flowers bloom between June and September. The plant is dioecious, meaning the pollen-producing and seed-producing flowers are borne on separate individuals.

Where it grows: Found along roadsides, alpine meadows, ditches, creeks, and streams.

When and how to harvest: Harvest the aerial parts in mid-to-late summer when the pearly buds are still compact. If harvested too late in the season, the dried parts will turn to fluff, which, although less ideal for medicinal purposes, makes an excellent natural fire starter.

How to work with it/ Medicinal use: Pearly Everlasting can be enjoyed as a tea to support the relief of colds and coughs. The tea or tincture helps break up mucus while soothing the mucous membranes. It is also a mild sedative that can soothe headaches and reduce fevers. With its antihistamine properties, it can alleviate allergy symptoms. A poultice of the leaves soothes sunburn, blisters, and boils. An oil infusion can be applied to stiff and aching joints to relieve inflammation and improve mobility.

Healing constituents/ Therapeutic actions: Pearly Everlasting is antibacterial, antihistamine, anti-inflammatory, anti-rheumatic, antiseptic, antiviral, astringent, diaphoretic, expectorant, sedative, and vulnerary.

Historical connections: Native Americans of the Pacific Northwest added this woodsy, fragrant herb to their smoking blends to treat tuberculosis. Chippewa Indians blended it with mint as a smudge to treat paralysis. Mohawk Indians infused the entire plant to treat asthma. Early American settlers and pioneers also used this plant to remedy colds and flu.

Jessica's notes: When I moved to the mountain, I noticed this lovely plant and immediately sensed that it was special. I have found that whenever I focus on a plant and think of it, it seems to come into my life for a reason. As soon as I spotted Pearly Everlasting blooming along the dirt road by the creek, I learned it was helpful for headaches, allergies, and colds. Learning its poetic name—*Pearly Everlasting*—made me fall in love with it even more. I enjoy combining Pearly Everlasting with Yarrow, Mullein, and Mountain Mint to create a tea blend that helps combat colds, fevers, and flu.

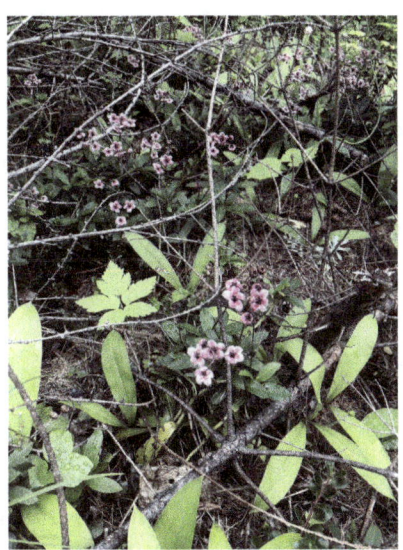

Pipsissewa

Chimaphila umbellata

Ericaceae (Heath) Family (previously classified in the Pyrolaceae (Evergreen) Family)

Other common names: Umbellate Wintergreen, King's Cure, Ground Holly, Rheumatism Weed, Prince's Pine, Butter Winter, Pyrola Umbellation, Love in Winter

Description: Pipsissewa is an evergreen flowering perennial herb that grows from 4 to 14 inches in height. The dark green, variegated leaves are lance-shaped, ranging from 2-7 cm in length and 0.2-1.0 cm in width. Reddish-brown stems emerge from creeping rhizomes beneath the forest floor. The waxy, pink flowers appear on tall stalks in summer, each with five petals and five sepals, measuring approximately 0.5 to 0.75 inches in length. As the flowers mature, they form small capsules that release seeds, which are dispersed by the wind.

Where it grows: A shade-loving forest plant, Pipsissewa thrives in the rich, thick loam beneath pine and cedar trees. It is native to North America, Europe, Eurasia, and Asia.

When and how to harvest: Harvest the leaves and aerial parts throughout the summer and into early fall. Be conservative in your harvesting, taking only a small amount from each plant colony to ensure its long-term survival.

How to work with it/ Medicinal use: Pipsissewa is traditionally prepared as a tea or tonic to stimulate urination and help flush toxins from the bladder and kidneys. The plant contains quinine-like compounds, making it a natural urinary antiseptic useful in treating urinary tract infections (UTIs). It is a safe and effective remedy for cystitis and other bladder disorders. Its diuretic properties also aid in the treatment of rheumatism and gout. A fresh leaf poultice can be applied topically to sore, rheumatic joints and muscles, as well as to blisters, sores, and swelling. Pipsissewa has also been used to make delicious root beer and soft drinks. Sadly, it has been overharvested in some regions of the United States for commercial use as a "secret" ingredient in soft drinks.

Healing constituents/ Therapeutic actions: Pipsissewa's active components include phenols, terpenes, salicylates, phenolic glycosides, flavonoids, resins, lignans, and the antimicrobial quinones chimaphilin and arbutin, along with other beneficial phytochemicals. Research has demonstrated Pipsissewa's antioxidant and antifungal properties, with case studies highlighting its efficacy against multidrug-resistant bacterial species.

Historical Connections: The name *Chimaphila* means "winter-loving," a fitting title for this hardy little plant that stays green through the coldest months. For generations, Native American tribes turned to Pipsissewa for its many healing gifts. It was used to ease kidney stones, soothe bladder inflammation, and help regulate menstruation. The leaves were steeped to make washes for inflamed eyes and skin conditions, including smallpox. In childbirth, it was called upon to aid difficult labors, and it was also valued in the treatment of respiratory troubles, rheumatism, stomach cancer, constipation, venereal diseases, and heart ailments. Among the Okanagan-Coleville, Iroquois, and Delaware peoples, Pipsissewa was known for its ability to promote sweating and reduce fevers, particularly in cases of typhus.

European settlers soon recognized the plant's worth as well, adopting it as a remedy for rheumatism and disorders of the kidneys and urinary tract. Its importance was solidified when it was officially included in the *U.S. Pharmacopoeia* from 1820 to 1916.

During the Civil War, Pipsissewa became an invaluable ally in the Confederate South, where shortages of imported medicines forced reliance on native plants. Confederate Surgeon-General Samuel Preston Moore tasked botanist and physician Dr. Francis Peyre Porcher with documenting local botanical remedies. In his 1863 work, *Standard Supply for the Table of Indigenous Remedies for Field Service and the Sick in the General Hospitals*, Porcher praised Pipsissewa as "aromatic, tonic, and diuretic... easily collected around our camps, in shady woods, in almost every part of our Confederacy" (p. 377). Amidst the hardships of war, this evergreen plant provided much-needed support to both soldiers and physicians alike.

Jessica's notes: Living near old-growth forests, I feel a deep sense of purpose in stewarding and protecting the land where this evergreen perennial grows in abundance. We harvest it sustainably each year, taking care to ensure that it will continue to thrive for future generations.

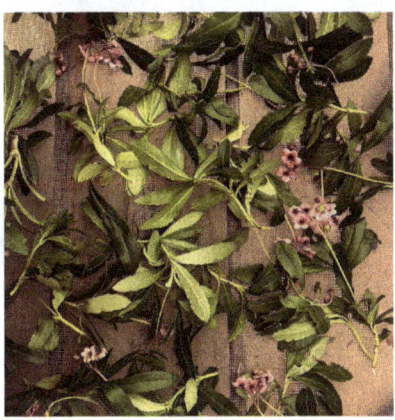

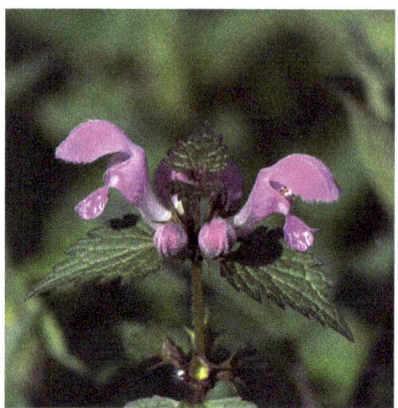

Purple Dead Nettle

Lamium purpureum

Lamiaceae (Mint) Family

Other common names: Dead Nettle, Purple Archangel, Red Dead Nettle, Velikdenche

Description: Purple Dead Nettle is an herbaceous annual weed that emerges in early spring, spreading in mats among other wild weeds. It is often mistaken for Henbit, as the two frequently grow side by side. One clear difference is that Henbit has stemless leaves, whereas Dead Nettle leaves have petioles. Although it shares the name "nettle," it is not a true nettle, but a member of the mint family. The fuzzy, spade-shaped green leaves are often tipped in purple hues, giving the plant its name. Delicate, tubular flowers are purple to pink in color. Purple Dead Nettle typically grows to a height of 8-10 inches.

Where it grows: Originally native to Asia, Purple Dead Nettle can now be found on nearly every continent. It thrives in gardens, disturbed soil, fields, meadows, and along roadsides.

When and how to harvest: Harvest the tops and aerial parts in early spring, continuing through spring and into summer.

How to work with it/ Medicinal use: Purple Dead Nettle is highly nutritious and can be added to a variety of culinary creations, including pesto, smoothies, salads, soups, and used as a garnish on various dishes. The leaves can be infused in oil to create a soothing ointment or salve for wounds, similar to the use of Yarrow or Plantain. Enjoy Purple Dead Nettle as a tea to support kidney function and help ease seasonal allergies.

You can also tincture the fresh plant and use it throughout allergy season. Another preparation is an infusion of the greens in apple cider vinegar, which can be taken as a tonic for sore muscles and inflammation, or used as a salad dressing. The plant also yields a beautiful natural green dye for wool or yarn. Purple Dead Nettle is a nutritious early food source for chickens and an important nectar source for bees and pollinators in the early spring.

Healing constituents/ Therapeutic actions: Purple Dead Nettle is rich in vitamins C and iron, as well as fiber and flavonoids. Therapeutic actions include anti-inflammatory, antibacterial, antifungal, diuretic, astringent, diaphoretic, and purgative properties.

Historical connections: A classic pioneer plant, Purple Dead Nettle is one of the first green allies to appear after a mild winter, growing robustly through spring. Traditionally, it has been used like Henbit—as a mild astringent and topically for wounds.

Jessica's notes: I find it fascinating—and not at all coincidental—that many of the weeds flourishing in springtime, such as Purple Dead Nettle, Stinging Nettle, Henbit, and Chickweed, are anti-inflammatory and help ease seasonal allergies. It feels like our Creator designed this perfect spring apothecary for us, right when our bodies need it most after the winter months.

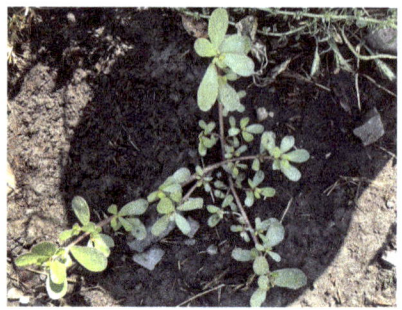

Purslane

Portulaca oleracea

Portulacaceae (Purslane) Family
Other common names: Common Purslane, Little Hogweed

Description: Purslane is a low-growing annual weed that spreads in mats, characterized by its succulent, juicy leaves, which may appear either in an alternate or opposite arrangement along reddish stems. The leaves form on a single taproot and form a sprawling mat. Tiny yellow flowers emerge in late summer.

Where it grows: Purslane thrives in sandy soil, lawns, gardens, roadsides, ditches, and other disturbed areas. It is a hardy plant and often appears in abundance once established.

When and how to harvest: Harvest the plump, juicy leaves from spring through summer and into early fall.

How to work with it/ Medicinal use: Purslane is a highly nutritious and versatile plant that can be enjoyed both raw and cooked. Steam, boil, or sauté it as you would spinach. It makes a delightful addition to fresh salads and sandwiches, adding a juicy crunch. The crushed leaves can be applied topically to soothe skin conditions such as acne, eczema, and minor irritations. Infusing the leaves in oil creates a nourishing skin oil rich in antioxidants and omega fatty acids.

Healing constituents/ Therapeutic actions: Purslane is packed with healing nutrients. It is high in vitamins A and C, beta-carotene, and omega-3 fatty acids. It also provides significant amounts of calcium, magnesium, potassium, folate, choline, and iron. Consuming Purslane supports heart health, thanks to its omega-3 content, and may help prevent cancer and other diseases through its antioxidant properties. Therapeutic actions include anti-inflammatory, purgative, emollient, muscle-relaxant, and cardiac-tonic effects.

Historical connections: Purslane has been eaten for over 2,000 years. Although its exact origins are debated, most scholars agree that it is native to the Middle East and its neighboring regions. The Ancient Egyptians cultivated it, while the Romans and Greeks valued it as both a culinary vegetable and a medicinal plant. Purslane may have reached Europe as early as the 13th century and was recorded in Massachusetts as early as 1672. Over time, this hardy plant has become naturalized and domesticated worldwide.

Jessica's notes: How can anyone consider this a weed when it offers such a powerhouse of nutrition? I love the idea of welcoming Purslane into the garden and the yard rather than trying to fight it. If you cannot beat them, why not eat them? This hardy little plant reminds me that sometimes the most overlooked and humble "weeds" can be among our greatest allies in nourishment and health.

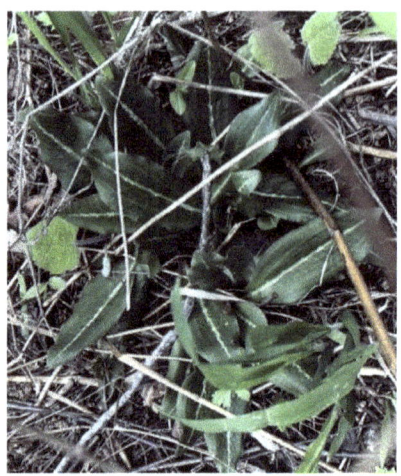

Rattlesnake Plantain

Goodyera oblongifolia

Orchidaceae (Orchid) Family

Other common names: Giant Rattlesnake Plantain, Green-leaved Rattlesnake Plantain, Western Rattlesnake Plantain, Rattlesnake Orchid

Description: Rattlesnake plantain is a low-growing forest herb, recognized for its distinctive, beautiful leaves. It spreads via rhizomes, often forming dense clusters of succulent, dark green, waxy basal leaves. The pale veining on the leaves resembles the pattern of rattlesnake skin, giving rise to its common name. Tiny white flowers bloom on upright stalks and are bilaterally symmetrical—a hallmark of the orchid family. The flowers appear in mid-to-late summer.

Where it grows: Rattlesnake plantain thrives in the shaded understory of conifer forests, preferring the mosses, spongy humus, and cool, moist soil of old-growth woodlands.

When and how to harvest: Harvest the entire plant—roots, shoots, and leaves—in late summer or early fall, though respectfully and with restraint, as it is a slow-growing forest dweller. A small shovel may be required to lift the roots if the soil is compacted carefully. Take only what you need and leave plenty behind to ensure its continued presence.

How to work with it/ Medicinal use: Known affectionately as an "Indian band-aid," rattlesnake plantain has long been used as a field remedy for minor wounds. Its soothing, emollient, and analgesic properties make it ideal for burns, cuts, scrapes, and insect bites. To use as a poultice, pick a fresh leaf, gently crush it to soften, split it open, and apply it directly to the skin. The leaves can also be dried and incorporated into healing salves, oils, and ointments. Gargling a warm tea made from the leaves helps soothe sore throats, hoarseness, and mouth sores. When consumed as tea, it can calm stomach upset and reduce intestinal inflammation. Following the "Doctrine of Signatures," its snake-skin patterned leaves were traditionally believed to soothe snakebites.

Healing constituents/ Therapeutic actions: Orchids generally contain alkaloids, flavonoids, sterols, carotenoids, and anthocyanins. Therapeutic actions include emollient, anti-inflammatory, and analgesic properties.

Historical connections: Numerous Native American tribes have used rattlesnake plantain since ancient times. Among the Salish, its name translates as "splitting open easily," a reference to how the leaves can be prepared for poultices. Coastal tribes used names meaning "it has got spots" or "medicine for childbirth." East of the Cascades, it became known as "Indian band-aid" and sometimes "frog leaves." Its reputation as a soothing and versatile forest remedy has earned it an honored place in traditional herbal practices.

Jessica's notes: One day, I was out exploring in the old-growth forest, and I noticed this evergreen plant with a white strip in the middle. I took a photo of it because it seemed important to know. Sure enough, I found its name and historical significance. Once you start to observe the plants that grow around you, you will find that many of them are forgotten medicine.

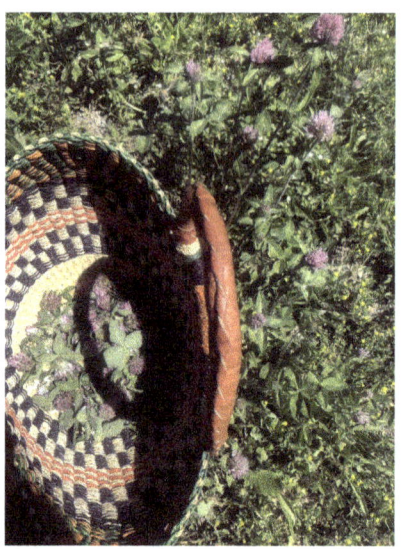

Red Clover

Trifolium pratense

Fabaceae (Legume) Family

Description: The genus name *Trifolium* reveals one of red clover's identifying characteristics: its leaves are composed of three leaflets (*trifolium meaning "three leaves"*). Each leaflet often has a distinctive pale crescent or "water stain" near the edge. The red-purplish flowers grow in dense, dome-shaped clusters, occasionally in pairs. A low-growing, charming perennial, red clover blooms from early spring to late summer, adding a splash of vibrant color to fields and meadows.

Where it grows: A short-lived perennial and a welcome volunteer in the garden. It is an excellent nitrogen-fixing plant, enriching poor soils and improving fertility for future crops. You will often find it growing amongst grasses in fields, meadows, ditches, and prairies—wherever the earth offers space for its cheerful blooms.

When and how to harvest: Gather the flowering tops from May through August. Harvest in the morning after the dew has dried, when the blooms are vibrant and fragrant. They dry beautifully and retain their lovely purple-red hue, making them an attractive addition to winter teas.

How to work with it/ Medicinal use: Red clover is rich in minerals and makes a delicious, nourishing tea. It is excellent in sun teas during summer and makes a soothing, gentle tea for winter wellness. The flowers can be tinctured to keep on hand for menstrual support and for times when extra minerals are needed. A honey infusion of red clover is lovely for soothing sore throats and helping clear excess mucus. "Red Clover, Red Clover, send your medicine right over!" This cheerful plant is also an ally for healthy skin and bones due to its wealth of bone-building minerals. Red clover contains isoflavones—plant-based compounds that can mimic estrogen and, in certain studies, have shown the ability to inhibit the growth of cancer cells. The U.S. government's National Cancer Institute has acknowledged the potential anti-cancer and anti-tumor properties of red clover.

Caution: Use mindfully and for short durations. Those with estrogen-sensitive cancers should avoid red clover internally, as it is rich in isoflavones. It may also interact with birth control pills, blood-thinning medications, or Tamoxifen. Always listen to your intuition and body, and consider your personal and family medical history before incorporating red clover medicinally.

Healing constituents/ Therapeutic actions: Red clover is packed with nutrients: vitamins A, C, E, K, and B12, along with minerals such as calcium, magnesium, chromium, iron, manganese, niacin, phosphorus, potassium, selenium, silicon, thiamine, and trace amounts of zinc. It also contains a small amount of protein. Therapeutic actions include alterative, antioxidant, antispasmodic, astringent, bitter, cholagogue, diuretic, expectorant, galactagogue, nervine, sedative, and tonic.

Historical connections: In Christian folk tradition, the three leaves of red clover symbolized the Holy Trinity. In England, the flowers were sometimes worn as amulets to ward off evil spirits. Among America's first professional herbalists—The Eclectics—red clover was valued as a powerful alterative and blood purifier. It remains a cherished herbal ally across many herbal traditions worldwide.

Jessica's notes: When I see red clover blossoming in the meadow, it always feels like a gift from the earth—a humble but powerful ally. I love adding their flowers to my Wild Woman tea blend, relying on their blood-building properties. To me, it is a plant for women: it symbolizes resilience, beauty, and nourishment.

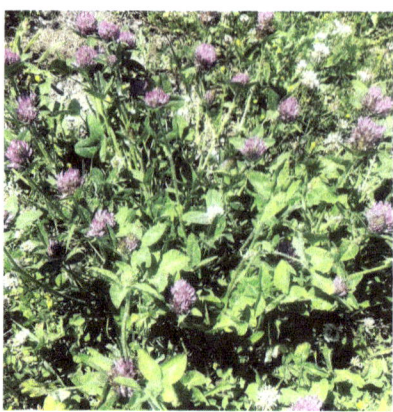

Red clover, red clover, send your medicine right over!

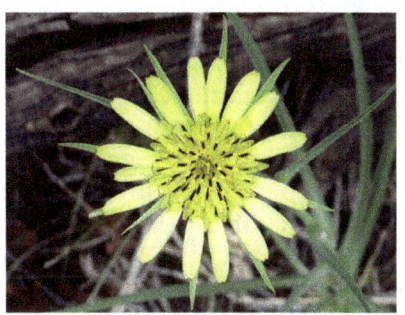

Salsify

Tragopogon dubius

Asteraceae (Daisy) Family
Other common names: Goat's Beard, Yellow Salsify, Wild Oyster Plant, Oyster Root
Description: Salsify grows as an annual or occasionally as a biennial forb and can reach heights of up to 3 feet. The buds are bluish-green, large, and elegantly tapered. Its yellow flower head resembles a small sunflower and opens in the early morning, often closing by late afternoon. The flowers may remain closed on cloudy or rainy days. The seeds, known as achenes, are 2–4 centimeters long and disperse much like dandelion seeds. When the plant has gone to seed, its seed heads form enormous, puff-ball-like structures that resemble giant dandelions. The grass-like leaves are long (up to 12 inches), narrow (about ½ inch wide), and pointed. Its taproot is prominent and long, similar to that of parsnips.
Where it grows: Look for salsify in meadows, open fields, and prairies. It also thrives along roadsides, ditches, and in dry, rocky soils. Once you know what to look for, you will spot its dramatic seed heads standing tall and proud in the summer sun.
When and how to harvest: Harvest the taproots in early spring or autumn, when they are tender and flavorful. Flower buds can be harvested just before they open in late spring or early summer.
How to work with it/ Medicinal use: Salsify was introduced to the Americas as a root vegetable. Of the standard varieties, *T. dubius* (yellow) tends to be more bitter and fibrous, while *T. porrifolius* (purple) is more flavorful. The buds can be eaten raw or cooked—sautéed, steamed, or added to stir-fries. Cultivated salsify roots are especially delicious, with a mild flavor reminiscent of parsnips. Some varieties earn the nickname

"Oyster Root" for their subtle, shellfish-like flavor when cooked. The roots can also be roasted and ground to make a coffee substitute, while the young shoots can be steamed or sautéed, much like asparagus. The seeds can be sprouted and added to salads as a nutritious ingredient. Historically, powdered root has even been added to cakes.

Healing constituents/ Therapeutic actions: Salsify is rich in potassium, calcium, and sodium, which help regulate blood pressure. The root provides about 82 calories per 100 grams—comparable to sweet potatoes—and is an excellent source of both soluble and insoluble dietary fiber, particularly inulin. Inulin acts as a prebiotic nutrient, promoting the absorption of minerals, regulating blood sugar levels, aiding in weight control, and supporting healthy digestion. Like other members of the Asteraceae family, Goat's Beard contains powerful polyacetylene antioxidants such as falcarinol, panaxydiol, and methyl-falcarinol. The fresh roots are also a good source of vitamin C and B-complex vitamins.

Historical connections: Some Native American tribes would gather the rubbery sap from broken stems and leaves, dry it, and roll it into balls to chew like gum. Salsify has long been used to relieve heartburn, stimulate urination, and aid in the elimination of kidney stones. The plant's milky juice was traditionally used to treat wounds by stopping bleeding and to soothe indigestion. A tea made from salsify was consumed—and sometimes applied externally—as a treatment for bites from rabid coyotes, for both humans and livestock (Kershaw, 2000).

Jessica's notes: We love to make wishes on salsify's giant seed heads, much as one does with dandelions. There is something magical about watching those feathery seeds drift on the wind. Their larger size makes the experience feel even more dramatic and satisfying! It reminds me of the playful joy that nature offers, if we only take the time to notice.

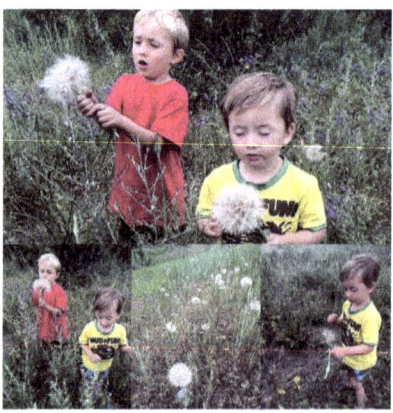

Make a wish!

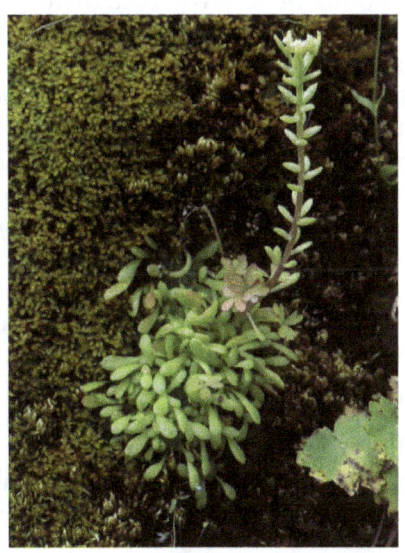

Sedum

Sedum spp.

Crassulaceae (Stonecrop) Family
Other common names: Roseroot, Stonecrop, Wormleaf Stonecrop

Description: Sedum is a succulent, low-growing perennial. The leaves are small, usually smaller than ½ inch long, and are either cylindrical (*Sedum stenopetalum*) or flat (*S. oregonense*), lance-shaped, or oval. The flowers are generally yellow and star-shaped, but some species bear white, red, or purple flowers. The roots are creeping stolons (roots that creep above ground) or rhizomes. These succulent plants grow as mats and seldom exceed 12 inches in height. The name *Sedum* is derived from the Latin *sedeo*, meaning "to sit," referencing the plant's compact, ground-hugging nature. Sedum flowers in July and sets seed in August.

Where it grows: Sedums thrive in rocky outcrops and banks. They prefer sunny hillsides and subalpine elevations.

When and how to harvest: Harvest the succulent, tender greens beginning in late spring and continuing throughout summer. Sedum can be eaten raw, even during the winter, making it an important survival food to remember.

How to work with it/ Medicinal use: The entire plant is edible. The leaves have a light, cucumber-like flavor. Add them to salads or enjoy them while grazing along the trail. Topically, the juice of Sedum can be applied to insect bites, burns, and skin rashes to soothe and cool the skin.

Healing constituents/ Therapeutic actions: Sedum is rich in vitamin C. Therapeutic actions include mucilaginous, slightly astringent, hypotensive, laxative, rubefacient, vermifuge, and vulnerary properties.

Historical connections: Nicholas Culpepper recommended the juice of Sedum to quench thirst during fevers. In his *Complete Herbal* (1652), he writes: "It is under the dominion of the Moon, cold in quality, and binding, and therefore very good to stay defluctions, especially such as fall upon the eyes. It stops bleeding, both inward and outward, helps cankers, fretting sores, and ulcers; it abates the heat of choler (bile)." Native Americans also prepared a decoction from Sedum to soothe sore throats and eye irritations.

Jessica's Notes: Drum roll, please... when you find Sedum, you eat 'em! This is a favorite trail snack at forest school. I can truly feel the hydrating effects when I nibble on a few of the fleshy leaves. I like to call Sedum *nature's Gatorade*!

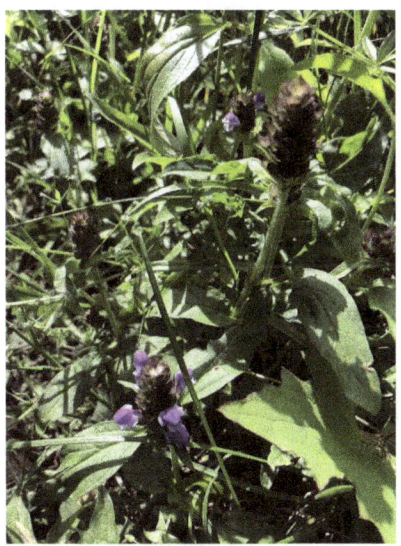

Self-Heal

Prunella vulgaris

Lamiaceae (Mint) Family

Other common names: Heals-All

Description: Being in the mint family, Self-Heal has the characteristic square stem. What distinguishes it from other members of the mint family is its unique terminal flowers, which are whorled together into a compact, pill-shaped purple head. The leaves are opposite, lance-shaped, and discreetly toothed. The plant varies in size depending on its location and soil conditions. I have seen Self-Heal grow as large as 12 inches in high-elevation subalpine meadows.

Where it grows: Heal-All is found in meadows, lawns, roadsides, pastures, and subalpine meadows. It is widespread throughout North America.

When and how to harvest: Harvest the flowers and aerial parts of Self-Heal from May to August, when the plant is in full bloom.

How to work with it/ Medicinal use: The entire plant is edible, either cooked or raw. The tender young greens are best and taste somewhat similar to bland romaine lettuce. When taken internally as a tea or decoction, Self-Heal can help alleviate symptoms of gastritis and diarrhea and may soothe digestive ulcerations. Topically, Heal-All is an excellent addition to healing salves, ointments, and lotions intended to soothe and promote the healing of minor burns, wounds, and other skin irritations.

Healing constituents/ Therapeutic actions: *Prunella vulgaris* contains ursolic acid, betulinic acid, D-camphor, delphinidin, hyperoside, manganese, oleanolic acid, and tannins—compounds shown to have antitumor and diuretic properties. It also contains vitamins A, C, and K, as well as flavonoids and rutin. Topically, Self-Heal acts as an emollient, astringent, and vulnerary. It is known for its anti-inflammatory, antiviral, antibacterial, and anti-allergenic therapeutic actions.

Historical connections: Heal-All has been used as medicine and a cure for almost everything. It was first mentioned in Chinese medical literature during the Han Dynasty (206 BC – AD 23). Self-Heal is also found in Druidic folklore. The druids gathered it in the same way as Vervain—picked at night during the dark phase of the moon, dug up with the druid's sickle, placed in the left hand, and followed by words of thanks. The plant was then separated into its components for drying: flowers, leaves, and stems. In medieval Europe, Self-Heal tea was used to treat quinsy and complications from tonsillectomy. John Gerard praised the properties of Self-Heal, as did Nicholas Culpepper, who wrote, "The juice used with oil of roses to anoint the temples and forehead is very effectual to remove the headache, and the same mixed with honey of roses cleanseth and healeth ulcers in the mouth and throat." John Gerard (1545–1612) wrote that Self-Heal "serveth for the same that Bugle doth, and in the world there are not two better wounde herbes as hath often been proved."

Jessica's notes: When I worked at Pilgrim's Market, my favorite summertime lunch break spot was under the shade of the maple trees in the market garden behind the store. I often read plant identification and foraging books while munching on lunch. One day, I paused midway through a book I was reading and looked down at the ground (a normal foraging habit of mine), and to my happy surprise, I discovered Self Heal growing right there on the lawn! I was so excited that I shared my discovery with Farmer Jeremiah, and he impressed me by calling it by its Latin name, *Prunella vulgaris*!

SELF-HEAL

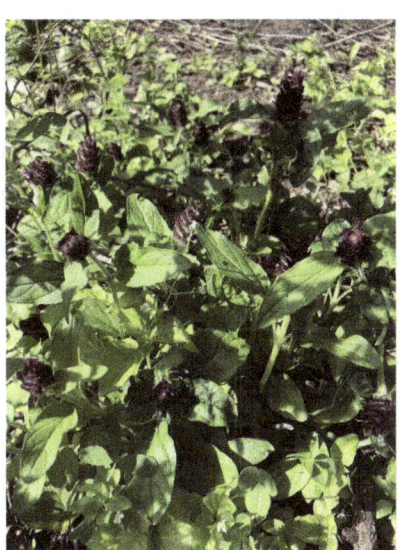

Self Heal, *Prunella vulgaris*

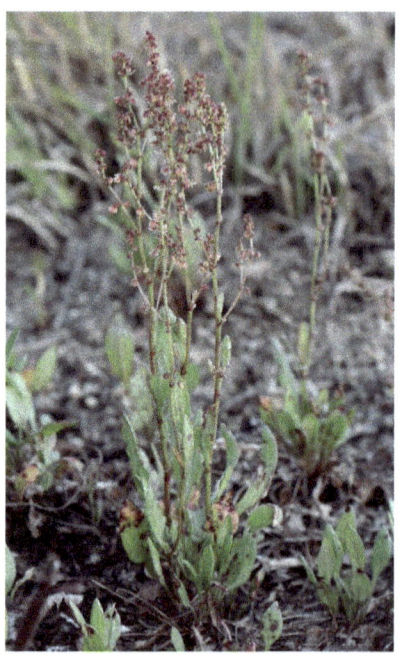

Sheep Sorrel

Rumex acetosella

Polygonaceae (Buckwheat) Family
Other common names: Field Sorrel, Wood Sorrel, Red Sorrel
  Description: Sheep Sorrel is a dioecious perennial weed that grows 10–60 cm tall. It has succulent stems with short petioles, and the basal leaves are long-petiolate. The flowers are tiny and grow in loose clusters. The reddish-brown seeded fruits are 1–2 mm long.
  Where it grows: Sheep Sorrel prefers disturbed soils and happily grows in gardens, meadows, and open, sunny fields. It is found growing all over the Northern Hemisphere.
  When and how to harvest: Harvest the leaves throughout spring and summer. The seeds can be harvested in late summer and early fall.
  How to work with it/ Medicinal use: Sorrel's claim to fame is its blood-cleansing, detoxifying, and cell-regenerative healing properties. An infusion of the fresh leaf can be used as an astringent mouthwash for sore gums and canker sores. Tea from the leaves can act as a vermifuge,

expelling intestinal worms. It is considered a beneficial herb for women. In Chinese medicine, sorrel is given after birth to help "cool" and tone the reproductive organs and prevent infection. It contains phytoestrogens that can bind to excess estrogen, much like those found in red clover, licorice, and soy.

Due to its rich tannins, tea can serve as a helpful remedy for excessive menstrual bleeding. Low doses of leaf tea can help alleviate diarrhea, while higher doses can help relieve constipation. Chilled tea is best to drink when you want to cool down on a hot day or help reduce a fever. Traditionally, Sheep Sorrel has been used by herbalists to help cool the body and promote detoxification through the skin. Its diuretic properties support kidney health and urinary function.

Sheep Sorrel is an ingredient in the renowned Essiac Tea formula, considered the most active ingredient in this cancer-fighting tea blend. Essiac Tea is a blend of herbs formulated by the late herbalist Rene Caisse (whose surname spelled backward gives "Essiac"). The tea includes Sheep Sorrel along with other healing herbs such as burdock root, slippery elm bark, and Indian rhubarb root.

The finely chopped leaves can be used as a face mask or in facial steaming to help decongest the sinuses. Its tangy lemon-like flavor is an excellent addition to many culinary dishes. In Europe, Sheep Sorrel is used to curdle the whey in the production of ricotta cheese.

Caution: Sheep Sorrel contains oxalates, the same acids present in spinach, rhubarb, and other leafy greens. Cooking and freezing the plant can help break down these oxalates.

Healing constituents/ Therapeutic actions: This tangy herb contains a wealth of antioxidant-rich vitamins and minerals, including vitamins A, B, C, D, E, and K, as well as calcium, beta-carotene, phosphorus, potassium, manganese, copper, and iron. Sheep Sorrel also contains several anthraquinones that are effective antioxidants and free-radical scavengers. Therapeutic actions include anti-inflammatory, antioxidant, antiseptic, astringent, diuretic, hepatic, laxative, and vermifuge.

Historical connections: Sheep Sorrel has a long history as a universal salad green and vegetable. Nicholas Culpepper (1616–1664) recommended it for its diuretic properties, suggesting an infusion made from 1 ounce of leaf to 1 pint of boiling water, taken in 2-fluid-ounce doses. He also praised sorrel leaf juice as a tonic for the kidneys and urinary tract. The Sámi utilized the acidic effect of sorrel leaves as a substitute for rennet in cheese making.

Jessica's Notes: I first discovered Sheep Sorrel growing wild along the edges of my garden beds. The bright, tangy flavor instantly delighted me! Now, each spring, I seek it out as one of the first greens to wake up my palate after winter. I am fascinated by its role in the Essiac tea formula and find it empowering to forage for this powerful little herb, which plays such a significant role in traditional healing. To me, Sheep Sorrel is a true people's plant—humble, widespread, and deeply nourishing.

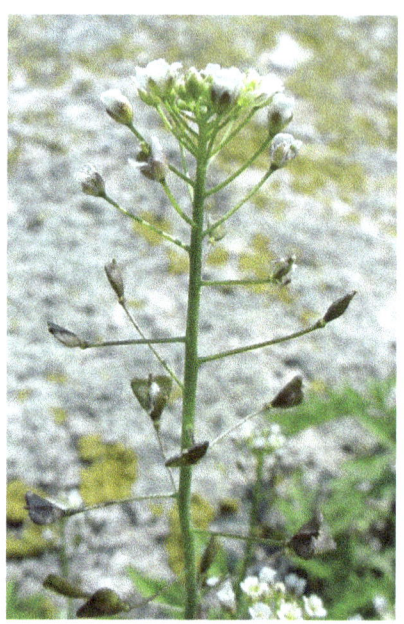

Shepherd's Purse

Capsella bursa-pastoris

Brassicaceae (Mustard) Family
Other common names *(get ready, there is a lot!)*: Witch's pouches, Poverty weed, Blind weed, Mother's heart, Shepherd's sprout, Casewort, Pickpurse, Pickpocket, St. James weed, St. James wort, Beggar's tick, Blindweed, Shepherd's bag, Shepherd's scrip, Shepherd's pouch, Rattle pouches, Case weed, Shovel weed, Pepper-and-salt, Sanguinary, Lady's purse, Clappedepouch (Irish), Hirtentaschelkraut (German), Patushya S umka (Russian)

Description: Shepherd's purse is a common weed in the western United States and worldwide. It is a hardy annual or sometimes biennial herb that emerges in early spring. The leaves form in a basal rosette and can either have smooth edges or be variously lobed or toothed. As the leaves mature, they are somewhat hairy underneath. From the rosette of leaves, clusters of tiny white flowers are born on long, upright stems. The white flowers have four petals and bloom progressively from the lower part of the stem upward. The seed pods, which develop on ½-inch stalks, are heart-shaped or triangular, giving the plant its well-known name.

Where it grows: *Capsella bursa-pastoris* grows abundantly in fields, gardens, pastures, meadows, ditches, disturbed sites, and roadsides.

When and how to harvest: Harvest the aerial parts of Shepherd's purse in early spring and summer. The roots can be dug in early to late fall.

How to work with it/ Medicinal use: The *Doctrine of Signatures* suggests that this is a woman's herb, as the seedpod is shaped like a uterus. A tincture can be prepared from the entire fresh plant, including roots, leaves, and flowers. Shepherd's purse tincture is renowned for helping with heavy menstrual bleeding and afterbirth hemorrhage. Richo Cech, founder of Strictly Medicinal Seeds, notes that the tincture has a shelf life of approximately one year before it loses potency.

The tea can be used as a remedy for chronic nosebleeds and excessive bleeding, both internally (in the kidneys and uterus) and externally (on wounds). Its vitamin K content may help promote blood coagulation. Midwives have used Shepherd's purse for centuries to stimulate uterine contractions during active labor. Postpartum, tea or tincture can help expel the placenta, shrink the uterus, and reduce lochia. Austrian herbalist Maria Treben recommends it topically for engorged breasts, much like cabbage leaves.

For hemorrhoids, brew a strong tea and add it to a shallow, lukewarm sitz bath. In homeopathy, *Capsella bursa-pastoris* is used to treat nosebleeds and urinary stones.

Warnings and contraindications: Shepherd's purse should be avoided during pregnancy due to its oxytocic (uterine-contracting) effects, except during the last weeks or active labor and only under the supervision of an experienced midwife or medical professional.

Healing constituents/ Therapeutic actions: Studies have found Shepherd's purse to contain a broad range of compounds: flavonoids, alkaloids, polypeptides, choline, acetylcholine, histamine, tyramine, fatty acids, sterols, organic acids, amino acids, sulforaphane, trace minerals, vitamins, and more (Al-Snafi, 2015). Pharmacological studies have demonstrated that Shepherd's purse exhibits anti-inflammatory, antioxidant, antihistamine, AChE-inhibitory, and anticancer properties (Goun et al., 2002). Russian research has explored its hemostatic and choleretic actions, though many studies remain untranslated. A Japanese study (1968) observed oxytocic effects on isolated rat uteruses. In vitro studies also demonstrate that Shepherd's purse has antioxidant, antibacterial, and AChE-inhibiting activity, suggesting potential use in treating Alzheimer's disease (Grosso et al., 2010-11).

Historical connections: The genus name *Capsella* means "little box," and *bursa-pastoris* translates as "purse of the shepherd." Shepherd's purse is an ancient remedy used worldwide. It appears in Chinese texts, such as Ben Cao Gang Mu and Ming Yi Bie Lu, and seeds have even been found at Çatalhöyük, a Neolithic site in Turkey.

The herb was well-known to Greek and Roman physicians and was widely used throughout the Middle Ages. Once in North America, colonists and Native Americans used it for diarrhea, dysentery, worms, stomachaches, and as a food source. The peppery seeds were added as a spice and roasted into flour for traditional breads such as pinole. Colonists observed that milk from cows grazing on Shepherd's purse acquired an off taste, but it was prized as a supplement for chickens.

In Philadelphia, it was cultivated and sold as a spring green. Historically, Shepherd's purse was used for blood in the urine, hemorrhoids, nosebleeds, wounds, bruises, strains, and rheumatic joints. Culpepper wrote, "If bound to the wrists or soles of the feet, it helps the jaundice... a good ointment may be made of it for all wounds, especially wounds in the head."

Maud Grieve (*A Modern Herbal*, 1931) called it "one of the best specifics for stopping hemorrhages of all kinds—of the stomach, the lungs, or the uterus, and more especially bleeding from the kidneys." During World War I, when supplies of Hydrastis and ergot were short, Shepherd's purse became a preferred hemostatic herb.

An 1892 text, *The Pharmacology of the Newer Materia Medica*, suggested that for stubborn nosebleeds, merely holding a handful of Shepherd's purse on the same side as the bleed could help stop it.

Jessica's Notes: As I was researching this humble but powerful herb, I stumbled across a fascinating fact—Shepherd's purse is considered *protocarnivorous*! When the soil is moist, its seeds produce a mucilaginous slime that emits a sweet scent, attracting and killing insects and nematodes. This enriches the surrounding soil, benefiting not only Shepherd's purse but also neighboring plants—and the foragers, mothers, midwives, and wildlife that rely on this resilient herb. It is incredible how such a common "weed" can offer so many gifts: healing, nourishment, and a living example of life's ingenious designs. Shepherd's purse reminds me that nature's simplest plants often hold the most profound wisdom.

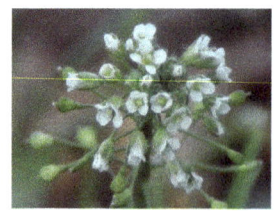

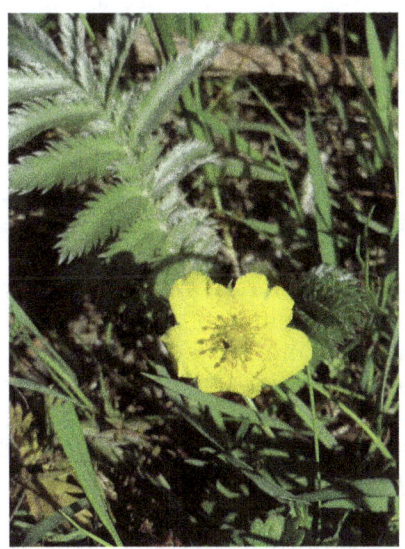

Silverweed

Potentilla anserina

Rosaceae (Rose) Family

Other common names: Cinquefoil, Silver Cinquefoil, Common Silverweed

Description: Silverweed is a low-growing herbaceous perennial with well over fifty species found throughout the western United States. Its creeping red stolons can be up to 80 cm long and spread like strawberries quite invasively. The leaves are 10-20 cm long, evenly pinnate, and have saw-toothed leaflets. Young leaflets have five leaves that are shaped like a maple leaf. The leaves are covered with white, silver hairs, which are more prominent on the underside. The white hairs also cover the stems and stolons, giving the plant a silvery appearance, which is why it is known as silverweed. Each leaf is borne on a petiole up to 5 cm in length. The petite yellow flowers have five petals and are produced singly on stems that range from 5 to 15 cm in length.

Where it grows: Silverweed is commonly found in sandy or rocky soils, often along trails, open fields, and meadows.

When and how to harvest: Harvest the leaves, flowers, and stems from spring to summer.

How to work with it/ Medicinal use: Silverweed can be a mild astringent, similar to wild roses. The tea or infusion can address urinary tract infections and is found to be soothing to the urethra, bladder, and renal tissues. Silverweed tea can help alleviate painful urination and reduce the cloudiness caused by mucus in the urine. It can also address the early stages of incontinence. Cinquefoil can curb heavy menstruation and midcycle bleeding. Silverweed decoctions can be soothing to inflamed tissue and used as a sitz bath for postpartum healing. Gargle Silverweed decoction for sore throats and inflamed gums. You can place fresh leaves in your shoes to dry out wet feet.

Healing constituents/ Therapeutic actions: Chemical constituents include flavonoids, ellagitannins, and gallotannins. Therapeutic actions include astringent, anti-inflammatory, and soothing.

Historical connections: Since at least the Roman Era, Silverweed has been used as a medicinal plant. Historically, it has been used as a wound remedy for various ailments, including fever, sore throat, and stomach cramps. Its Latin name, *Potentilla*, indicates it is a potent astringent medicine. Culpepper writes in *The Complete Herbal* (1653), "It is an especial herb used in all inflammations and fevers, whether infections or pestilential; or among other herbs to cool and temper the blood and humours in the body." In Europe, since prehistoric times, the root has been eaten like a potato, either cooked or raw. Cinquefoil was so astringent that it was used in the tanning leather industry when other tannin-rich trees were difficult to come by. There is rich folklore behind Silverweed. The plant bears the common name "richette" in French, which translates to "rich through silver and gold." The five leaflets represented love, money, health, power, and wisdom; carrying a leaf granted these. When hung at the door, Cinquefoil was believed to protect the dwelling against evil. Legend has it that Silverweed grew along the dusty streets of Palestine, where Jesus walked, and it has been called "the Footsteps of Our Lord." Native Americans used cinquefoil medicinally. The Chippewa administered *Potentilla arguta* to treat dysentery. *Potentilla arguta* was used by the Gosiute for swellings, and the Cherokee used common silverweed as a mouthwash. There is a very ancient fossil record of the species *Argentina anserina*, commonly found in the Pleistocene Era.

Jessica's notes: I was unfamiliar with Silverweed by name, though I noticed it everywhere and was curious to learn more. One day at Forest School, a student brought me a mystery leaf. I admitted I did not know the plant, but I promised to find out. Later, while browsing a botanical encyclopedia gifted by a friend, I discovered it was *Cinquefoil*! I was thrilled to learn about its astringent properties.

One day, on a mountain hike, the Freeborn family and our neighbor, Jeffrey, were exploring the vast canyon that cuts between our properties. As we traversed the rocky ledges, we noticed Silverweed growing in abundance. We nibbled on a few leaves—and wow! They dried out our mouths immediately. You can taste and feel the astringency.

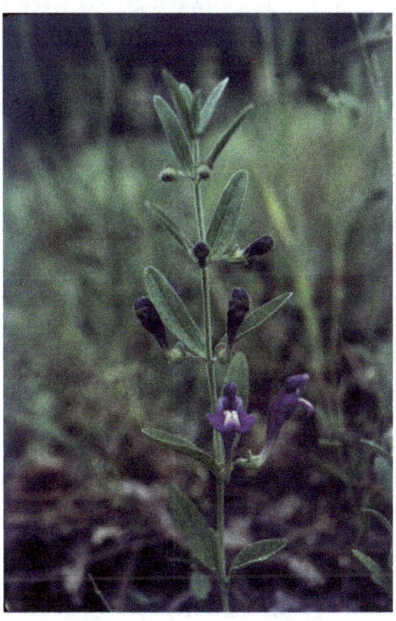

Skullcap

Scutellaria angustifolia, Scutellaria galericulata

Lamiaceae (Mint) Family
Other common names: Narrowleaf Skullcap, Helmet Flower, Hoodwort, Mad-dog Skullcap, Quarter Bonnet, American Skullcap
  Description: *Scutellaria angustifolia* is a herbaceous perennial that often forms colonies through the growth of creeping rhizomes. The leaves are narrow and oval to lance-shaped, measuring 2-3 inches long. The violet to dark blue flowers are solitary and form from axils on the upper stems. It reaches approximately 1 foot in height. *Scutellaria galericulata* grows to a height of 1 to 2 feet. Its distinguishing difference from *S. angustifolia* is its square stems and opposite leaves. The individual leaves are lance-shaped with toothed margins. The flowers intermingle with the upper leaves. The flowers are tubular, with two lips, and are a dark violet-blue.
  Where it grows: Unlike other moisture-loving members of the Skullcaps, *S. angustifolia* prefers more rocky and drier soil. It can be found in

prairies and on the outskirts of mountain meadows. *S. galericulata* can be found in wetlands and along the banks of grassy streams. It grows alongside medicinal plants such as St. John's Wort and mountain mint.

When and how to harvest: Harvest the aerial parts when in flower. Drier climate skullcaps are more straightforward to gather as they form in clumps. Wetland skullcaps are more tedious to collect. Snip a sprig here and there as you meander in the meadow.

How to use it/ Medicinal use: Skullcap's medicine supports the nervous system and acts as a mild sedative. Clinical research highlights Skullcap's stimulating effects on GABA (gamma-aminobutyric acid) receptor sites, which calm the brain. Take a full dose of tea or tincture before bed as a sleep aid. Use for a restless mind with racing thoughts that then keep the body awake. Use a lower dose during the daytime for anxiety. Consider taking a dose ten minutes before performing to reduce stage fright. It can help reduce social anxiety and alleviate stress and unease in social situations. Skullcap pairs nicely with Kava, making a nice 'mocktail.'

Where small doses help relax the anxious mind, large doses can support epilepsy and seizure-like symptoms. Take 3 to 4 times a day for epilepsy as a preventative.

Skullcap is bitter and can help stimulate appetite and digestion. However, please do not take it on an empty stomach because it can cause heartburn. The more bitter the plant is, the more effective the medicine. The more resinous a species is, the more apt it will be to encourage a sweat (diaphoretic). These resinous skullcaps can serve as a sedative and help induce sweating to break a fever, especially when stress and lack of sleep prolong the fever.

Healing constituents/ Therapeutic actions: Contains flavones (baicalein, baicalin, chrysin, wogonin, oroxylin, genkwanin), flavonols (quercetin, rutin), flavones (hesperitin, hesperidin, naringenin), isoflavone (daidzein), and neo-clerodane diterpenoids. These compounds contribute to its diaphoretic, mild sedative, nervine, trophorestorative, and anticonvulsant effects.

Historical connections: Skullcap has been traditionally used by many Native American tribes, who taught European settlers and folk herbalists about its medicinal properties, including its use to soothe nerves, support women's health, and facilitate ceremonies. Herbal physicians reintroduced Skullcap to Great Britain in the 19th century and have continued to use it for its relaxing properties to the present day. *Scutellaria lateriflora* appeared in the first American Materia Medica, published in 1785.

Jessica's notes: Skullcap has been one of my greatest herbal allies when life feels overwhelming. When I first began my deep dive into nervous system herbs, Skullcap stood out as a plant that gently calms frazzled nerves without dulling the senses. I often turn to a Skullcap tincture when I feel that fluttery heart, jittery feeling before teaching a class or leading an herbal walk. It helps me shift from nervousness to grounded presence.

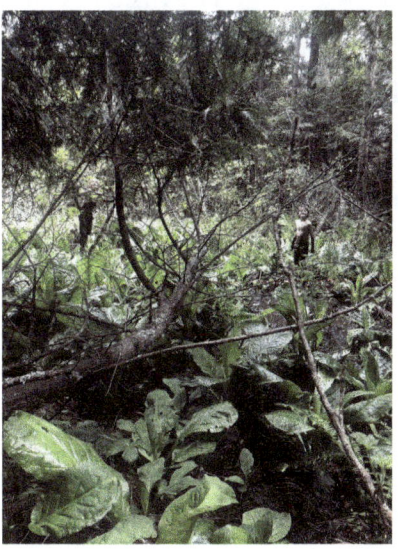

Skunk Cabbage

Lysichiton americanus

Araceae (Arum) Family

Other common names: Western Skunk Cabbage, American Skunk Cabbage, Swamp Lantern

Description: In early spring, out of the mucky earth, Skunk Cabbage rhizomes give rise to a spike of small, densely arranged, greenish-yellow flowers on a 12- to 20-inch-long stalk. A bright yellow, leaf-like bract enfolds the skunky-smelling flower spike, attracting pollinating insects. The flowers emit a strong odor which is why it is called skunk cabbage. The waxy-coated leaves can grow to massive sizes—up to three feet long—and teleport you to a prehistoric forest scene. The leaves are short-stalked, fleshy, and broadly egg-shaped or lanceolate, emerging after the Skunk Cabbages have produced their flowers. The egg-shaped fruits, greenish to reddish, remain embedded in the flower spike after maturing. The roots and rhizomes resemble tiny octopuses. This semi-aquatic perennial can live up to 80 years.

Where it grows: Skunk Cabbage inhabits swamps, bogs, marshes, and springs.

When and how to harvest: Harvest the rhizomes and side roots in late summer and mid-fall. **Warning:** The rhizomes and roots are difficult to remove. One plant can take several hours to uproot!

How to work with it/ Medicinal use: Where Skunk Cabbage grows—in the muck and swampy earth—indicates how it can work in the body. The root and rhizome-prepared tincture can help clear and remove mucus from the lungs. It can also calm spasmodic coughing, especially when the force of coughing causes gagging and nausea. Skunk Cabbage can be used for winter colds, asthma, and bronchitis.

Topically, a balm made from the root can be powerful in alleviating the pain of open sores, wounds, blisters, fungal infections, and skin tumors. You can use the leaves as a "primitive tinfoil" to cook food over a campfire.

Caution: Do not consume fresh plants or eat the cooked leaves. All parts of Skunk Cabbage contain needle-sharp calcium oxalate crystals that can injure the digestive tract when ingested. Eating the plant raw will cause a burning sensation in the mouth and throat. In extreme cases, the throat may swell shut. Additionally, use the prepared rhizome and root medicine in small quantities, as consuming large amounts can cause nausea and digestive upset.

Healing constituents/ Therapeutic actions: *L. americanus* contains Scopoletin, a coumarin compound that exhibits anti-inflammatory, antioxidant, and antimicrobial activities. It contributes to the plant's therapeutic effects, particularly in respiratory and inflammatory conditions. Skunk Cabbage also contains **salicylates**, which may account for its use in alleviating pain and inflammation. Therapeutic actions include antispasmodic, diuretic, expectorant, and narcotic.

Historical connections: Skunk Cabbage has been used by many Native American tribes, including the Abnaki, Chippewa, Delaware, Haudenosaunee, Malecite, Menominee, Meskwaki, Micmac, Mohegan, and Nanticoke. Its host of medicinal uses included treating epilepsy, being used externally as a gynecological aid, and treating worms. The Haudenosaunee cooked the young leaves and used a wash of the powdered root as a deodorant.

Jessica's notes: Skunk Cabbage always makes me pause in awe when I see it emerging from the muck in early spring. There is something primal about its presence, as though it belongs to an older era of the Earth's story. One day, while walking through the swampy edges of our mountain creek, my son spotted one of the giant yellow bracts glowing in the dappled light. We crouched down to get a closer look and were surprised by the warmth of the plant—it was one of those rare early bloomers that can generate its own heat! When I make tincture from the roots, I am reminded of how this plant, which thrives in decay and muck, can help us clear our own internal "swamp" of stuck mucus and chronic cough. It teaches me that beauty and medicine can emerge from the darkest and most murky places.

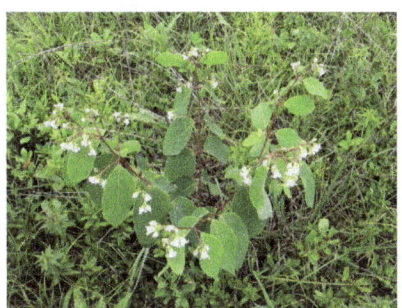

Spreading Dogbane

Apocynum androsaemifolium

Apocynaceae (Dogbane) Family
Other common names: Bitter Root, Dog's Bane, Werewolf Root

Description: Spreading Dogbane is a low-growing perennial with reddish-brown branching stems that spread 7–8 inches from a rhizomatous network of narrow, woody, dark-barked roots. Smooth-edged, oval to egg-shaped, dark green leaves (1½ to 3 inches long) are arranged oppositely on the stem. The leaves droop downward and have a lighter underside. Dogbane flowers from early summer to early fall. The pink, bell-shaped, five-lobed flowers bloom at the ends of stems or from the stalks that form in the upper leaf axils. The fragrant flower lobes fan out or curve backward. Sometimes the flowers can be pinkish-white with pink stripes.

Pollinated flowers produce pairs of thin, 2- to 5-inch-long, pincer-like pods. Fluffy, cotton-tufted seeds ripen inside these curving pods, eventually taking flight on the wind. When cut or broken, the stems and leaves ooze a milky sap.

Where it grows: Spreading Dogbane is often found on south-facing roadcuts and sunny meadows throughout much of North America.

When and how to harvest: Gather the roots and rhizomes in early fall, after the seeds have ripened and the tops have died back. Dig deep from the crown of the rhizome until you find the junction between the vertical and horizontally running rhizomes. Follow these roots as far as possible before uprooting a section.

How to work with it/ Medicinal use: Early American botanical doctors worked with Spreading Dogbane to stimulate weak bile secretion. The bitter root tincture was thought to strengthen and tone the bile ducts. It was especially recommended for jaundice, liver swelling, or any symptoms indicative of deficient bile duct function. It was also considered an effective laxative.

Today, Dogbane is often overlooked or misunderstood—many modern sources label it as toxic. However, more profound herbal wisdom holds that Dogbane is a potent medicine for psychological and emotional healing. In small doses, the tincture can support releasing addictions to substances and toxic relationships and help break habits that contribute to depression and despair. Once these negative patterns are cleared, Spreading Dogbane is said to bring clarity of life purpose and inner truth.

The milky sap that oozes from the stems and leaves can be applied directly to remove warts. Because this plant is such a powerful medicine, it is also well-suited for use as a flower essence. The essence supports self-confidence and encourages us to trust our wild, rebellious instincts.

Healing constituents/ Therapeutic actions: Spreading Dogbane is a bitter stimulant and contains cardiac glycosides, which, in large doses, can slow the heart.

Caution: Do not take large doses of the root, which may cause nausea and vomiting. Do not use during pregnancy or alongside prescription medications. Do not ingest the milky sap. Work with this plant under the guidance of an experienced herbalist.

Historical connections: Native North American peoples worked with Dogbane for many conditions, including headaches, convulsions, and digestive complaints. The Chippewa used a decoction of the root for heart palpitations. The Iroquois used a compound infusion of the roots to treat stomach cramps. The Potawatomi used the root as a diuretic and prepared a decoction of the green berries to treat kidney infections.

In addition to spreading the medicinal uses of Dogbane, women of several Native American tribes used its strong stems to make fine thread for sewing, as well as twine for nets, fabric, and bowstrings.

Jessica's notes: Spreading Dogbane is one of those plants that seems to call to me from the edges of the trail, asking not to be forgotten. I first noticed it when hiking a sunny, south-facing slope alongside Spirit Lake, and was drawn to its dainty pink flowers swaying in the breeze. Once I learned of its deep, bitter medicine and emotional healing gifts, I felt a new respect for this unassuming plant. I view it as a guide for releasing old patterns and stepping more fully into my authentic self. It is strong medicine, both physically and spiritually, and reminds me to approach it—and life—with reverence and care.

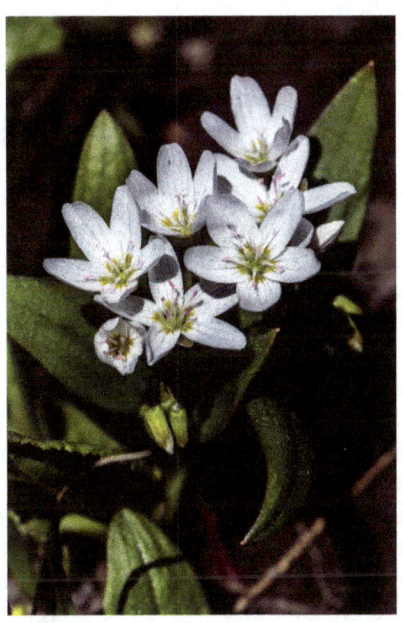

Spring Beauty

Claytonia lanceolata

Montiaceae (Miner's Lettuce) Family
Other common names: Virginia spring beauty
Description: Spring Beauty is a small and delicate plant that graces the forest floor and mountain hillsides as one of the first heralds of spring. It features succulent green, lanceolate leaves and pink to red stems. The petite spring flowers are white with a soft pink tinge, featuring five petals and two stamens. You can tell the plant is several years old when more than one stem emerges from the underground tuber. The roots are round and resemble miniature potatoes, rarely exceeding an inch in diameter.
Where it grows: Spring Beauty appears as soon as the snow melts, arriving as a spring ephemeral in mountain meadows, forest floors, and between valleys. It is one of the first showy wildflowers of the north.
When and how to harvest: Harvest the tender green leaves and flowers in early spring, but only when you encounter a well-established colony. The roots can also be harvested in early spring, but only in areas with

nutrient-dense soil and abundant plant life. Seek out the older plants with multiple stems, leaving younger ones to thrive.

How to work with it/ Medicinal use: The succulent leaves add a citrusy-sweet flavor to salads and are beautiful as a garnish for many dishes. Finely minced, they elevate chilled soups, such as gazpacho. The tender shoots can be used in stir-fries and sautés, and the dainty flowers make an enchanting garnish for poultry or wild game dishes.

The crisp, starchy tubers can be eaten raw for a sweet crunch or cooked like creamy baby potatoes. Like other wild tubers, Spring Beauty roots are a rich source of fiber, supporting healthy digestion and weight management.

Healing constituents/ Therapeutic actions: The corms contain vitamins A and C and are rich in calories and carbohydrates for such a small root vegetable.

Historical connections: Spring Beauty has deep roots in human history and forest folklore. Indigenous Americans and early European settlers used it as both food and medicine. The corms were often stored like root vegetables for use during the winter. The greens were made into poultices to treat wounds and skin irritations. The Thompson Indians applied poultices of Spring Beauty to the eyes to aid vision (Turner et al., 1990).

The Cowlitz, Snohomish, Quileute, and Skykomish used the plant as a hair tonic to create glossy hair, while the Skagit used it to treat sore throats (Gunther, 1973). Quinault women would chew the entire plant during pregnancy to ensure the baby would be soft (Gunther, 1973). The Iroquois used powdered root as a remedy for colds and flu, or prepared it as a cold infusion to treat convulsions.

A Chippewa story tells of its origins: "Thus the spirit of Winter departed, and where he had melted away, there the Indian children gathered the first blossoms, fragrant and delicately pink… The modest Spring Beauty." (indiananativeplantsociety.com)

Jessica's notes: Spring Beauty is one of my favorite signs that the forest is waking from its winter sleep. I am always delighted to see its dainty flowers scattered like confetti across the ground. Knowing how important this plant is for early pollinators makes me all the more careful and mindful when harvesting. A fascinating study from 1978 observed that 22 species of insects visited Spring Beauty over two years. The flower filaments reflect UV light, guiding pollinators like a runway—a beautiful example of nature's intelligence at work (Schemske et al., 1978). To me, this plant symbolizes the fragile yet persistent hope of spring.

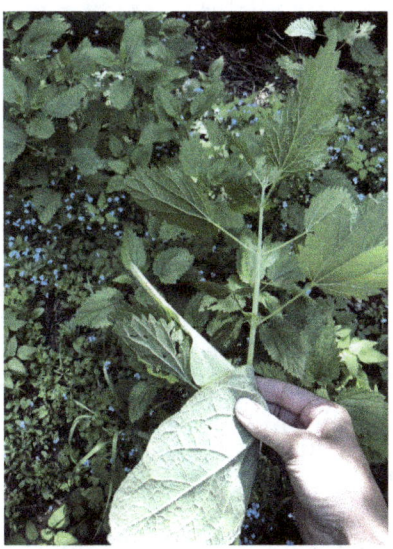

Stinging Nettle

Urtica dioica

Urticaceae (Nettle) Family
Description: Stinging Nettles bear tiny, needle-like hairs on the stems and leaves that can cause contact dermatitis and a painful stinging rash in humans and animals—hence the name. The sting can last up to 12 hours. Hunting dogs running through a nettle thicket have sometimes been poisoned, even lethally. The stinging trichomes have bulbous tips that break off when brushed against, revealing sharp tubes that pierce the skin and inject a mix of acetylcholine, formic acid, histamine, and serotonin. This is a powerful defense mechanism against large herbivores. Heating or cooking the fresh leaves eradicates the sting.

Nettle is a robust perennial that can grow up to 6.5 feet tall. It spreads vegetatively through yellow, creeping rhizomes and often forms dense colonies. The dark green, toothed leaves grow opposite each other along stout, square, fibrous stems. The leaves are lance-shaped, oval, or heart-shaped. Tiny green or white flowers form in dense, drooping clusters on the leaf axils. Nettles are wind-pollinated. After pollination, the female flowers develop into tiny green seeds that ripen during the summer months.

Where it grows: Nettles thrive along creeks, springs, streams, brooks, and rivers, preferring damp, rich soils. They also grow in shady forest clearings, mountain slopes, disturbed sites, garden groves, and near human habitation.

When and how to harvest: Harvest the greens with gloves in early spring through late summer, before the plants flower. If you do not have gloves, pinch the top tip of the plant, which often lacks stinging hairs. Clip stems with shears or scissors, and place them carefully in your harvesting bag. Gather ripe green seeds from late summer into early autumn. Harvest dormant roots and rhizomes once the tops die back.

How to work with it/ Medicinal use: Modern herbalist Robin Rose Bennett calls stinging nettle "herbal health insurance." A daily cup of nettle tea supports the body with essential minerals and helps repair and restore balance. Nettle tea or cooked greens can build the blood, strengthen hair, skin, nails, and connective tissues, and increase breast milk production. It is recommended during pregnancy to support the healthy growth and development of the baby.

The iron content helps combat anemia and alleviate menstrual cramps and heavy bleeding. Nettle tea soothes gout, eases seasonal allergies, asthma, and respiratory complaints. Historically, intentional stinging with fresh nettles was used to restore nerve function and alleviate arthritis and rheumatism. The seeds and greens nourish the adrenals and kidneys and may help restore failing kidney function. Nettle root is a well-known remedy for benign prostatic hyperplasia (enlarged prostate) in aging men.

Healing constituents/ Therapeutic actions: The juice of stinging nettle hairs contains acetylcholine, a neurotransmitter, and formic acid, also found in ant venom. This combination enhances cellular response and promotes circulation and lymphatic flow. Nettles are rich in minerals—iron, calcium, magnesium, potassium, zinc—and contain more protein and chlorophyll than most wild plants. They also provide vitamins A, B1, B2, C, and K.

Therapeutic actions include antihistamine, antibacterial, anti-inflammatory, astringent, diuretic, tonic, anodyne, pectoral, rubefacient, styptic, anthelmintic, nutritive, alterative, hemetic, anti-rheumatic, anti-allergenic, anti-lithic/lithotriptic, depurative/nephritic, galactagogue, hypoglycemic, expectorant, and anti-spasmodic.

Historical connections: Nettle's botanical name, *dioica*, means "two houses," referring to its male and female flowers. Nettle use is documented across Europe and Asia as far back as the Late Bronze Age (1570–1200 BCE). Julius Caesar's troops reportedly rubbed themselves with nettles to stay awake and alert during cold northern campaigns (Schneider, 2024).

Throughout history, nettle stalks were dried and pounded to extract textile fibers, similar to those obtained from flax or hemp. Nettle fabric dates back to the Late Bronze Age and was used for fine linens in 16th- and 17th-century Scotland. During wartime, Germans mixed nettle fiber with cotton for use in underclothes, stockings, and tarps. Nettle leaf was also used to curdle milk in the cheese-making process.

Native American tribes have utilized nettle for food, medicine, clothing, and ceremonial purposes since time immemorial. The Winnebago, Coastal Salish, Omaha, Cupeno, Menominee, and Subarctic peoples wove nettle fiber into clothing, fishing nets, and bowstrings. Warriors and hunters used nettle stings to stay alert. Nevada tribes burned nettle leaves in sweat lodges to treat pneumonia and flu (Hatfield, 2004).

The Kawaiisu tribe viewed nettle as a plant of dreams: walking barefoot through nettle fields was believed to prepare one for powerful "medicine dreams" (D'Azavedo & Sturtevant, 1986). In Indigenous folklore, nettle is often portrayed as a trickster plant, associated with Coyote. One story suggests that nettle's sting serves as a reminder to pay respect to this powerful medicine.

Jessica's notes: Nettles have been a part of my life since my teenage years, when I first discovered the healing properties of plant medicine. I used to suffer from miserable seasonal allergies, and nettles worked better for me than Claritin! I now add nettles to pesto, soups, teas, and baked goods. One of my favorite herbalists, Rosemary Gladstar, teaches that if you harvest nettle with mindful attention, gloveless, you will not get stung. I put this to the test one day, harvesting while my baby boy played beside me. I was on a roll-no stings!—until the baby distracted me and *zap*! I was stung. To this day, I harvest stinging nettles without gloves and often barefoot. This practice reminds me, and my students, to move through the wild with careful presence and deep respect for the plants we gather.

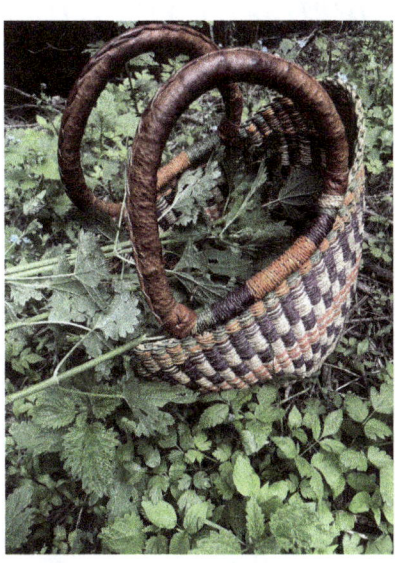

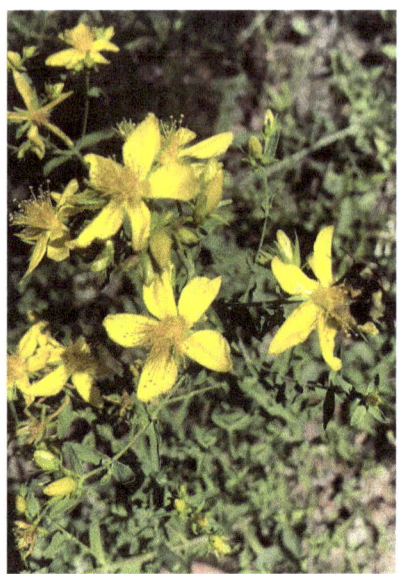

St. John's Wort

Hypericum perforatum

Hypericaceae (St. John's Wort) Family

Description: A sturdy perennial often regarded as an invasive weed by some. St. John's wort can grow up to 3 feet tall. Members of this genus have simple, opposite, or whorled leaves that may develop red dots in late summer. The stems and leaves usually have smooth margins. Its bright yellow flowers resemble small, rounded stars, each with five petals and numerous stamens, and often bloom in dense clusters. The fruits are dry, brownish-green capsules.

Where it grows: St. John's wort thrives in disturbed soils, sunny fields, meadows, roadsides, and pastures.

When and how to harvest: Gather the yellow blooms and aerial parts from late July to August. Gently dry the flowers for winter teas and medicines.

How to work with it/ Medicinal use: This beautiful summer flower brings a little sunshine to a dark mind. When infused in oil or alcohol, it transforms into a bright ruby red. Its medicine can help alleviate depression, particularly seasonal depression. St. John's wort also acts as a liver tonic, helping relieve stagnation, especially helpful during the sedentary winter months. Enjoy it as a tea or tincture for depression and mood support. It promotes restful sleep and relaxation when taken before bedtime. I have also found that St. John's wort can help balance and regulate hormones and menstruation. An oil infusion makes an excellent wound-healing salve for cuts, scrapes, and minor skin irritations due to its antibacterial and vulnerary properties. As a field poultice, rub the crushed flowers on bug bites and minor skin irritations. St. John's wort has the remarkable ability to heal both physically and emotionally.

Caution: Do not consume if taking prescription antidepressants or birth control, as it may reduce their effectiveness.

Healing constituents/ Therapeutic actions: St. John's wort contains several active constituents, including cyclopseudohypericin, hypericin, hyperforin, protohypericin, pseudohypericin, and various flavonoids. These components contribute to its antidepressant effects and other healing actions. Therapeutic actions include vulnerary (wound-healing), vermifuge (parasite-clearing), nervine, and anti-inflammatory.

Historical connections: The medicinal properties of St. John's wort have been recognized for thousands of years, mentioned by Dioscorides and Hippocrates. Herbalists have long used it to treat nervous system injuries and chronic depression.

In Gaelic tradition, wearing an amulet of St. John's wort was believed to ward off evil. Sprigs of the flowers were burned for good luck during Beltane, coinciding with the time of their bloom. After the rise of Christianity in Europe, the plant became associated with St. John the Baptist, as it blooms profusely around his feast day, which is June 24. The red spots that appear on the flowers and leaves in August were said to symbolize the blood of the Baptist, martyred in that month.

In *The Herbal* (1597), Gerard called it "a most precious remedy for deep wounds." He recommended steeping the flowers and leaves in olive oil and exposing them to the hot sun until they turned deep red. Thus came its folk names "Touch and Heal" and "Balm of the Warrior's Wound."

In North America, related Hypericum species were used by Indigenous peoples. The Iroquois used it for fever and reproductive health, while the Cherokee used it for diarrhea, venereal sores, and snake bites.

St. John's wort, St. John's wort. *My envy whoever has thee! I will pluck thee with my right hand./ I will preserve thee with my left hand. Whoso findeth thee in the cattle field. Shall never be without kine.* — Gaelic poem

Jessica's notes: St. John's wort has healed my life on many levels—emotionally and physically. I have come to appreciate its medicine deeply. One cold fall day, facing the icy, dark approach of my first northern winter after moving from California, I felt despair settling into my heart. Seeking solace, I walked to the Welsh Woods. In the open prairie behind the woods, a single St. John's wort flower was still in bloom. It felt like encountering an old friend. I put the flower in my mouth and lay on the earth. Suddenly,

I felt warmth and comfort, as if receiving a hug from my Papa (Father Richard Ballew).

"Papa, is that you?" I asked. "Yes, it is me," came the reply. "I wanted to let you know that I love you, and you will be taken care of."

Not long after, our family moved into our first Idaho home, where we lived happily for many years.

I often add St. John's wort to tea blends when I have been cooped up indoors for too long and need a little sunshine in my cup. It never fails to lift my mood. My kids also love St. John's wort, especially for soothing itchy bug bites, cuts, and scrapes with its healing oil and salve.

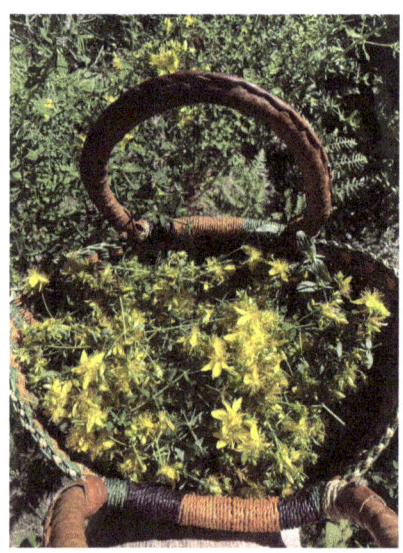

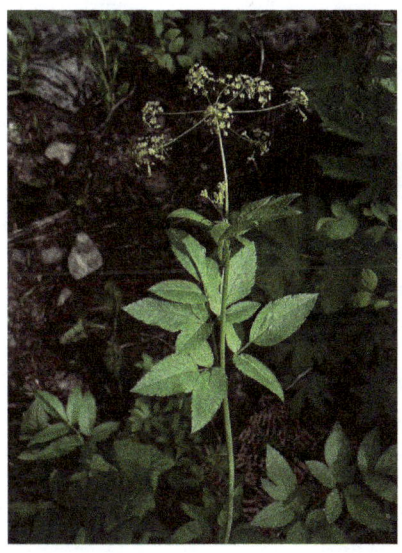

Sweet Cicely

Ozmorhiza occidentalis

Apiaceae (Carrot) Family
Other common names: Western Sweet Cicely, Sweet Root

Description: Sweet Cicely is a mountain-hardy perennial with dense, dark-green foliage. The compound leaves grow in threes, pointed and serrated, arising from the base of the plant, while a few smaller leaves cling to the stem. Sweet Cicely can reach heights of up to 4 feet. Its yellow flowers, sometimes with a greenish hue, bloom in umbels, resembling the flower heads of fennel, dill, and other members of the carrot family. The long, slender, dark green seed pods are slightly arched and ripen in late summer. The roots are light brown to gray, with a creamy interior, and grow in a tangled, fragrant mass. When exposed, the sweet aroma of the root greets the eager forager.

Where it grows: Sweet Cicely prefers shade and clean mountain soil. It thrives in high mountain forests and blooms in late spring to early summer, with seeds ripening in late summer.

When and how to harvest: Harvest seeds as soon as they ripen in late summer; older seeds tend to lose their aromatic flavor. The roots of mature plants are most fragrant and are best harvested in the fall. Leaves and flowers can also be gathered in spring and summer for teas and other preparations.

Caution: Sweet Cicely has several look-alikes that are deadly, including Water Hemlock (Cicuta species) and Poison Hemlock (Conium maculatum), which can be fatal. Hemlock roots can smell sweet like celery. Be 100% certain of your identification. If you are unsure, always consult an experienced herbalist or forager.

How to work with it/ Medicinal use: Sweet root is a warming, carminative herb used similarly to fennel. The root tincture has a rich, fennel-like flavor with a gentle warmth that soothes the stomach. Traditionally, Sweet Cicely was used to treat internal and external fungal infections, as well as to act as a vermifuge. The whole plant—leaves, seeds, flowers, and roots—can be infused in vinegar to create a medicinal tonic such as Fire Cider. The aromatic leaves can be used fresh or dried in teas to ease digestive upset and bloating, or to stimulate bowel movements gently.

The seed pods are a favorite trail nibble with their sweet, licorice-like flavor. They can also be added to honey, vinegar, or alcohol to extract their warming qualities. Sweet Cicely's carminative action can help soothe menstrual cramps and gas.

Healing constituents/ Therapeutic actions: Sweet Cicely is carminative and aromatic. Its signature licorice scent indicates the presence of anethole, a compound also found in plants such as anise, licorice, hyssop, and basil. Therapeutic actions include carminative, digestive stimulant, antispasmodic, and warming.

Historical connections: Many Native American tribes used Sweet Cicely as a panacea herb. The root was considered a tonic to ease childbirth. Decoctions of the root were used as eyewash and applied as poultices for wounds and boils. *Ozmorhiza* species have been used in American folk medicine as expectorants and tonics for digestive troubles.

The Greek genus name derives from *osmo* ("smell") and *rhiza* ("root")—"good-smelling root." The species name *occidentalis* means "western." Western Sweet Cicely was collected by the British botanist Thomas Nuttall in the early 1830s during his explorations in what is now the state of Oregon. He originally named it *Glycosma occidentalis* in 1840. Its current botanical name, *Ozmorhiza occidentalis*, was assigned by American botanist John Torrey in 1858.

Jessica's notes: Sweet Cicely is one of those hidden mountain treasures that reveals itself only to the patient and observant. Its licorice scent is unforgettable—comforting, grounding, and instantly recognizable once you know it. I love nibbling on a fresh seed pod while walking the alpine trails. When I work with the root, I feel connected to generations of healers who turned to this plant for everything from childbirth to broken skin to bellyaches.

*Photo by Walter Siegmund, CC□BY-SA/ GFDL

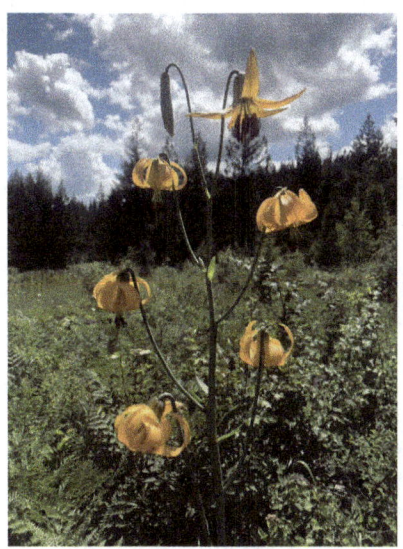

Tiger Lily

Lilium lancifolium

Liliaceae (Lily) Family

Description: Tiger Lily is a perennial wildflower that grows up to 3 feet tall, bearing clusters of bright orange flowers adorned with purplish-brown spots. The petals gracefully curl back toward the base, capturing the image of a stalking tiger mid-pounce. The tepals measure 3 to 6 cm long. Like many true lilies, the leaves are arranged in whorls around the plant's stem. The smooth, slightly lanceolate leaves measure approximately 3 to 7 cm long. The flowers exude a heavenly, intoxicating scent that fills the air in summer.

Where it grows: Tiger Lily graces the foothills, mountain fields, and high-elevation meadows.

When and how to harvest: Lilies are seldom found in abundance, and harvesting them often leads to the plant's demise. It is best to leave this stunning wildflower in place, allowing it to thrive and admire its beauty. When we harvest from the mountain, we pluck only the petals, leaving the pollen-loaded stigmas intact. Consider cultivating Tiger Lilies in your garden to enjoy their beauty and potential medicinal gifts without impacting wild populations. Although this plant must be protected, understanding its medicinal uses is beneficial for future sustainable harvests.

How to work with it/ Medicinal use: The cooked bulbs are high in starch and can serve as a substitute for potatoes, thickening soups and stews. The tubers, young shoots, and flowers are all edible, either cooked or raw. The roots and shoots have been used in the treatment of breast cancer. A decoction of the bulb can help address edema and kidney issues, while a decoction of the flower buds has been used to treat jaundice. A poultice of the plant may soothe hemorrhoids.

In Korean traditional medicine, Tiger Lily is used to treat coughs, sore throats, heart palpitations, and boils. It also holds a place in traditional Chinese medicine for respiratory support; its expectorant properties help expel phlegm and relieve symptoms of coughs, bronchitis, and other respiratory ailments. Tiger Lily also contains carminative and anti-inflammatory compounds that may relieve gas, bloating, and inflammatory pain.

Tiger Lily flower essence is worked with to release outdated ancestral beliefs and emotional patterns. The six petals peeling back represent the symbolic shedding of layers that no longer serve, while the long stamens reaching outward suggest the act of seeking new understanding and growth.

Healing constituents/ Therapeutic actions: Tiger Lily bulbs are considered to have anti-inflammatory, antibacterial, vermifuge, diuretic, emmenagogue, emollient, and expectorant properties. The flowers are carminative and possess a pleasantly peppery flavor.

Historical connections: Northern Native peoples traditionally used Tiger Lily roots to make medicinal teas for stomach disorders, coughs, tuberculosis, fevers, and as a labor aid and postpartum tonic. Decoctions were also used as washes for swellings, bruises, wounds, and sores. Pacific Northwest tribes, including the Salish and Nuu-chah-nulth, steamed, boiled, or pit-cooked the bulbs, often adding them to soups alongside meat and fish.

Globally, Tiger Lily carries rich cultural symbolism. In Chinese tradition, it is a symbol of wealth, prosperity, and good fortune, frequently associated with the Lunar calendar and traditional celebrations. The Chinese name for Tiger Lily, *Baihe*, translates to "a hundred kinds of blessing."

In Western cultures, the Tiger Lily is emblematic of courage, passion, and strength. It is associated with the Divine Feminine, representing nurturing, protective instincts, and resilience.

Jessica's notes: Tiger Lily reminds me to forgive and let live. She teaches me the power of reserved strength and graceful endurance. Her vibrant return each summer is a fierce, feminine declaration of resilience, urging me to embody both softness and power. I have come to regard her as sacred medicine—one to be revered and protected, not taken lightly. Tiger Lily is a bold, fragrant teacher with deep roots in both cultural and emotional healing.

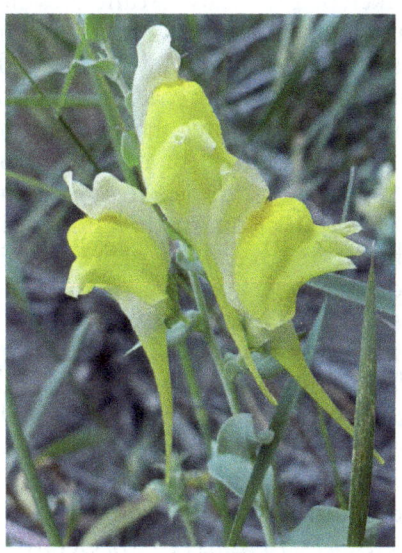

Toadflax

Linaria dalmatica and Linaria vulgaris

Plantaginaceae (Plantain) Family

Other common names: Dalmatian Toadflax (*L. dalmatica*), Butter and Eggs (*L. vulgaris*)

Description: Both species are cold-hardy, small, weedy perennials with alternating leaves. *L. dalmatica* has ovate leaves that clasp the stem, giving the plant a tidy and upright appearance. In contrast, *L. vulgaris* displays looser leaves that do not clasp the stem. The flowers of both species are cheerful, two-tone yellow, with five lobes and two lips, ending in a funnel-shaped spur that resembles a tiny snapdragon. The small round seed capsules form as the flowers fade. Toadflax spreads vigorously through an extensive network of horizontal rhizomes, often forming colonies.

Where it grows: Toadflax thrives in moist soil and is commonly found in prairies, along roadsides, in disturbed soil, and throughout open meadows.

When and how to harvest: Gather the aerial parts of Toadflax, ideally when the plant is in full bloom. It typically flowers in late summer.

How to work with it/ Medicinal use: Toadflax is a highly functional bitter tonic. When taken before meals, it stimulates digestion and improves the absorption of nutrients. Like other bitters, Toadflax pairs beautifully with aromatic herbs, such as Mountain Mint or Bee Balm, to help calm a range of gastrointestinal complaints. Toadflax tea or tincture supports the liver and kidneys and can be taken regularly to soothe dry or allergy-reactive skin. It is slightly more stimulating to the gastrointestinal tract than other bitters and can serve as a gentle laxative. Swishing Toadflax tea in the mouth increases saliva production, further aiding digestion. Those who struggle to digest rich, fatty meals and experience poor lipid assimilation may find relief with Toadflax.

Healing constituents/ Therapeutic actions: Toadflax contains a wealth of flavonoids, including aureusin, bracteatin, cyanidin, linarin, and pectolinarin, as well as iridoids such as aucubin, antirrinoside, antirride, and procumbide. Its therapeutic actions include cholagogue (stimulating bile flow), purgative, hepatic, and astringent properties.

Historical connections: Toadflax is native to the Mediterranean region and escaped cultivation during the colonization of North America. In *The Herball or Generall Historie of Plants* (1636), Gerard notes, "the decoction openeth the stopping of the liver and spleen, and is singular good against the jaundice which is of long continuance," adding that "a decoction of Toadflax taketh away the yellownesse and deformitie of the skinne, being washed and bathed therewith." In *A Modern Herbal*, Maude Grieve comments that when boiled in milk, Toadflax makes an effective fly poison.

Jessica's notes: Toadflax reminds me of the Doctrine of Signatures—its bright yellow blossoms mirror the color of bile, hinting at its natural affinity for the liver and gallbladder. There is a kind of divine intelligence in this symmetry between form and function. It teaches me to trust the deeper order in nature's medicine. While not the most glamorous of herbs, Toadflax is a true workhorse—bright, persistent, and quietly powerful.

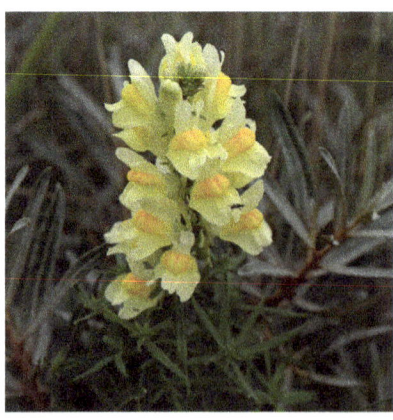

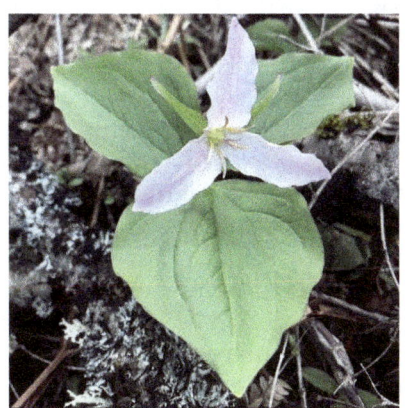

Trillium

Trillium ovatum

Trilliaceae (Trillium) Family, formerly classified in the **Liliaceae** (Lily) Family

Other common names: Western Trillium

Historical common names: Wake Robin, Tri-Flower, Birthroot, Birthwort

Description: Trillium is a long-lived perennial that emerges in early spring with an unmistakable presence. Its stems rise from an underground rhizome, topped with oval bracts that resemble and function as leaves. These are borne in graceful whorls of three—a pattern echoed throughout the plant. The sepals, petals, stamens, and stigmas all appear in triads, which gives the plant its name *tri*-llium. Each solitary, tri-petaled flower is most commonly white but matures to soft pink or deep purple with age. Occasionally, you may find a rare pink blossom among a cluster of white. The yellow reproductive parts sit at the heart of the bloom, while the seeds, encased in winged capsules, emerge as small red eggs nestled like treasures. Trillium is extraordinarily slow-growing. Counting leaf scars on its rhizome can reveal an age of 80 years or more. In its first 5–10 years, only a single genuine leaf may form, and it may not produce its first flower until 15 years of age or older.

Where it grows: Trillium is a widely distributed forest perennial, found in low to mid-elevation meadows and the wet, shaded terrain of rich forest floors.

When and how to harvest: Wild Western Trillium relies on us for its survival. Due to its slow growth, ethical harvesting is crucial. If you plan to harvest, wait until late summer, just before the tops turn brown and die back. This timing allows the plant to store energy for the coming year. Never harvest the rhizomes. If you wish to work with Trillium more freely, consider cultivating it in your garden, remembering to gather soil from an established patch to provide the specific mycorrhizae it requires to thrive.

How to work with it/ Medicinal use: Trillium is a revered women's herb, traditionally used during childbirth and postpartum care. Its astringent tannins help staunch bleeding and dry excess discharges. A tincture made from Trillium leaves can help stop postpartum hemorrhage, bleeding from miscarriage, or bleeding caused by uterine fibroids. It is also helpful in addressing vaginal discharges such as leukorrhea. Taken in the final week of pregnancy, a small daily dose may help tone the uterus in preparation for labor and delivery. Trillium tincture can also be used for lung-related bleeding and, for men, to reduce prostate inflammation and ease painful urination.

Healing constituents/ Therapeutic actions: Trillium contains tannins, including gallotannin and aucubin, as well as phenolic acids such as caffeic and ferulic acid. These constituents contribute to its anti-inflammatory, antibacterial, astringent, and wound-healing properties.

Historical connections: The Indigenous peoples of North America have long regarded the Trillium as a sacred women's plant, used to aid childbirth, afterbirth care, and address various female concerns. According to Ojibwa legend, Trillium originally bore four petals, but a Jesuit priest altered the plant while attempting to teach the concept of the Trinity to Native people. In subsequent seasons, the plant returned with three petals, leaves, and bracts. Those who encounter a rare four-petaled Trillium today may recall this tale. Mrs. Grieve, in *A Modern Herbal* (1931), describes Trillium as "antiseptic, astringent, and tonic expectorant, used principally in hemorrhages, to promote parturition, and externally, usually in the form of a poultice for skin disease or gangrene." The genus name *Trillium* comes from the Swedish word meaning "triplet."

Jessica's notes: Trillium is a holy flower to me, representing the Holy Trinity with its flowers of three and emerging from the snow-laced forest floor with a quiet yet profound declaration of new life. While exploring a historical stagecoach road tucked into the South Central coastal hills of California, the Freeborn family and I were tuning into our surroundings. As we slowly drove down the dusty, old road, my eye caught the delicate shimmer of a single trillium in bloom—like a lantern lit in the understory. It felt like a signpost left by the homesteaders of old, whose footsteps once echoed down this same path. The fragility of life, it seems, does not fade but waits patiently—stored like a whisper in the hidden depths of a trillium bulb, ready to bloom again a hundred years later. In that fleeting blossom, the past and present danced together, reminding us that wild things remember.

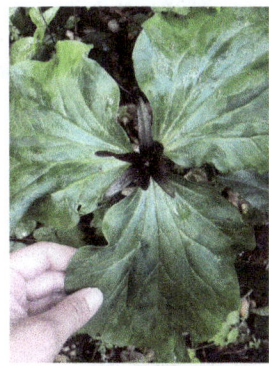

Trillium found on a historical stagecoach road

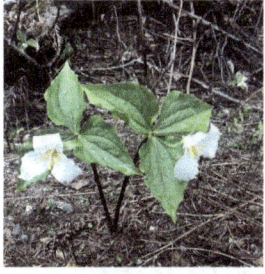

Double bloom

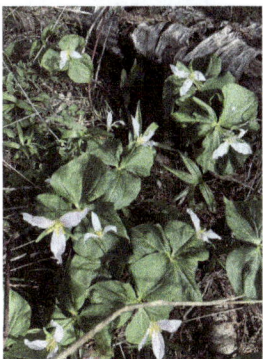

A blanket of trillium

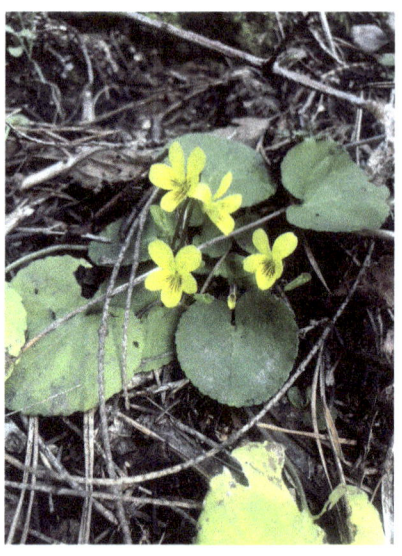

Violet

Viola adunca (Purple), Viola biflora (Yellow)

Violaceae (Violet) Family
Other common names: Purple Violet, Hookedspur Violet, Early Blue Violet, Western Dog Violet
  Yellow Violet: Alpine Yellow Violet, Two-Flower Violet, Arctic Yellow Violet
  Description: In early spring, as the earth begins to warm, Violets unfurl their tender leaves and cheerful blossoms. The round to egg-shaped leaves are hairless to slightly hairy, with subtly blunt, toothed edges, emerging from branched stems attached to hairy rhizomes. These delicate herbs grow to about 4 inches tall. Their violet flowers appear in late spring, with five petals, purple veins, and white bee-guiding patches at the center. A slender spur extends behind the central petal. After pollination, smooth, three-valved pods burst open, flinging seeds far across the forest floor. Yellow violets display five-petaled flowers marked with dark brown, bee-guiding veins—sunny spots of color in the shaded understory.

Where it grows: Violets favor meadows, woodlands, and disturbed sites. They are shade-loving plants that brighten the forest floor each spring and are widely distributed across North America.

When and how to harvest: Harvest the aerial parts in early to mid-spring, when they are in bloom. All violet species possess healing qualities, although the purple variety is most highly regarded for medicinal purposes. The yellow variety, however, makes a delightful garnish and refreshing trail nibble.

How to work with it/ Medicinal use: Violets offer cooling and moistening properties, making them ideal for relieving dry, inflamed tissues and easing pain. They are a superb spring tonic for moving winter's lymphatic stagnation. Violet tea or tincture is helpful for respiratory complaints such as whooping cough, asthma, and bronchitis, and can soothe bloodshot, tired eyes. This gentle herb supports lymphatic flow, helping to clear skin conditions linked to internal stagnation. It can help ease swollen glands, particularly in the ears and throat, and its diuretic and laxative effects aid the body in releasing waste and excess heat. The yellow variety tends to be the more potent laxative. A honey infusion makes a soothing cough syrup, and a fresh herb poultice may be applied to aching joints or inflamed skin. Traditionally, violets have been used to help reduce breast and lymphatic tumors. Violet-infused lotions and balms soothe bruises, rashes, eczema, and boils.

Caution: Use in moderation. While the flowers and leaves are safe, consuming large quantities may cause an upset stomach due to the presence of saponins. Avoid ingesting the roots or seeds, which can be toxic.

Healing constituents/ Therapeutic actions: Violets are remarkably nutrient-dense, containing more vitamin A than spinach and vitamin C equivalent to four oranges. They also offer flavonoids, saponins, salicylates (up to 4,000 ppm), and rutin, which strengthens capillary walls. Their therapeutic actions include anti-inflammatory, antispasmodic, astringent, lymphatic, and mildly sedative properties.

Historical connections: Violets have been a staple in medicine chests for centuries. In folk traditions, they were regarded as blood purifiers and gentle nerve tonics. Hildegard von Bingen, in her *Physica* (1150–1158), wrote: *"Anyone oppressed by melancholy with a discontented mind, which then harms his lungs, should cook violets in pure wine... When he drinks it, it will check the melancholy, make him happy, and heal his lungs."* Indigenous peoples used violet roots to induce vomiting after poisoning and recognized the plant's soothing and cleansing properties.

Jessica's notes: Violets always bring me back to my mother, Mary. They bloom in abundance near Mother's Day, blanketing the wild lands with yellow and purple flowers. Each spring, I pick these tender flowers from the meadow near my mom's driveway, adding them to festive drinks and dishes. Their ability to return each year, fragile yet resilient, mirrors my mother's gentle strength. Violets ask us to be present, to notice the small and beautiful, and to honor spring's awakening with reverence and delight.

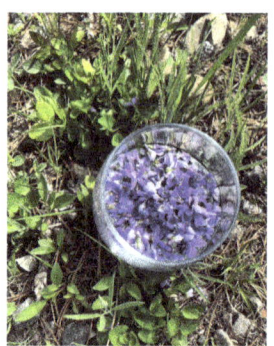

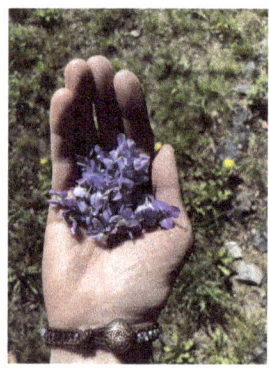

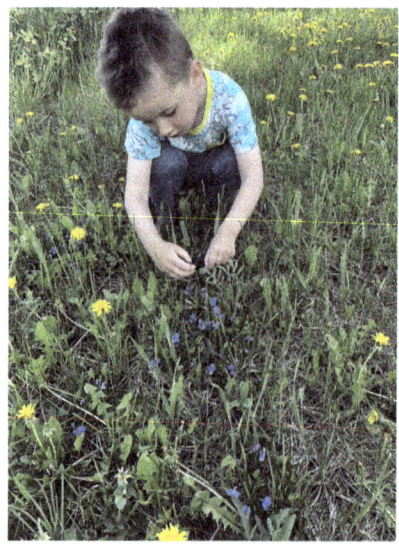

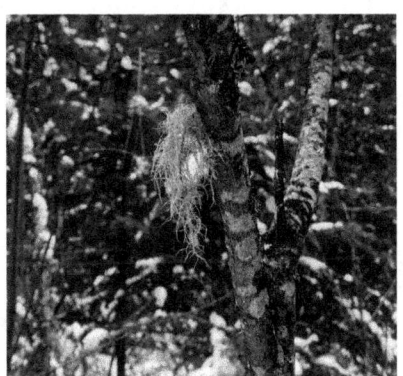

Usnea Lichen

Usnea longissima

Parmeliaceae (Lichen) Family
Other common names: Beard Lichen, Methuselah's Beard
Description: Usnea is not an herb or a flower, but I include it here as a true forest medicine—a lichen, meaning it is a living symbiosis of algae and fungi. To me, Usnea resembles delicate lace draped across the shoulders of ancient trees, its pale green strands swaying gently in the breeze. It grows in stringy, trailing tufts, often 6 to 14 inches long. To confirm a true Usnea, gently pull one strand—if you find a white, stretchy inner core, you have found the real thing. Without that inner cord, it is likely another, non-medicinal lichen. Usnea grows incredibly slowly, at a rate of less than 1 mm per decade. A five-inch strand could be over 200 years old, a quiet testament to its ancient wisdom.
Where it grows: Usnea lichen graces trees and shrubs in old-growth forests, shaded woodlands, and areas with dense, moist air and clean skies. It serves as a bioindicator of healthy ecosystems.
When and how to harvest: Because Usnea is such a slow-growing organism, it is best to leave it undisturbed. I only gather Usnea when I find it fallen on the ground or after a storm, when branches have been naturally shed. This ensures a sustainable and respectful harvest.
How to work with it/ Medicinal use: This is a plant that can quite literally save your life. Usnea is a powerful natural antibiotic and antifungal, especially effective against gram-positive bacteria. In the field, you can apply fresh Usnea directly to wounds as a dressing to prevent infection. The white inner core acts like a built-in bandage. I prepare a tincture to

extract the potent usnic acid, which works internally to fight bacterial and fungal infections, supporting cases of Candida, E. coli, foodborne illness, and urinary tract infections. Studies have shown Usnea to be more effective than penicillin against several strains of Streptococcus, Pneumococcus, and even tuberculosis. It is also an immune stimulant, helping increase white blood cell count and resistance to infection. In Chinese medicine, Usnea is used for tuberculosis and lung conditions, and it is traditionally valued for its antitumor and immune-stimulating properties. Topically, it excels in salves and sprays for wounds, burns, fungal infections, and sore throats. I especially love using it in an All-Purpose Healing Salve and a throat spray for travel and cold season.

Caution: Some individuals may be sensitive to usnic acid and develop a rash when using it topically. Internally, large quantities of lichen can cause kidney damage. While it would take a significant amount to cause harm, this is something to keep in mind, particularly in survival situations. Moderation is key.

Healing constituents/ Therapeutic actions: Usnea contains a remarkable array of compounds: usnic acid, sterols, terpenes, depsides, fatty acids, flavonoids, depsidones, polyphenols, benzofurans, phenolic acids, diffractaic acid, norstictic acid, and polysaccharides. Its actions include: antibiotic, antifungal, antiprotozoal, antipyretic, anticancer, antiseptic, antioxidant, antiviral, antiulcer, anti-genotoxic, anti-inflammatory, laxative, digestion-stimulating, and immune-stimulating.

Historical connections: Usnea's use as medicine dates back thousands of years. It was employed by ancient Chinese, Egyptian, and Greek healers as early as 1600 B.C. In medieval Europe, "old man's beard" was used to treat tuberculosis, lung ailments, and scalp disorders, guided by the Doctrine of Signatures. In Scandinavia, Usnea was boiled and used to treat chapped baby skin and cracked feet. It has long been a sacred ally of forest peoples around the world—an indicator of clean air and a healthy, living f orest.

Jessica's notes: I hold a deep reverence for Usnea. It is sacred medicine—one of the most cherished gifts from the old-growth forest. I always teach my students that respect and restraint are essential when working with it. I love preparing a Usnea throat spray for travel and keep its tincture in our home apothecary throughout cold and flu season. It is also a key ingredient in our All-Purpose Healing Salve, where its potent antiseptic powers can shine. Whenever I find Usnea strewn across the forest floor after a storm, I see it as a gift-a wise offering from the trees.

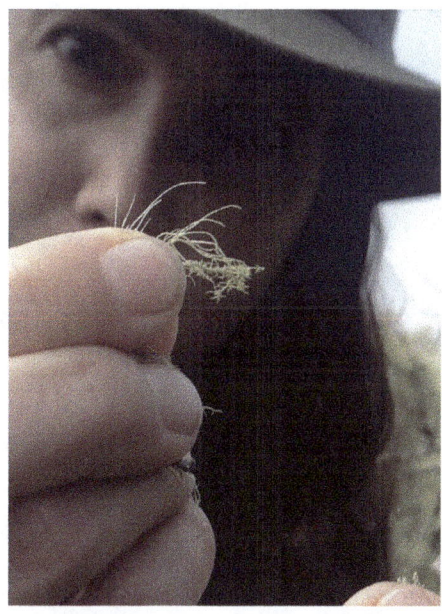

Inner white thread of Usnea Lichen

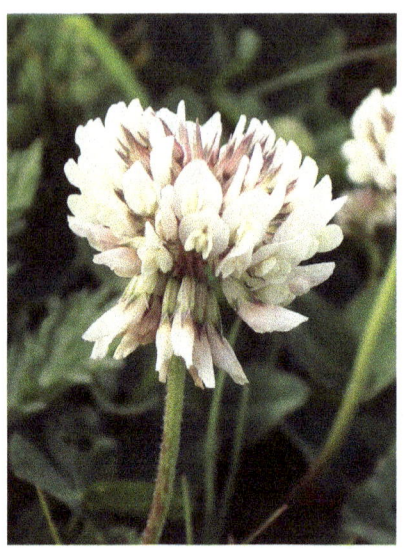

White Clover

Trifolium repens

Fabaceae (Legume) Family

Description: White clover is easy to distinguish from its clover cousins by its nearly round flower heads, composed of many small individual blossoms. Each flower has five petals fused at the base to form a tube-like structure. The blooms are white but often blush with a pinkish hue. The sweet fragrance of the flowers fills late spring and early summer meadows. Each flower head measures about 1 cm across. White clover is a prolific bloomer and "re-seeder," producing a great abundance of seed heads that help it persist even in grazed fields. White clover's creeping stems, or stolons, allow the plant to root at nodes along their length, enabling it to spread and thrive in pastures and mixed plant communities. The leaves are trifoliate—three heart-shaped leaflets—each marked with a distinct white V-shaped watermark. Like its relative red clover, it is polymorphic, meaning its form, leaf size, and spread vary depending on location and conditions.

Where it grows: White clover is a low-growing groundcover commonly found in meadows, pastures, fields, lawns, and open spaces. It is a nitrogen fixer, pulling nitrogen from the air and enriching the soil, making it a valuable companion in regenerative agriculture.

When and how to harvest: Harvest the flowers and leaves from spring through early summer. As summer progresses, the flowers lose some of their vanilla sweetness, so earlier harvests yield the most flavorful tea and infusions.

How to work with it/ Medicinal use: While red clover often receives more attention in herbal literature, white clover is a gentle, versatile ally for the kitchen and the family apothecary. It is a cooling herb that helps reduce fever and supports the body in recovery from colds and flu. The tea or tincture may also be used to alleviate symptoms of gout. The flowers make a delicious and refreshing tea, especially iced in the summertime, and they can be dried for winter use. White clover has detoxifying and circulatory-supporting properties. Regular clover tea is believed to aid in improving blood circulation and supporting healthy cholesterol levels—an ally for heart health. White clover also supports the respiratory system. Taken as a tea or tincture, it can help loosen phlegm and ease congestion. Its antimicrobial properties may help combat respiratory infections. Topically, white clover can soothe inflamed skin. Its anti-inflammatory and antimicrobial properties make it helpful in oils and balms for eczema, rashes, minor cuts, and scrapes. In the kitchen, the young leaves can be eaten raw in salads or cooked as a nutritious green, providing a good source of vitamins and minerals. Moreover, of course, this humble little flower is beloved by bees and pollinators, and clover honey is rich in antioxidants.

Healing constituents/ Therapeutic actions: White clover is rich in vitamins A, B1, B2, B3, and C, along with minerals such as calcium, chromium, cobalt, magnesium, manganese, phosphorus, potassium, selenium, silicon, sodium, and zinc. Its therapeutic actions include anti-inflammatory, antimicrobial, and analgesic properties.

Historical connections: White clover was introduced to the Americas by European colonists. Many Indigenous peoples called it "white man's foot grass," as it seemed to follow the footsteps of settlers. In Irish folklore and history, the clover holds deep symbolic significance. The Druids believed that clovers held mystical powers, particularly in relation to the sacred number three. St. Patrick is said to have used the three-leaf clover to illustrate the Holy Trinity. Later, wearing green, particularly a shamrock or clover, became a symbol of Irish resistance to British rule. The word "shamrock" comes from the Irish *seamróg*, meaning "summer plant." Finding a four-leaf clover has long been a symbol of good fortune. Whether the legendary shamrock referred to red clover or white clover is still debated, but both share this powerful symbolism. In Christian tradition, the three leaves represent faith, hope, and love; the fourth, when present, represents luck or divine grace. One old legend says that Eve carried a clover from the Garden of Eden as a remembrance of paradise lost.

Jessica's notes: I spent many hours of my childhood searching for the lucky four-leaf clover. The few I did find, I would press between pages of my favorite books . White clover is such a humble, abundant plant—a flower of the earth that quietly supports life all around it. I love adding blossoms to summer sun teas for their light, sweet fragrance. I think of white clover as an everyday ally-a plant of peace, of nourishment, of gentle healing.

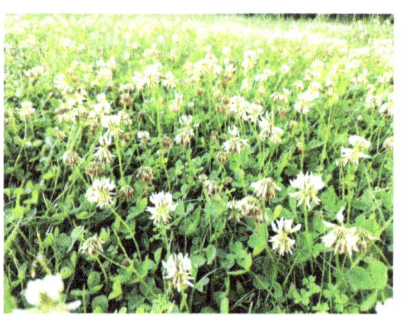

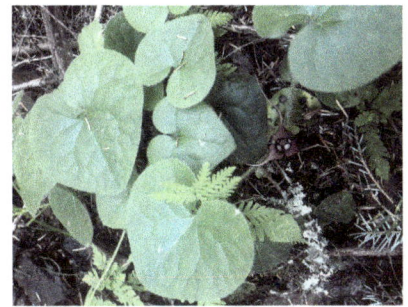

Wild Ginger

Asarum caudatum

Aristolochiaceae (Birthwort) Family
Other common names: British Columbia Wild Ginger
Description: Heart-shaped to kidney-shaped green leaves, 2 per node, attach to creeping rhizomes that spread on the forest floor in loose mats. The leaves are hairy and have prominent veins. The petal-less flowers are made of 3 maroon sepals, 1-3 inches long. The flowers ripen into capsules filled with seeds and fleshy appendages. These seed capsules contain an oil that attracts ants who carry the seeds back to their nest. When crushed, the entire plant has a spicy, ginger-lemony aroma.
Where it grows: Commonly found in wet and shady forests near creeks, springs, and streams. It often grows along the roots of cedar trees.
When and how to harvest: Harvest the roots and rhizomes in early to late fall.
How to work with it/ Medicinal use: Wild ginger is warming, pungent, and stimulating. It warms the skin and promotes sweating. Steep the roots in hot water and drink to speed up the healing process of acute respiratory infections, colds, and flu. Both the tea and tincture can relieve intestinal gas and cramping. For delayed menstruation with lower back pain, take wild ginger tea or tincture to lessen the pain and stimulate bleeding. A chest poultice can promote sweating and help break up mucus and phlegm, aiding in their removal from the body.
Caution: Large amounts of wild ginger can be emetic, causing vomiting. Due to its uterine-stimulating effects, wild ginger should not be taken during pregnancy. This plant should not be consumed for extended periods as it contains aristolochic acid (like other members of the birth-

wort family), which is reported to cause kidney damage and cancer-causing effects.

Healing constituents/ Therapeutic actions: Wild ginger essential oil contains bioactive compounds such as β-caryophyllene, β-sesquiphellandrene, β-bisabolene, B-Sesquiphellandrene, B-Bisabolene, neral, etc. Wild ginger's therapeutic actions are stimulant, carminative, diuretic, and diaphoretic.

Historical connections: Native Americans and early Euro-American settlers used wild ginger root as a spice. They dried the roots and ground them into a powder. The early settlers also cooked pieces of the roots in sugar water for several days for a candied root. The leftover water was then boiled down into syrup. Native Americans and Euro-American settlers also used wild ginger poultices to treat wounds.

Jessica's notes: I sometimes like to nibble on wild ginger root when I am out foraging. Its earthy and spicy aroma connects me to the land and grounds, sparking my inner fire. Its heart-shaped leaves decorate the forest floor like cookie-cutter shapes, inviting a childlike imagination.

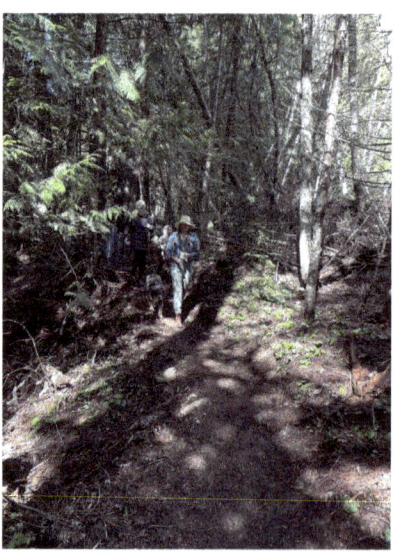

Wild Ginger under the cedar grove

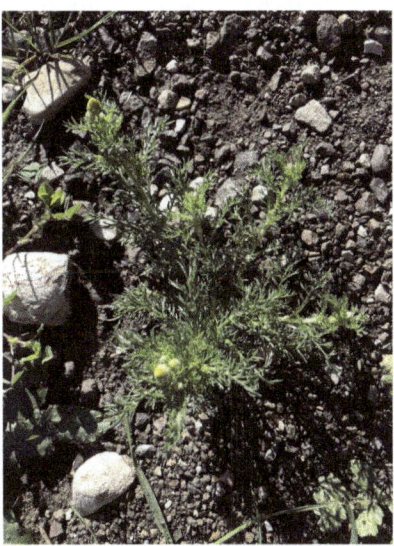

Wild Chamomile

Matricaria discoidea

Asteraceae (Daisy) Family

Other common names: Pineapple Weed, Disc Ragweed, May Rayweed

Description: A humble, low-growing perennial weed, Wild Chamomile blends easily into grasses and pathways. However, its unmistakable sweet fragrance gives it away—step on it, and a burst of pineapple and chamomile scent rises to greet you. The cone-shaped flower heads resemble tiny green-yellow Q-tips, composed of densely packed disc flowers without the white rays characteristic of its more familiar chamomile cousins. Its finely feathery, pinnately dissected leaves are aromatic and grow alternately along slender stalks. Multiple leafy stems emerge from the root, giving this little plant a bushy appearance despite its miniature size.

Where it grows: Wild Chamomile thrives where others may not—along lake shorelines, sandy soils, driveways, trails, ditches, and disturbed ground. It thrives in compact soils where few other plants can compete, earning its reputation as a resilient little survivor.

When and how to harvest: Gather the fragrant flowers during the heat of summer when their aroma is at its strongest. You may also harvest leaves, though they become increasingly bitter once the plant begins to flower.

How to work with it/ Medicinal use: Matricaria offers many of the same gifts as common chamomile. Its gentle, calming properties make it a beloved ally for the nervous and digestive systems. Infusions of flowers and leaves serve as a mild sedative, promoting relaxation, easing digestion, and relieving colic and gas. Drink as a tea to soothe tension and prepare the body for restful sleep. The fresh flowers can also be cold-infused in water to create a refreshing summer tea. Try freezing the flower tips into ice cubes for a beautiful and functional addition to cool drinks. Dried flowers and leaves can be added to winter teas to help alleviate upset stomachs and bloating, especially when paired with aromatic allies like mountain mint or bee balm. The leafy greens can be tossed into a salad when young, though they grow quite bitter once the plant flowers. Externally, wild chamomile can be prepared as a soothing wash for irritated skin, sores, or itchy rashes.

Healing constituents/ Therapeutic actions: Wild chamomile contains polyphenols, flavonoids, and coumarins, which contribute to its antispasmodic, carminative, and anti-inflammatory effects.

Historical connections: Originally native to Eurasia, wild chamomile spread rapidly across North America after being introduced by European settlers. It is now found in abundance across the continent. John Hutchinson (1887–1973) remarked in one of his botanical writings, "The more it is trodden on, the better it seems to thrive." True to its spirit, this humble little plant responds to adversity with resilience and fragrance. Traditionally, wild chamomile has been used to alleviate colds, support digestive health, and soothe the nerves.

Jessica's notes: This was the very first wild medicinal plant I was ever introduced to. I must have been about four years old, attending daycare in Isla Vista, California. The caregivers would take us to the park each day in a wooden wagon we affectionately called The Goat Cart. Some of the littlest ones would nap inside the cart while others, like me, walked alongside. One day, on our way to the park, I noticed this cheerful little plant growing along the dusty path. One of the hippie teachers told me its name—Wild Chamomile—and explained that you could eat it to soothe an upset stomach. I tasted a bit, and sure enough, it settled my tummy. I was captivated: here was a wild plant, growing free, that could *help* me! That experience sparked a lifelong love of plants and natural healing. I have since noticed a beautiful pattern—that often, the plants I most need appear in my life when I need them most. Wild Chamomile was the first to teach me this lesson, and I remain grateful for that early moment of plant magic, as well as to all the unexpected teachers who have guided my herbal path ever since.

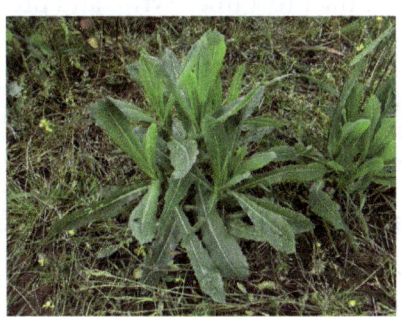

Wild Lettuce

Lactuca virosa

Asteraceae (Daisy) Family
Other common names: Opium Lettuce, Bitter Lettuce
  Description: Wild Lettuce is a tall, weedy biennial with a remarkable presence and potent medicine. In its first year, it forms a basal rosette of leaves. In its second year, it shoots up a tall stalk—sometimes reaching six feet or more—and produces small yellow flowers. One of the easiest ways to identify Wild Lettuce is by its milky latex, which oozes when the stalk is cut. Another telltale feature is the line of small hairs along the underside of the midrib on the leaves, as well as the triangular cross-section of the stem. The leaves themselves vary in shape but are generally simple, alternate, and often clasp the stem. Trichomes (hair-like structures) are present on the undersides of the leaves.
  Where it grows: Wild Lettuce prefers sunny spaces. It thrives along roadsides, near riverbeds, springs, and creeks—places where the soil is disturbed and the sun shines freely.
  When and how to harvest: The best time to harvest is after the plant bolts, when the latex is most concentrated. Strip the leaves from the stalk and either use them fresh or dry them for future preparations.
  How to work with it/ Medicinal use: Wild Lettuce contains compounds with sedative and pain-relieving properties akin to opium, though much milder and non-addictive. The tincture can ease pain, calm restlessness, and promote sleep. It is also known for producing vivid, dream-rich sleep—an aspect honored in Native American medicine, where Wild Lettuce was used for dreamwork and visions. A tea can be prepared from the leaves. However, the most potent extraction comes from a concentrated tincture made through a meticulous process: dry the leaves, macerate in

strong alcohol to extract the bitter compounds *Lactucin* and *Lactucopicrin*, then cook down the extract to a thick syrup and preserve it. Though this process is time-consuming, it yields a concentrated medicine with powerful sedative and analgesic properties.

Healing constituents/ Therapeutic actions: The primary active compounds in Wild Lettuce are *Lactucin* and *Lactucopicrin*. These bitter chemicals have been shown to have both sedative and pain-relieving effects. *Lactucin* enhances the action of adenosine in the body, naturally inducing relaxation and sleepiness. *Lactucopicrin* is an acetylcholinesterase inhibitor, further contributing to its calming effects. In studies, these compounds demonstrated analgesic effects comparable to ibuprofen at proper doses. Therapeutic actions include sedative, analgesic, antitussive (cough-suppressing), and mild antispasmodic effects.

Historical connections: The lore of Wild Lettuce stretches far back into ancient times. The Ancient Egyptians valued it both as an aphrodisiac and a sacred plant, often depicting the fertility god *Min* with stalks of Wild Lettuce behind him. However, they also warned that consuming too much would dull the mind. Emperor Augustus of Rome was reportedly cured of a serious illness by an infusion of Wild Lettuce, after which he dedicated an altar to the plant. In the 19th century, *Lactucarium* (the dried latex extract of Wild Lettuce) was an everyday pharmacy staple, sold as a remedy for headaches, coughs, and as a mild sedative.

Jessica's notes: Wild Lettuce fascinates me—it is a plant that bridges ancient wisdom with modern herbal practice. Its milky latex and tall, commanding stalk speak of deep, hidden medicine. When I need a more potent, plant-based pain reliever, I reach for Wild Lettuce. It also holds a special place in dreamwork rituals. When life feels mentally restless or I need clarity through my dreams, a dose of Wild Lettuce before bed helps open those doors. I always teach students to approach this plant with patience and care, as its medicine is subtle but powerful. Like the dreams it encourages, Wild Lettuce invites us to surrender to a quieter, more introspective space, where healing happens not through force, but through deep rest.

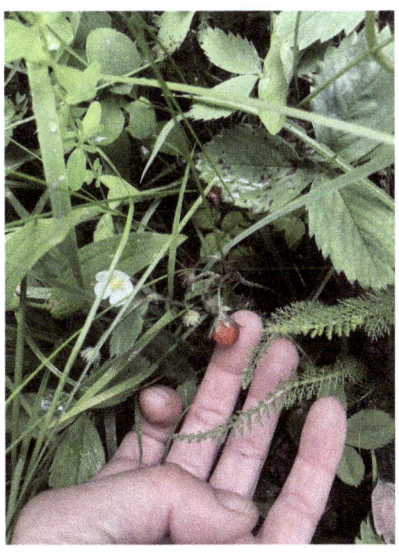

Wild Strawberry

Fragaria vesca

Rosaceae (Rose) Family

Description: Wild Strawberry is a charming, low-growing perennial herb that spreads gracefully through above-ground runners. It produces three dark green, toothed leaflets on hairy green to reddish stems. In spring, it offers delicate white flowers with five petals, followed by heart-shaped, ruby-red berries that resemble miniature cultivated strawberries. These little gems are rare and precious when found ripe in the summer.

Where it grows: You will find Wild strawberries along grassy woodland edges, sunlit meadows, and the banks of streams, springs, and creeks. It prefers full sun but will tolerate dappled shade.

When and how to harvest: Harvest the young leaves in spring through midsummer. The berries ripen from late spring into early summer, though finding an abundance is always a special treat!

How to work with it/ Medicinal use: The tender leaves of Wild Strawberry offer gentle astringent and diuretic properties. Brewed as a tea, they soothe digestive complaints such as diarrhea and bloating, ease urinary imbalances, and offer a caffeine-free tonic alternative to green tea. Rich in Vitamin C, this tea also bolsters the immune system. A folk method for preparing strawberry leaf tea involves "sweating" the leaves in a sunny window to enhance their flavor, then drying them for storage. The tannin-rich leaves make an effective wash for sunburn and irritated skin. Powdered leaves can be incorporated into toothpaste to help treat bleeding gums and reduce plaque, or used as an eyewash for conditions such as pink eye and conjunctivitis. The berries themselves—when you are lucky enough to find them—burst with sweet flavor and are packed with antioxidants, Vitamins B, C, and E. They can be eaten fresh or transformed into a luscious jam.

Healing constituents/ Therapeutic actions: Wild Strawberries are rich in anthocyanins, quercetin, potassium, vitamins B, C, and E, folate, and fiber. The leaves, rich in tannins, tone and strengthen both the digestive and urinary tracts. Therapeutic actions include astringent, diuretic, tonic, anti-inflammatory, and immune-boosting.

Historical connections: Wild Strawberry has nourished and healed people since ancient times. Carl Linnaeus once prescribed the leaves for rheumatic gout. In Native American tradition, the heart-shaped Wild Strawberry symbolizes love and reconciliation. One tale tells of the first man and woman, who quarreled and parted in anger. The Great Spirit laid blueberries, raspberries, and other berries in the woman's path, but she did not stop until Wild Strawberries appeared. Their sweetness slowed her, allowing her husband to catch up and offer an apology, thus healing the rift between them. The English name "strawberry" may have come from the Anglo-Saxon *streoberie* (strewn berry), or the old practice of mulching plants with straw, or even from the custom of stringing berries on straw to sell them at market. Mrs. Grieve's *Modern Herbal* shares an elaborate recipe for a turkey cooked with strawberry leaves and a blend of fragrant herbs—a culinary glimpse into the plant's long history in European kitchens.

Jessica's notes: The first Wild Strawberry I ever tasted was shared with Jason during our early courtship days. We had been hiking together and stumbled upon two perfect little berries on a sunny hillside. I will never forget how unbelievably sweet that first bite was—it was as though nature had crafted the perfect candy. The burst of energy and joy we felt afterward carried us bounding up the hill with laughter. Even now, whenever I come upon Wild Strawberries, I am struck by their potent sweetness, so much richer than anything cultivated. They remind me of life's little gifts and the unexpected delights that await us in nature if we walk slowly and attentively.

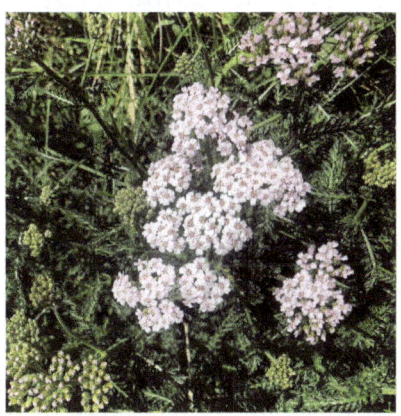

Yarrow

Achillea millefolium

Asteraceae (Daisy) Family

Other common names: Milfoil, Staunchweed, Soldier's Woundwort

Description: An attractive and hardy perennial, Yarrow can reach up to three feet in height. Its feathery, soft green leaves resemble delicate ferns. The name *millefolium* means "a thousand leaves," and a close look at Yarrow's foliage will reveal its many finely divided leaflets. The alternate leaves, 3 to 5 inches long, are composed of numerous smaller leaflets arranged along each side of the midrib. Yarrow's flower heads bloom in large, compact clusters at the tops of the stems. In the wild, they are typically yellowish-white, though they sometimes display a soft pink hue.

Where it grows: Yarrow thrives in meadows, sandy slopes, dry open areas, gardens, and waste places. In North Idaho, we are blessed with its bright white blooms, while in the suburban yard we once had, pink and purple varieties would form cheerful rings each spring.

When and how to harvest: I harvest the flowers in summer as soon as they bloom, gathering them in bunches and snipping the stems with scissors. I tie the bunches at the base and hang them to dry in the kitchen or living room. When time allows, I strip the leaves and flowers for future medicinal use.

How to work with it/ Medicinal use: Yarrow is sometimes called the "Echinacea of the North"—and for good reason. I love adding its flowers to my winter tea blends. Though a bitter herb, it pairs well with other flavors. I use Yarrow to support female balance and promote a smoother menstrual cycle. It also stimulates perspiration, helping the body break fevers and clear toxins during colds and flu. Yarrow is an immune stimulant and mild expectorant, which helps eliminate excess phlegm. Crushed leaves will staunch a nosebleed; I often powder the dried leaves to use as a wound dressing. Though it stings when applied, the results are miraculous! I also use Yarrow-infused oils in our family's healing balms and salves. The roots are helpful for soothing mouth sores and may even help prevent cavities. A Yarrow leaf decoction makes an excellent sitz bath for postpartum healing or afterbirth hemorrhage.

Healing constituents/ Therapeutic actions: Yarrow contains numerous potent healing compounds, including isovaleric acid, salicylic acid, asparagine, sterols, and flavonoids. It also offers a rich array of phenolic acids (chlorogenic, vanillic, caffeic, syringic, p-coumaric, sinapic, ferulic, cinnamic) and flavonoids (myricetin, hesperidin, quercetin, luteolin, kaempferol, apigenin, rutin, hyperoside). Its many actions include analgesic, antibacterial, anticatarrhal, anti-inflammatory, antiseptic, astringent, bitter, carminative, diaphoretic, digestive, diuretic, emmenagogue, expectorant, febrifuge, hepatic, hypoglycemic, hypotensive, stimulant, styptic, tonic, and vulnerary properties.

Historical connections: Yarrow has been valued as a medicinal herb for thousands of years, especially for battlefield wounds. It was found among the grave goods in a Neanderthal burial in the Zagros mountains (near Turkey and Iraq), a testament to its ancient use. In Greek mythology, Yarrow's powers were so esteemed that it was believed to bestow immortality. Legend says Achilles was dipped in Yarrow-infused waters as an infant, rendering him nearly invincible save for his heel—hence the genus name *Achillea*. According to Homer's *Iliad*, the centaur Chiron taught Achilles to use Yarrow to heal the wounded on the battlefield of Troy. In the Middle Ages, Yarrow was used both for brewing (as part of gruit, before hops were common) and for love spells. In Victorian flower language, Yarrow symbolized everlasting love. Native American tribes revered Yarrow as a sacred "life medicine." The Navajo used it for toothaches and earaches. The Miwok used it for analgesia and head colds. The Plains Indians employed it as a sleep aid and pain reliever. The Ojibwe used Yarrow leaves in steam baths to treat headaches and root decoctions for skin applications. In Ancient Chinese tradition, Yarrow was regarded as a plant of great luck and wisdom, its dried stalks used in I Ching divination. During the American Civil War, soldiers carried Yarrow in their pockets to staunch battlefield wounds.

Jessica's notes: Yarrow is one of my favorite plants—one that has healed my life in profound ways. Its earthy, fragrant aroma is a deep comfort to me. I love its versatility: it can stop bleeding both internally and externally, ease fevers, and promote rapid wound healing. I have many personal testimonials of its power. One example: My mother-in-law once sliced her hand badly while cooking. The bleeding would not stop, and she was preparing to head to urgent care. I ran out to the yard, grabbed fresh Yarrow, and insisted she apply it. By the time she arrived at urgent care, the bleeding had stopped entirely. I always keep Yarrow in our home apothecary. I hang it in bunches in the kitchen and living room, using it as both a medicinal aid and a fragrant blessing. To me, Yarrow is a plant of fierce protection and profound wisdom—one of the great gifts of the green world.

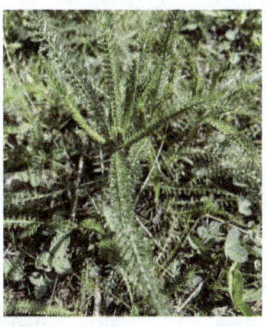

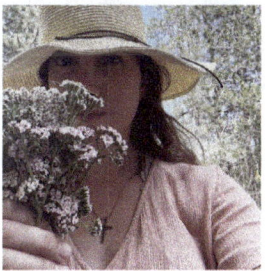

Then

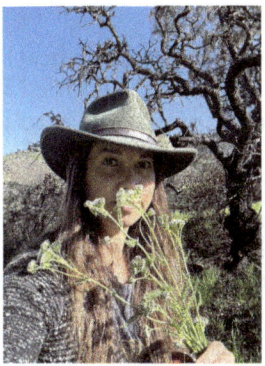

and now

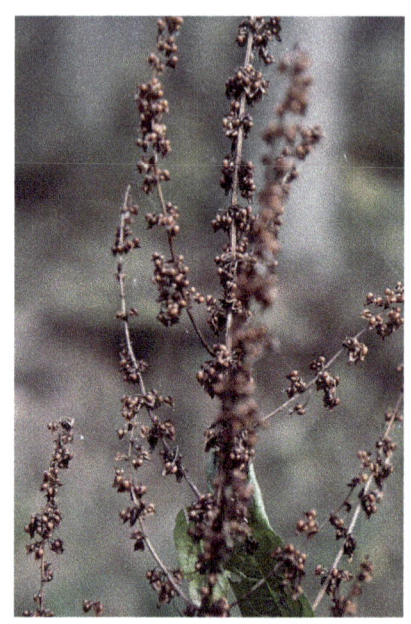

Yellow Dock

Rumex crispus

Polygonaceae (Buckwheat) Family
Other common names: Curly Dock, Curled Dock
Description: This familiar weed is easy to identify and incredibly resilient. Yellow Dock is a long-lived perennial with a strong presence. Its lance-shaped leaves form a basal rosette; they are smooth, dark green, and curled along the edges, typically measuring 5 to 10 inches in length. The plant produces a tall flowering stalk that can reach up to five feet. Its distinctive yellow taproot is forked and resembles an oversized carrot. The flowers and seeds form dense clusters along the stalk, with the most significant clusters at the apex. Each shiny brown seed is enclosed within a calyx, which allows it to float on water or cling to animal fur and clothing—nature's clever way of ensuring widespread dispersal. The seeds can remain viable for 50 to 80 years, and each plant can produce as many as 60,000 seeds!

Where it grows: You will find Yellow Dock thriving in sunny meadows, wastelands, prairies, and roadside ditches—anywhere disturbed soil offers it a foothold.

When and how to harvest: Harvest young greens in the spring and early summer. The root is best dug in the autumn or early spring, when the plant's energy is stored below ground.

How to work with it/ Medicinal use: Yellow Dock is an exceptional herbal ally for sluggish liver function and skin conditions often linked to poor detoxification. The tinctured root or a decoction can stimulate the liver, aiding digestion and helping flush out toxins. It can also ease pain and inflammation in the sinuses and respiratory tract and serve as a gentle laxative to promote regular elimination and healthy bile flow. Yellow Dock is renowned for its ability to soothe chronic skin issues such as acne and eczema, and its iron-rich root is often used to support those with anemia or iron deficiency. Its anti-inflammatory and purifying effects can further benefit those dealing with arthritis or systemic inflammation. The young, tender greens (rich in vitamins A and C) can be cooked like wild spinach. Because the leaves contain oxalic acid, it is best to consume them in moderation—cooking helps break down some of this compound. The young stalks can be cooked like asparagus or added to soups, stews, and stir-fries. The root itself can also be prepared like other root vegetables. The plant's brown seeds, rich in fiber, can be ground into flour and used in baking. Though a valuable food and medicine for humans, Yellow Dock is toxic to livestock.

Healing constituents/ Therapeutic actions: Yellow Dock contains glycosides with hepatoprotective properties that support and protect liver function. It is also rich in iron, potassium, calcium, and vitamins A and C, making it an excellent blood-building and nutritive herb. Its therapeutic actions include liver stimulant, mild laxative, blood purifier, anti-inflammatory, and skin tonic.

Historical connections: Yellow Dock has been used as both food and medicine since ancient times. Remarkably, the body of the *Tollund Man* (4th century BCE, Denmark), found preserved in a peat bog, revealed his last meal included a gruel made from dock seeds. The Ancient Greeks and Romans valued Yellow Dock for its purifying properties. Its seeds were soaked to treat dysentery, while the roots were used to cleanse the skin. Nicholas Culpepper, in *The Complete Herbal* (1653), wrote: "The roots boiled in vinegar help the itch, scabs, and breaking out of the skin, if it be bathed therewithin. The distilled water of the herb and roots have the same virtue, and cleanses the skin from freckles, morphews, and all other spots and discoloring's therein." Native Americans traditionally mashed the root for poultices to soothe sores and wounds.

Jessica's notes: Yellow Dock came into my life when I was a teenager struggling with painful acne. The conventional treatments prescribed by dermatologists only worsened the problem, so I began seeking natural solutions. In my research, Yellow Dock consistently appeared as a liver-supporting herb that can help cleanse the blood and improve skin health. I began taking it daily, and, along with other holistic practices, I was able to heal my skin. I remain deeply grateful for plants like Yellow Dock—gifts of creation that offer such targeted healing. Its yellow root, echoing the color of bile, is another beautiful example of the *Doctrine of Signatures*—a subtle teaching that plants often reveal their purpose through their characteristics. Though many now dismiss Yellow Dock as a useless weed, I hope to help restore its reputation and reconnect people with the ancestral plants that once nourished and healed us.

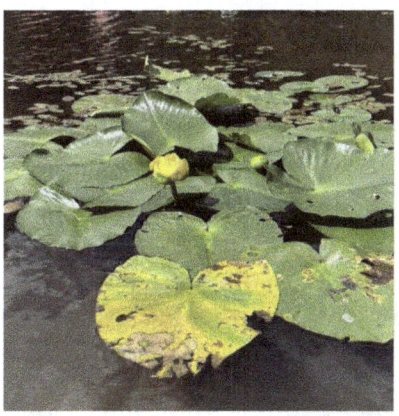

Yellow Pond Lily

Nuphar lutea subsp. polysepala, Nymphaea polysepala

Nymphaeaceae (Water Lily) Family

Other common names: Yellow Pond Lily, Pond Lily, Spatterdock, Bullhead Lily

Description: Yellow Pond Lily is a water-bound perennial, an ancient plant that has remained essentially unchanged for millions of years. Its large, heart-shaped to oval leaves float serenely on the water's surface, tethered to thick, submerged rhizomes hidden deep in the mud below. These rhizomes resemble giant, waterlogged pinecones or tree branches resting at the pond's bottom, anchoring the plant in place. The plant's single yellow flowers rise elegantly on long, submerged stalks, blooming about a foot above the water. Each flower consists of 5 to 12 sepals surrounding numerous smaller inner petals. The fruits form as multi-seeded capsules, and the whole plant has an aura of ancient resilience.

Where it grows: Look for Yellow Pond Lily in shallow, still bodies of water—ponds, lake margins, and slow-moving streams—often in mountain settings. They thrive in nutrient-rich, stagnant sections where other plants might falter.

When and how to harvest: Harvest the rhizomes in summer when the water is warmer and more inviting. This task is not for the faint of heart! Retrieving the rhizomes requires balancing on top of the submerged log-like structures while using a handsaw to cut through a section carefully. Once freed, the rhizomes can be broken or sawn off entirely. It is a wildcrafter's challenge and a rite of passage for those who seek this ancient medicine.

How to work with it/ Medicinal use: Yellow Pond Lily is a remarkable reproductive tonic, beneficial to both men and women. For women, a decoction or tincture of the rhizome can ease painful menstruation, polycystic ovarian syndrome (PCOS), and cycle-related ovulation sensitivity. For men, it can soothe prostatitis, relieve the dull ache of epididymitis, and support other irritations in the reproductive tract. It also addresses painful, burning urination, whether caused by infection or the after-effects of spicy foods or beverages. Yellow Pond Lily tea can help soothe intestinal disturbances, including spastic diarrhea, colitis, and food poisoning. Pairing the tea with Bee Balm or aromatic conifers such as Pine, Spruce, or Fir adds a complementary antimicrobial and soothing action. As a gargle, Yellow Pond Lily tea calms sore throats. Externally, a sitz bath made from the tea provides relief for cervical and vaginal irritations, acting as both an anti-inflammatory and an astringent. Its sulfur-based alkaloids have drawn the attention of researchers for their antimicrobial properties. Yellow Pond Lily inhibits the growth of bacteria, such as Staphylococcus aureus, and rivals pharmaceutical antifungals, like Amphotericin B, in its ability to combat fungal overgrowth (Bate-Smith, 1968). As food, Yellow Pond Lily seeds can be popped like popcorn or ground into a meal. The rhizomes are edible but require soaking and multiple rinses to temper their bitterness; they are best used as a survival food. Interestingly, when the mud around its rhizomes becomes oxygen-deprived, the plant naturally produces alcohol in place of carbon dioxide, a fascinating quirk of this ancient aquatic plant.

Healing constituents/ Therapeutic actions: Yellow Pond Lily rhizomes contain a variety of fatty acids (arachidic, behenic, palmitic, and trans-cinnamic acids), unique alkaloids (nupharolidine, nupharcristine, nupharidine, nupharamine), and polyphenols (ballotins, ellagitannins). Therapeutic actions include anti-inflammatory, analgesic, sedative, astringent, and antimicrobial effects.

Historical connections: Nuphar has been a vital food and medicine for countless generations. Native American tribes, particularly in the Pacific Northwest, valued the Yellow Pond Lily as an emergency food source. The Klamath Indians of California harvested seed pods from vast marshlands, drying them and pounding them to release the seeds. Another method involved burying pods in underground pits until they fermented, at which point the softened seeds were washed free for use (Schofield, 1989). Historically, the rhizome has been utilized in both European and Indigenous herbal traditions for the treatment of gastrointestinal and reproductive health issues, as well as for topical applications to wounds and infections.

Jessica's notes: I love the name *Nuphar*—it carries an exotic resonance that perfectly suits this ancient and mysterious plant. The Doctrine of Signatures whispers here: this water-bound plant supports the watery systems within the human body so beautifully. The rhizomes, submerged in cool, dark mud, offer cooling, calming, and grounding medicine to tissues that are hot, inflamed, or overstimulated.

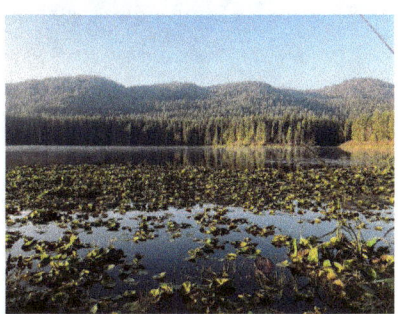

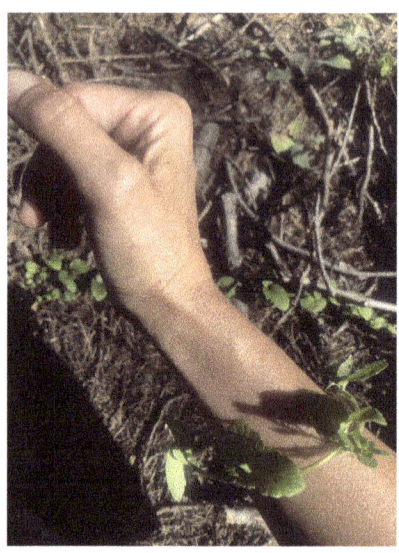

Yerba Buena

Micromeria douglasii (formerly Satureja douglasii)

Mentha (Mint) Family

Description: Yerba Buena, meaning "The Good Herb," spreads gracefully across the forest floor, reaching up to 3 ¼ feet and rooting at its nodes to send out new runners. Its glossy, bright green leaves are oppositely arranged along square, four-sided stems. The leaves are unevenly round-toothed, slightly hairy, and dotted with tiny glands that release a tantalizing minty fragrance when touched. Each leaf measures between ⅜ and 1 ⅜ inches long. In late spring to midsummer, delicate, single, tubular flowers appear, white or tinged with purple, blooming on slender stalks. The lower lip of each two-lipped flower is three-lobed, while the upright upper lip stands like a little crown. After blooming, four shiny brown seeds form within five-toothed calyces. In winter, the evergreen leaves and stems often turn a deep purple from frost.

Where it grows: Yerba Buena thrives throughout the Northwest, from British Columbia to Southern California. It is commonly found weaving through the forest floor alongside companions such as Kinnikinnick,

Oregon grape, and other ground covers. A hearty and adaptable plant, Yerba Buena also tolerates drier soils, making it a delightful find in many woodland habitats.

When and how to harvest: Harvest the leaves from late spring through late summer. I love to gather leaf stalks and weave them into wreaths to hang in my kitchen—a beautiful way to enjoy their aroma year-round and have them on hand for tea and medicinal purposes.

How to work with it/ Medicinal use: Yerba Buena makes a delicious and soothing tea, perfect on its own or blended with other herbs to enhance flavor and harmonize their effects. It brings many of the same benefits as other mints—relieving gas, soothing an upset stomach, and promoting digestion. It is also a gentle diaphoretic, helping to stimulate sweating and break fevers during colds or flu. As a refreshing iced tea, it cools the body on hot summer days. In winter, a warm infusion soothes the digestive tract and kindles inner warmth during the cold season. Topically, Yerba Buena is a lovely insect repellent. I often craft necklaces and bracelets from its leaf stems when foraging in the forest—both functional and beautiful! It also makes an excellent addition to a garden as a natural insect deterrent.

Healing constituents/ Therapeutic actions: Yerba Buena contains *mentha lactone*, a compound known for its pain-relieving (analgesic) properties. Its actions include carminative, diaphoretic, digestive aid, mild analgesic, cooling, and soothing.

Historical connections: The plant's beloved name, *Yerba Buena*, comes from the California Spanish settlers and Catholic missionaries of Alta California, who learned of the herb from local Native peoples. The Spanish phrase *hierba buena* means "the good herb." Yerba Buena grew so abundantly around the early settlement near Mission San Francisco de Asís that the area itself became known as Isla Yerba Buena. In 1846, during the Mexican-American War, the United States seized the town and renamed it San Francisco. Even today, Yerba Buena Island remains a part of the San Francisco-Oakland Bay Bridge. Yerba Buena has long been valued by Indigenous peoples for both ceremonial and healing purposes, offering gentle medicine for body and spirit alike.

Jessica's notes: We rejoiced when we first identified this minty plant, Yerba Buena—*The Good Herb!* While foraging on the mountain one day, I instinctively picked a sprig and fashioned it into a bracelet. Suddenly, the name surfaced from my memory like an old friend calling out. Since then, this plant has become a dear companion. I always seem to find it along my journey, from the coastal trails to the inland Northwest. There is something about its cheerful presence and vibrant aroma that lifts the heart. Every time I work with Yerba Buena, I am reminded of the gifts of nature and the joy of rediscovering the ancient wisdom of plants that surrounds us. The forest school students absolutely love the addition of yerba buena to our wild teas!

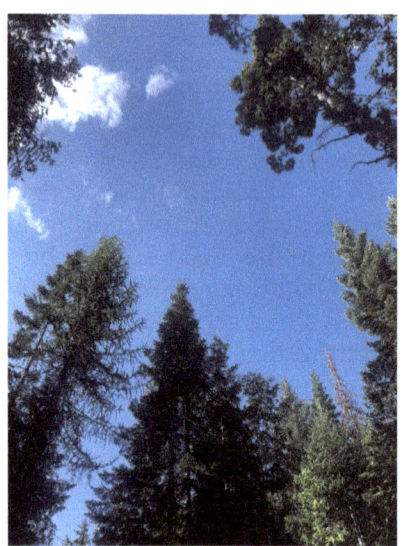

Trees and Shrubs

 Welcome to the section dedicated to the mighty and vigorous trees and hardy shrubs of the forest. The trees offer a wealth of medicinal gifts to the people. Year-round, we can harvest vitamin C-rich pine needles. Resin-rich cottonwood buds, like jeweled ornaments, decorate fallen limbs brought down by heavy snowfalls and windstorms—collected in the depths of winter, when we most need their medicine for colds, flu, and chapped cheeks. The trees of the North shelter us and cool the land on long, hot summer days. Thanks to these generous perennials, there is always a bounty to gather when fruits ripen. Their perennial endurance connects us to the past as they stand like living relics. The language of the trees reminds us to care for one another, provide shelter, protect the little ones, and stand strong.

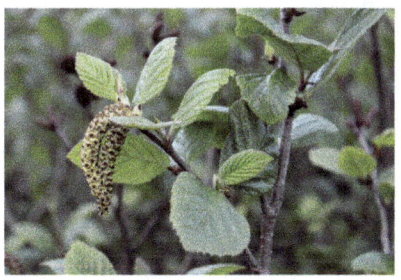

Alder

Alnus sp. (including A. glutinosa, A. rubra)

Betulaceae (Birch) Family

Description: Alder bark is greenish-gray to reddish-brown, thin and smooth on younger trees, growing scaly at the base of larger trunks. The leaves are toothed, with revolute margins (edges slightly rolled under) and a sticky feel in the spring. Alder is hermaphroditic, bearing both male catkins and female cones. The long catkins appear in spring, decorating the tree like ornaments at an Easter-themed party. In summer, small brown cone-like strobiles (less than 1 inch long) develop, remaining on the limbs through winter like natural ornaments. The bark is aromatic, with a bitter, astringent taste. The tree typically reaches 15 feet in height and lives around 5 0 years.

Where it grows: Where there is water, there is Alder. It grows alongside willows, aspens, and cottonwoods near streams, springs, and seeps. A key player in ecosystem restoration, Alder is a nitrogen fixer, forming a symbiotic relationship with *Frankia alni* bacteria, which enriches the soil. Quick to colonize disturbed areas, it stabilizes and heals the land.

When and how to harvest: Gather bark any time of year, harvesting respectfully. Cut thin strips sparingly from each tree—never girdle it. The developing cones can be harvested in spring; they remain shelf-stable for up to three years. Alder leaves are best gathered in mid-spring.

How to work with it / Medicinal use: Alder is an ancient and sacred medicine for both people and land, embodying the elements of earth, water, and fire. In alignment with the Doctrine of Signatures, Alder's role in rebuilding soil mirrors its ability to rebuild the immune system and calm inflammation. Internally, Alder tincture or decoction acts as an alterative, cleansing the blood and draining the lymph, while balancing bile. It is both astringent and mucilaginous, tightening and toning inflamed tissues while soothing them. Alder is also an immunostimulant, supporting white blood cell production and helping to fight infections such as candida overgrowth. Due to its antibacterial and antifungal properties, it is most effective for the short-term treatment of chronic infections.

Topically, Alder soothes itchy, inflamed skin conditions, including weeping eczema, athlete's foot, psoriasis, poison oak/ivy rash, scabies, and lice. An Alder salve or liniment supports wound healing. The bark's analgesic properties make it ideal for a sore foot soak, and soaking feet in an Alder decoction helps "toughen" them for barefoot foraging and gardening. Alder decoction or tincture can also be used as a gargle for canker sores, tonsillitis, and sore gums. Bark powder can be used as a natural tooth whitener and may also help treat diarrhea (a slight pinch in warm water, taken up to three times daily for no more than three days). For women's health, Alder helps regulate menstrual flow. Alder cones decocted in water address internal bleeding and soothe digestive tract inflammation. To aid nutrient absorption and fat digestion, take a decoction of dried bark powder before meals.

Emerging research suggests that Alder's antiviral properties may be beneficial in treating HIV, SARS, and even coronavirus by mitigating cytokine storms (Park et al., 2012). For optimal immunostimulant extraction, macerate fresh bark in 40–50% alcohol; for dried bark, use 70% alcohol.

Caution: Fresh bark is emetic and can cause vomiting; dry it first unless you are using it for that purpose.

Healing constituents / Therapeutic actions: Alder contains alnincanone, brassinolide, castasterone, taraxerone; leaves contain three-beta-hydroxyglutin-5-en, alnusfoliendiolone, delta-amyrenome, L-ornithine, and sucrose; bark contains alnulin, beta-sitosterol, citrullin, emodin, glutinone, hyperoside, lupeol, phlobaphene, protoalnulin, tannin, and taraxerol. Therapeutic actions include immunostimulant, antiviral, antibacterial, anti-inflammatory, alterative, diaphoretic, and (fresh bark) emetic.

Historical connections: A true people's plant, Alder is rich in lore and ancient use. In Norse and Greek mythology, Alder is associated with Loki, the trickster god, due to its terrain-shifting properties. Its wood was used for boats, bridges, and structures over wetlands, hardening when wet—thus also used for shields and associated with warfare. In Irish folklore, Alder was considered unlucky and associated with death, as the cut wood "bleeds" red. However, in Celtic mythology, Alder symbolizes balance, embodying both male and female energies with its catkins and cones.

Scottish lore tells of a groom stolen by fairies, whose body was replaced with an Alder branch. Evidence suggests the Inca used Alder to restore Andean soils. The Nez Perce applied heated Alder leaf poultices to wounds and sores, and fresh leaves were tucked into moccasins for long journeys.

Jessica's notes: Alder fascinates me deeply. Its myriad medicinal and practical uses, coupled with its vital ecological role, create a strong bond with this remarkable tree. From boat building to powerful medicine in bark, leaves, and cones, Alder is truly a people's plant. The sight of its "bleeding" wood and the rich folklore it carries inspire visions of enchanted forests alive with ancient magic.

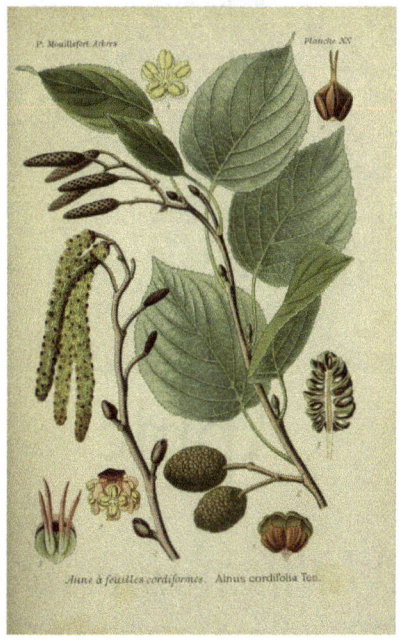

Italian alder (Alnus cordata), after Pierre Mouillefert, Planche XX from his tree atlas (public domain).

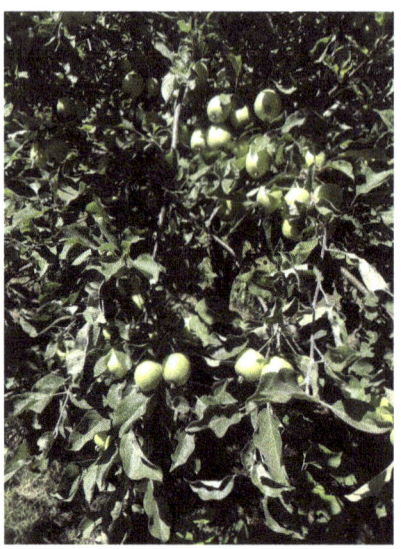

Apple

Malus domestica

Rosaceae (Rose) Family

Description: Apple is a deciduous tree that sheds its leaves at the end of each growing season. Domesticated apple trees reach about 16 feet, while wild apple trees can grow up to 32 feet. The leaves are alternate, oval, and serrated at the edges. Blossoms appear in spring as the leaves emerge—five-petaled, white with a pinkish blush, 3–4 cm in diameter. The fruit of wild apples ranges in color from green to pink to deep red, with whitish flesh that is sometimes tinged with yellow or green.

Where it grows: Often found along forest edges, lake shores, rivers, and creeks, apple trees frequently stand as living markers of long-forgotten homesteads.

When and how to harvest: Harvest fruit in late summer into early fall, before the first frost. Leaves can be harvested in the spring, before the tree bears fruit. Bark can be gathered throughout the year.

How to work with it / Medicinal use: Apple is truly a people's plant—its fruit, leaves, and bark all provide healing nourishment.

Apples are rich in pectin, which helps the body remove heavy metals and toxins. Pectin powder, made from dehydrated apples, has been used effectively in detox protocols, including with Chernobyl victims, to draw radioactive cesium from the system. Pectin also assists in clearing mercury and aluminum. Apples aid digestion, support liver function, and improve cardiovascular health by lowering blood pressure, reducing cholesterol, and protecting against stroke.

A raw apple poultice can soothe eye inflammation, slow-healing wounds, and sore muscles. Fresh apples regulate the bowels, helping both constipation and diarrhea. Sour apples have a diuretic action and support urinary tract health. Stewed apples can soothe inflamed bowels caused by food intolerance or IBS. Apple peel is traditionally used in France for the treatment of rheumatism, gout, and urinary disorders. Grated raw apple, taken first thing in the morning, can ease morning sickness. Eating apples before bed can help alleviate insomnia and support digestive health.

Apple cider vinegar (ACV), made from wild apples, is an excellent natural remedy in its own right, promoting weight loss, appetite stimulation, blood sugar regulation, and detoxification. ACV's acetic acid enhances the extraction of minerals from herbs (such as stinging nettle) and helps pull alkaloids from roots like Oregon grape in tincture making.

Leaves and bark are mildly bitter and astringent. A decoction supports digestion, soothes diarrhea and IBS, and when used externally, can calm bug bites, cuts, and abrasions.

Beyond its medicinal properties, applewood is a valued tool-making and cooking wood—burning hot and slow, it is perfect for high-heat cooking and smoking foraged meals.

Healing constituents / Therapeutic actions: Apple fruit contains flavonoids, vitamins A, B1, and C, minerals, pectin, acids, and sugars. Its therapeutic actions include diuretic, anti-diabetic, and digestive support. The leaves contain tannins, which make them astringent and antiseptic, and also possess antidiarrheal properties.

Historical connections: Sir John Hill (1716–1765) wrote: "Verjuice (pressed unripe crab apple juice) is made from the crab; and it is a remedy for the falling of the uvula, better than most other applications: it is also good, against sore throats, and in all disorders of the mouth."

Apples have long been used as eye compresses—Hildegard von Bingen provides a beautiful method using young apple leaves and grapevine sap to soothe foggy eyes. In Grieve's *Modern Herbal*, cider is noted for preventing kidney stones: "It is stated on medical authority that in countries where unsweetened cider is used as a common beverage, stone or calculus is unknown."

Apples have been an integral part of human culture since antiquity. In the Bible, they are linked to the Tree of Knowledge and the fall of Adam and Eve. Henry David Thoreau wrote in *The Wild Apple* (1862): "It is remarkable how close the history of the apple tree is connected with that of man."

The familiar phrase, "An apple a day keeps the doctor away," originated in Wales in 1866. The expression "You are the apple of my eye" is drawn from *Deuteronomy 32:10*: "He kept him as the apple of his eye."

No tree is more entwined with American folklore than the apple, thanks to the legendary Johnny Appleseed (John Chapman), who spread apple seeds across frontier America in the early 1800s. Pioneers primarily used apples for cider, as safe drinking water was scarce. Johnny Appleseed—barefoot, with his tin pot hat—helped root apple culture deeply in early American life.

Jessica's notes: Shaking wild apple trees and gathering their fruit at forest school fills me with joy and a deep sense of connection. It feels like a timeless ritual, practiced over many lifetimes. Apple medicine is for the people—past, present, and future. When I find a lone apple tree in the forest, it whispers stories of old homesteads and hands that once planted and cared for it, staking their claim to the land.

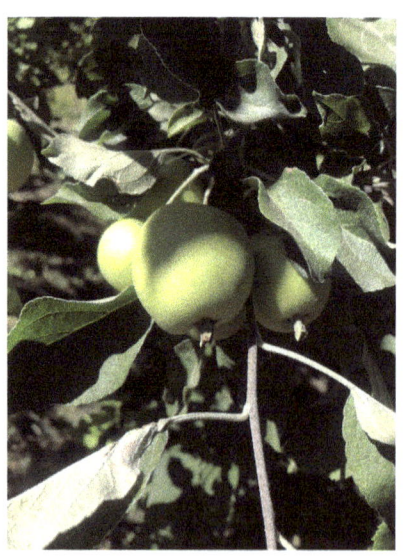

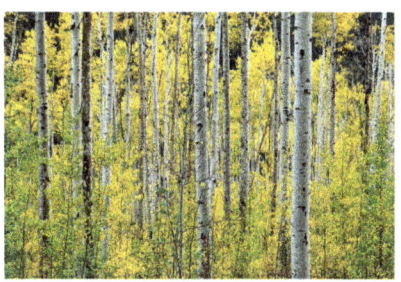

Aspen

Populus tremuloides

Salicaceae (Willow) Family
Other common names: Quaking Aspen
Description: Aspen is a tall, fast-growing deciduous tree, reaching heights of up to 60 feet with a slender trunk approximately 10 inches in diameter. The bark is smooth and whitish (light green when young), marked with black horizontal scars and bulbous black knots where branches once grew. Vertical scars may mark areas where elk have stripped the bark to reach the sugary cambium in winter. Rubbing the bark leaves a chalky white powder on the hands.

Leaves are rounded, heart-shaped, with finely toothed edges and long, flattened petioles, allowing them to quake and flutter with the slightest breeze. This trembling quality gives quaking aspen (*P. tremuloides*) its name. Leaves turn brilliant yellow in the fall. Younger trees and root sprouts bear larger, more triangular leaves.

Aspen is dioecious, with both male and female clones. Its catkin flowers appear in early spring, before the leaves emerge. Each fruit capsule contains tiny seeds surrounded by cottony fluff, aiding wind dispersal in early summer. Aspen reproduces prolifically by suckering—forming clonal colonies that can live for hundreds of years, with root systems that persist even if the visible trees die back.

Where it grows: Aspen thrives in groups in open meadows, fields, and near creeks and springs. They are one of the first trees to recolonize burned areas and disturbed land—virtually immortal beings of the forest.

When and how to harvest: Harvest leaves in late spring to early summer. Strip bark in late summer into fall, always harvesting sparingly. Flower buds can be gathered in winter as a source of survival food. The inner cambium is sweetest in late winter or early spring when sugars are flowing.

How to work with it / Medicinal use: Aspen bark and leaves contain salicin, a compound metabolized into salicylic acid, the same pain-relieving agent found in aspirin. Tinctures and decoctions of the bark can help ease headaches, fever, nerve pain, rheumatoid arthritis, and general inflammation. Aspen also aids digestive issues such as diarrhea and IBS, and its astringent, antiseptic qualities make it worthwhile for urinary tract infections.

Topically, aspen bark preparations can soothe acne, eczema, bug bites, sunburn, and other inflamed skin conditions. Add the flower buds to ointments or balms for enhanced effect. Aspen bark decoction (1–4 grams simmered for several hours) can be used both internally and externally. The chalky powder on the bark has mild sun-protective qualities, though it is not as effective as modern sunscreens.

The inner cambium can be eaten as a survival food, though it is bitter. Buds are also edible, although they are best left as a last resort for food. Aspen flower essence supports those dealing with vague fears or apprehension.

Aspen wood is valued for lumber, pulp, and paper—light, soft, and minimally shrinking. It is used for matches, plywood, particleboard, and renewable energy applications. There is a good chance this book was printed on aspen paper!

Healing constituents / Therapeutic actions: Aspen is rich in salicin (a phenolic glycoside), which inhibits inflammatory molecules such as cytokines, leukotrienes, and prostaglandins. These compounds reduce pain, swelling, and redness. Phenolic glycosides and tannins also provide antiseptic and astringent effects.

Historical connections: In Greek, *aspis* means "shield," and lightweight aspen wood was used to make shields for warriors. Greek heroes were crowned with aspen leaves. The shields were thought to offer both physical and magical protection.

Like the rowan, the aspen was often planted near homes as a protective tree and was believed to guard buried treasures. The Nuche (Ute) people used aspen bark for wound healing, while the Carrier people of British Columbia chewed the bark and applied it to wounds to stop bleeding. Warm aspen ash compresses were used to ease arthritic pain and swelling.

According to Ute legend, aspens tremble to this day as a sign of humility, having once refused to bow when the Great Spirit visited during a full moon. Angered, the Spirit decreed that aspen leaves would forever tremble before all eyes.

Jessica's notes: For me, aspens symbolize community—you never see one growing alone. They thrive in kinship with their brothers and sisters, standing together as allies in the forest. The golden, trembling leaves of fall seem to whisper ancient secrets of the land. I find great comfort in their resilience and in the quiet wisdom they offer to those who listen.

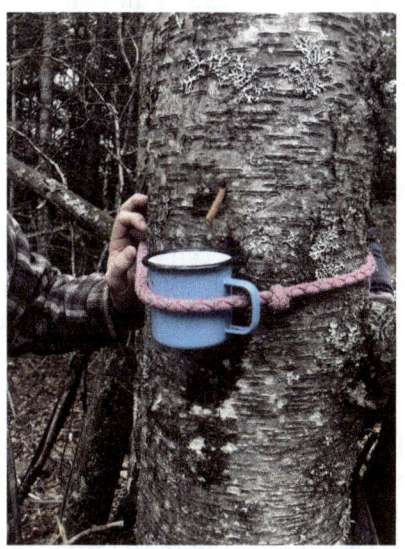

Birch

Betula spp.

Betulaceae (Birch) Family
Other common names: Paper Birch, Silver Birch
Description: In Celtic lore, the birch is known as the Lady of the Forest, characterized by her silvery bark, delicate flowers, and shimmering leaves. Birch species are generally small to medium-sized trees, often appearing in graceful pairs. The leaves are simple, alternate, serrate or doubly serrate, with feather-shaped veins and petioles. Female catkins disintegrate at maturity to release seeds, unlike the woody cones of alder (another genus in the Birch family).

Birch bark is soft, separating into papery plates, marked with long horizontal lenticels. Color varies with species, though the most common northern paper birch is a luminous white or pale grey.

Buds form in early summer, with flowering in catkins—male catkins drooping at maturity, female catkins remaining erect. Winged seeds are dispersed by wind in late summer. Birch is among the first deciduous trees to lose its leaves each fall.

Where it grows: Birch thrives in open woodlands near rivers, creeks, and damp meadows. It is often found in the company of cottonwood and aspen.

When and how to harvest: Harvest sap in late winter to early spring. Always seal tapped holes with beeswax after collection. Gather buds in early spring; leaves and branches can be harvested throughout spring and summer.

How to work with it / Medicinal use: Birch bark is a powerful pain reliever, rich in methyl salicylate, a compound with anti-inflammatory properties. Bark, leaves, and twigs can be used for muscle sprains, joint pain, and headaches. Betulin and lupeol, key compounds for wound healing, are best extracted in alcohol or fat, rather than water.

Steaming the leaves can help clear sinus congestion. Spring buds infused into oil make an excellent topical salve for inflamed skin conditions. Birch bark and leaves can be infused in oil or animal fat, blended with beeswax to create healing salves for rashes and wounds. An infusion of leaves and twigs can also soothe weeping rashes and wet eczema.

Birch is bitter and stimulates digestion—an apple cider vinegar infusion with birch leaves and twigs draws out both bitter compounds and minerals. Birch twig tea is a mild diuretic and cleansing tonic, high in vitamin C. Young spring leaves can also be crisp-fried for a flavorful wild snack.

Birch sap, tapped in late winter or early spring, is a highly nutritious drink rich in minerals, excellent for rehydration, blood sugar regulation, and gentle detoxification. Birch sap syrup, although more subtle than maple syrup, is a delicious and nourishing treat. Birch sap is also rich in manganese, magnesium, and vitamin C, which support bones, connective tissue, and skin. Birch trees host the medicinal chaga mushroom, a potent immunostimulant and adaptogen. Birch bark is highly flammable and an excellent natural fire starter.

Healing constituents / Therapeutic actions: Birch contains betulin (a triterpenoid), shown to support balanced glucose absorption and insulin secretion, as well as providing anti-inflammatory, analgesic, and antiviral effects. Leaves contain phenolic acids (chlorogenic, caffeic), flavonoids (rutoside, hyperoside), tannins, and methyl salicylate—all contributing to pain relief, astringency, and venolymphatic support.

Birch sap contains antioxidants, minerals, and antispasmodic properties.

Historical connections: The Latin name *Betula* derives from the Celtic *betul*. The Anglo-Saxon *beorc* or *birce* means "white" or "shining." Grieve's *Modern Herbal* notes that the name "birch" likely stems from the Sanskrit *bhurga*—"tree whose bark is used for writing." Birch bark was indeed an ancient writing surface.

Birch is a symbol of regeneration, new growth, and the arrival of spring in many cultures. Associated with the moon (silver bark) and sun (birch torches), birch was honored in rituals of renewal. In Norse mythology, birch was sacred to Frigg and Freya, goddesses of fertility and motherhood. The ancient Greeks associated the birch with Aphrodite.

At Beltane, birch was burned to light the bonfire and used as the Maypole in spring dances celebrating new beginnings. Later, birch switches were used in the Samhain ceremony of *Beating the Bounds* to sweep away evil spirits—a ritual later misrepresented as witchcraft. In the language of flowers, birch symbolizes modesty and grace. Among Slavic peoples, birch represents eternity and the return of spring.

In North America, Indigenous people used birch bark for wound healing, splints, and casts. The bark was prized for making containers, canoes, and snowshoes. Birch wood has long been used for making tools, baskets, bobbins, and firewood.

Jessica's notes: When I think of birch, gratitude fills my heart. It has kindled countless hearth fires, campfires, and bonfires that have kept my family warm through the seasons. Birch bark is our favorite kindling—we gather fallen bark, dry it in strips, and keep it ready for use.

As we have come to rely on birch for warmth, we have also discovered its potent medicinal gifts. The leaves and twigs have eased headaches, rashes, and sore muscles. Moreover, there is nothing more restorative than drinking fresh birch sap in late winter or early spring—a tonic for body and spirit alike. Although we have yet to make syrup, we tap enough sap each year to share with friends and neighbors. Birch feels like an old friend—generous, steadfast, and deeply woven into the life of the forest.

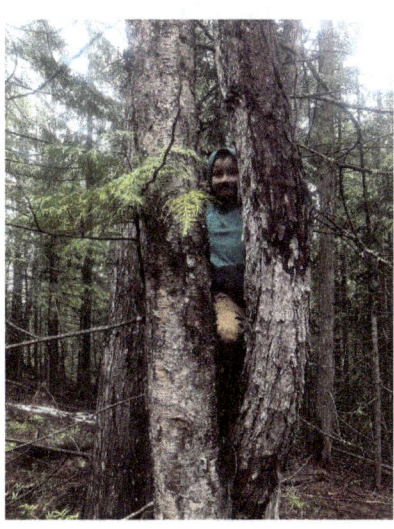

The Three sisters: Cedar, Birch, and Fir

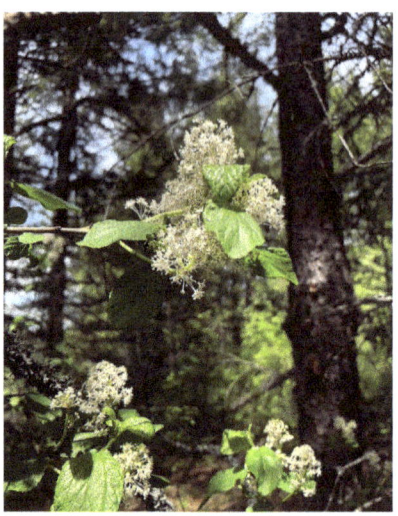

Ceanothus

Ceanothus velutinus, C. cuneatus, C. integerrimus, etc.

Rhamnaceae (Buckthorn) Family

Other common names: Redroot, Wild Lilac Bush, Snowbrush, Tobacco Brush, Deer Brush, Mahala Mat, Oregon Tea Tree, Sweet Birch, "See-and-Know-This"

Description: Ceanothus is a perennial, evergreen shrub easily identified by its glossy, often sticky leaves with three prominent veins. The oval to egg-shaped leaves, 3–10 cm long, are alternate, slightly toothed, and curled, giving off a rich, balsamic scent when crushed. Throughout summer, creamy-white, fragrant flowers bloom in pyramidal clusters, glowing against the dark green foliage. Snowbrush varieties grow 3–5 feet tall with stout, reddish-brown stems. At each leaf stalk, a tiny pair of stipules (1 mm long) can be seen. Fruits develop as three-lobed capsules that burst open forcefully, launching seeds into the soil, where they may remain viable in a seed bank for up to 200 years, awaiting the perfect conditions to sprout.

Where it grows: Ceanothus is abundant from British Columbia and Alberta down through Southern California. It thrives in dry soils along the edges of pine forests and high-elevation meadows, where summers are dry and winters are deep with snow.

When and how to harvest: Harvest the flowers and leaves throughout the summer when they are in full bloom. The roots are best gathered from midsummer through late fall. Roots from plants in harsher climates are the most potent. Look for red to wine-colored bark for the most medicinal strength.

How to work with it / Medicinal use: The reddish color of Ceanothus bark and roots signals its affinity for the blood and capillary systems—a classic example of the Doctrine of Signatures at work. A tincture of red root helps recharge the blood and support the lymphatic system. It is especially beneficial after rich or fatty meals, helping calm inflammation and reduce blood fats.

Fresh roots tincture best at a 1:5 alcohol ratio. A cold infusion can be sipped throughout the day to soothe post-tonsillectomy symptoms or used as a gargle for sore throats and mouth sores. Internally, red root can help relieve swollen lymph nodes and is particularly beneficial for conditions such as breast and ovarian cysts, varicose veins, hemorrhoids, and congestion in the cervical and prostate areas.

Because it strengthens and tones lymphatic tissues, red root is often used to support recovery from conditions such as hepatitis, mononucleosis, and chronic infections that involve enlarged lymph nodes or spleens. Michael Moore, in *Medicinal Plants of the Pacific West*, praises red root for treating menstrual hemorrhage, nosebleeds, hemorrhoids, ulcers, and capillary rupture from coughing or vomiting. It also helps soothe gastritis in heavy drinkers and can be used for fragile capillaries overall.

Red root tincture has been shown to increase T-cell counts and support the immune system against long-term infections.

The flowers themselves contain antibacterial properties, and when mixed with water, they lather like soap. Ceanothus flower wash can be used for wounds, cuts, scrapes, or as a gentle body cleanser in the wild.

Healing constituents / Therapeutic actions: Ceanothus contains cyclic peptide alkaloids, triterpenes, ceanothenic acid, tannins (10%), resins, bitters, and gums. Its therapeutic actions include hepatoprotective, hepatorestorative, lymphatic, astringent, antispasmodic, expectorant, and mild antiseptic.

Historical connections: Eastern cousins of our western Ceanothus—*Ceanothus americanus*—were known as New Jersey Tea, a beloved alternative to imported tea during the Boston Tea Party.

Native Americans long understood the blood-purifying and wound-healing powers of red root. The name "kikuki manito," meaning "spotted snake spirit," was shared among several Indigenous languages (Mesquakie, Potawatomi, Menomini, and Ojibwa), reflecting both the plant's deep spiritual significance and its practical value in treating snake bites, fevers, and inflammation.

The Choctaw of Louisiana used an extract for lung hemorrhages, while the Cherokee made a root lotion for skin cancer.

Jessica's notes: "See-and-know-this," Nova said, leading me down to the creek with a handful of Ceanothus flowers. I was nine years old. She showed me how to mix the flowers with water and lather them into a sweet-scented soap. That moment stayed with me forever. It was one of the first profound teachings that revealed the quiet magic of the plant world—a moment of wonder and connection that helped shape my life-long path with herbal medicine.

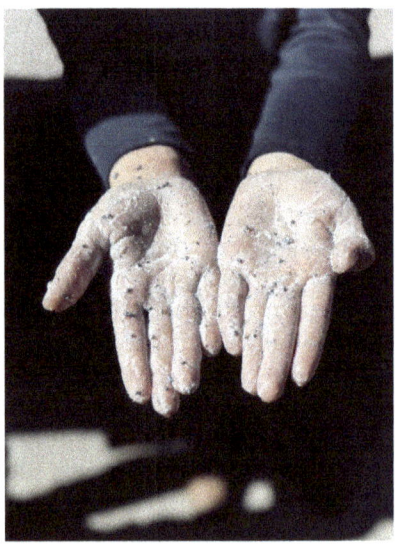

Ceanothus Soap

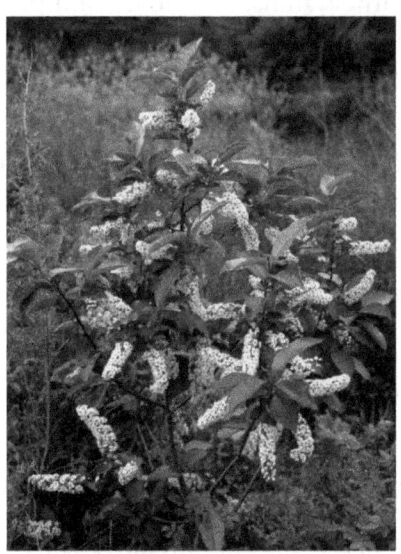

Chokecherry

Prunus virginiana

Rosaceae (Rose) Family

Description: *Prunus virginiana* is a fast-growing, deciduous, large shrub or understory tree that can reach up to 12 feet in height and often forms dense thickets. In spring, it adorns itself with fragrant, 5-lobed, cup-shaped white flowers arranged in cascading clusters that resemble delicate wedding bouquets. Come late summer, globular, pea-sized berries ripen from bright red to deep black, hanging like little jewels along the branches. The oval-shaped, dark green leaves display prominent veins and undergo a brilliant transformation in the fall, turning a brilliant golden yellow and vibrant orange.

Where it grows: You will often find chokecherry growing along roadsides, field edges, and the margins of woodlands—those liminal places where forest and meadow meet.

When and how to harvest: Harvest the bark in fall, once the energy of the tree begins to return to its roots. The berries are gathered when fully ripe in late summer to early fall.

How to work with it / Medicinal use: Though its name—*chokecherry*—may not immediately entice, do not be fooled. This plant offers an abundance of culinary and medicinal gifts. The berries are rich in potent antioxidants: anthocyanins, flavonoids, and proanthocyanidins—all known to help fight disease, cancer, viruses, and allergens. They also contain quinic acid, which has shown promise in preventing urinary tract infections and is being studied for its potential to lower blood pressure and reduce the risk of cardiovascular disease.

The inner bark carries antibacterial properties and can be used as a wash or poultice on wounds and cuts. Traditionally, wild cherry bark was brewed as a tea to treat coughs, colds, pneumonia, diarrhea, and sore throats.

Although separating the tiny seeds from the flesh is labor-intensive, it is not necessary for syrups—cook the berries whole, fresh or dried, and then strain them afterward. Chokecherries make a delicious, deep-flavored syrup, as well as homemade wines, jellies, and jams.

Beyond medicine and food, chokecherry wood is prized for its beauty and workability, making it ideal for crafting walking sticks, sculptures, furniture, and other handmade objects. When dried, the hardwood makes excellent fuel for cooking over high heat.

Caution: Chokecherry pits contain amygdalin, which the body can convert into cyanide, a dangerous poison. However, a toxic dose would require consuming far more than is pleasant, as the astringency would naturally limit intake. The bark also contains cyanogenic compounds and should be used under the guidance of a professional herbalist or approached with great care.

Healing constituents / Therapeutic actions: Chokecherry is packed with antioxidants—especially anthocyanins—and vitamins including niacin, pantothenic acid, thiamin, vitamin B6, vitamin C, vitamin K, choline, and riboflavin. Its therapeutic actions include antitussive, pectoral, expectorant, astringent, carminative, and sedative.

Historical connections: Native American tribes made brilliant use of chokecherry. They dried the berries and pounded them with elk, deer, and fat back to create *pemmican*—a high-energy, shelf-stable food for travel and survival. The berries also yielded a vibrant red dye. Dried chokecherries, along with other wild fruits, served as valued trade items between tribes, carried from one community to the next along ancient trade routes.

Jessica's notes: Another stunning and essential plant of the wild margins, where forest, meadow, and road meet. The rich taste of chokecherry syrup always takes me back to foraging adventures, fingers stained dark red from gathering the berries. There is something deeply satisfying about transforming what was once called "choke" into sweet medicine, just as nature herself transforms bitterness into balance.

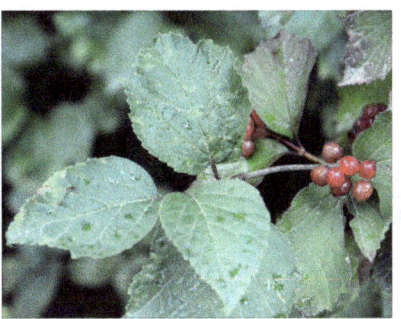

Crampbark

Viburnum edule

Caprifoliaceae (Honeysuckle) Family
Other common names: Highbush cranberry, American cranberry bush, mooseberry

Description: Crampbark is an upright, branching perennial shrub that can grow up to 6 feet tall, characterized by its dark grey bark. Its opposite leaves are petioled and roughly maple-shaped, with palmately three- to five-veined lobes and coarsely toothed edges that turn a brilliant red in autumn. In spring, creamy white, fragrant flowers bloom in axillary compound clusters, their airy form resembling floating lace among the branches. By late summer, bright red, one-seeded berries develop, offering a vibrant visual feast at the forest edge. The berries soften and sweeten after the first frost, though some foragers prefer their tart flavor when harvested earlier.

Where it grows: Look for crampbark along riverbanks, streams, thickets, and at the edges of woods. It thrives in cool, moist environments and stands as a bright beacon in the autumn landscape.

When and how to harvest: Harvest the bark either before or after the berries ripen. The berries themselves are ready in late summer into fall, and while they can be enjoyed when tart and firm, many choose to wait until after the first frost, when they become plumper and sweeter.

How to work with it / Medicinal use: As its name suggests, crampbark is famed for its ability to relieve cramps—whether in muscles, the uterus, or the digestive system. If you find yourself on a long hike with aching legs, you can gather a few twigs and simmer them into a tea right on the trail to soothe tired muscles. This same infusion can be used as a topical soak or compress for sore, cramping muscles.

Crampbark is also highly effective for uterine cramps. I like to keep a tincture on hand for fast relief of menstrual cramps, afterbirth pains, and digestive cramping. Midwives and herbalists have long used crampbark to ease postpartum cramping and even to help prevent miscarriage by calming an overactive uterus in late pregnancy. It is also used for easing pain from uterine fibroids, endometriosis, and testicular pain.

For menopausal women dealing with excessive bleeding or painful cramps, crampbark combined with yarrow makes an excellent supportive remedy.

Beyond cramps, crampbark's astringent and antibacterial properties lend themselves well to treating sore throats and gum issues—an infusion of the bark can be used as a gargle or mouth rinse for gingivitis, strep throat, and loose gums.

In the fall, the vitamin C-rich berries can be transformed into medicinal syrups, juices, jams, and jellies.

Healing constituents / Therapeutic actions: Crampbark contains viburnine (a bitter compound), hydroquinones, coumarins, valerianic acid, phenolic compounds, salicocides, and resins. Its therapeutic actions include: alterative, antispasmodic, astringent, diuretic, nervine, and sedative.

Historical connections: Crampbark has a long history of use by Native American tribes and Western herbalists alike. The Meskwaki of Wisconsin used it for menstrual cramps, back pain, and arthritis. The Penobscot of Maine turned to crampbark to treat swollen lymph nodes and gout, while the Iroquois valued it for treating uterine prolapse after childbirth.

Dr. William Cook, an Eclectic physician in the late 18th and early 19th centuries, was a great admirer of crampbark, recommending it for nervous irritability, leucorrhea, coughs, and bronchial irritation. In European folk medicine, it was used for afterbirth pain and menstrual cramping.

The herb is revered in Russian and Ukrainian folklore and was officially listed in the United States Pharmacopeia from 1894 to 1916, and in the National Formulary through 1960, as a recognized sedative and antispasmodic.

Jessica's notes: Crampbark was one of the first herbs to truly win me over to the world of natural healing. At 19, while recovering from illness in Guatemala, I promised that if I healed, I would dedicate my life to helping others through the gifts of nature. Returning home, I began working in the supplement department of New Frontiers. That is where I first learned about crampbark capsules and tried them for menstrual cramps—what a revelation! The pain melted away without side effects. Later, Jason began teaching me to recognize plants in the wild, and I was astonished to realize that many expensive supplements on store shelves could be harvested right from the land. That early "aha" moment continues to inspire my passion for plant medicine to this day.

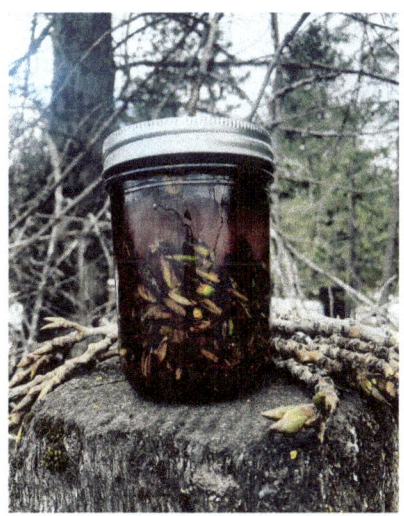

Cottonwood

Populus balsamifera

Salicaceae (Willow) Family
Other common names: Black cottonwood

Description: One of the forest's true giants, cottonwood trees can tower up to 120 feet tall, with broad trunks reaching 1 to 3 feet in diameter, and live for a century or more. These stately trees are dioecious, meaning that individual trees are either male or female. The female trees produce long, string-like seedpods that dangle like strands of a necklace, eventually releasing millions of cottony seeds into the air in midsummer, giving the tree its common name. The males grow deep purple catkins in early spring.

Though grand, cottonwoods often take on a half-dead appearance in old age, with inner branches hollowing or dying back long before the rest of the tree. Their massive limbs are prone to breaking during storms, leaving the forest floor littered with fallen branches, often rich with resin-laden buds.

Young trees have smooth, tawny-gray bark that darkens, roughens, and develops deep furrows as they mature. Their lustrous, dark green leaves are egg-shaped with notched edges, turning a brilliant yellow in fall before blanketing the ground. In late winter, ruby-red buds, rich with fragrant resin, swell and gleam like tiny jewels, protected from frost by their sticky coating. This sweet-smelling resin is beloved by honeybees, who collect it to make propolis, nature's powerful antimicrobial shield for the hive.

Where it grows: Cottonwood thrives along waterways—creeks, springs, rivers, and wetlands—where its thirsty roots draw deeply from the earth. It is a water-loving tree and vulnerable to drought.

When and how to harvest: The resinous buds are gathered in late winter into early spring, just before they begin to open. This is sticky work! Expect your fingers to be stained a fragrant red—a badge of honor that can be removed with alcohol and hot, soapy water.

How to work with it / Medicinal use: Cottonwood buds hold a wealth of healing properties. Their resin contains salicin, the same pain- and fever-relieving compound found in willow and aspen, along with tannins and flavones that lend antifungal and antimicrobial properties.

Applied externally, cottonwood resin is a wonder for promoting wound healing and easing joint pain and arthritis. It can be massaged into the chest to loosen stubborn mucus or spread onto cold sores, where its sting signals its potent antiviral action. The buds can be infused into oil and crafted into a balm known as Balm of Gilead, an ancient and revered remedy. This balm soothes menstrual cramps, backaches, chest pain, and sore muscles a like.

Internally, cottonwood resin tincture is an effective fever-reducer and expectorant. For sore throats and lung support, a honey infusion of the buds makes a delicious and soothing medicine—let the buds steep in honey for 4 to 6 weeks and stir into teas.

To tincture the resin, infuse the buds in high-proof alcohol (151 proof) for an effective extract. This can be taken at the onset of viral illness or used topically on wounds, cuts, scrapes, and herpes lesions.

Cottonwood's doctrine of signatures is charmingly evident—the gnarly branch tips resemble aged, aching fingers, hinting at its role in easing joint pain and stiffness.

Healing constituents / Therapeutic actions: Cottonwood buds and bark contain salicylates, tannins, and flavones. Their therapeutic actions include analgesic, anti-inflammatory, antiseptic, febrifuge, stimulating, and expectorant properties.

Historical connections: The legendary Balm of Gilead, derived from cottonwood buds, is mentioned throughout the Bible:

"An Ishmaelite caravan passes by on their way to Egypt from Gilead, carrying balm, spices, and myrrh." (Genesis 37:25)"Is there no balm in Gilead? Is there no physician there? Why then is there no recovery for the health of the daughter of my people?" (Jeremiah 8:22)

Sacred and healing, cottonwood was honored by many Native American tribes. The Hopi, Pueblo, and Navajo carved ceremonial Kachina dolls, masks, and sacred objects from the roots of Cottonwood trees. Plains tribes regarded cottonwood as a medicine tree—its trunks and branches used for Sun Dance poles and sacred artifacts. The buds were also used as glue and a yellow dye, and the bark and leaves were used to treat swelling and wounds.

Children fashioned toy tipis and moccasins from cottonwood leaves, and young women made a simple birdcall whistle from its flexible foliage. For early American pioneers crossing the parched prairies, the sight of cottonwood groves meant life-giving water was near; shade, shelter, and firewood awaited.

Jessica's notes: "Cottonwood, oh Cottonwood, would you be my love and medicine?" I sing this joyfully as I gather the sticky buds in late winter and early spring. Cottonwood offers one of the first medicines we can harvest each year when the forest is still slumbering beneath its winter blanket. There is nothing quite like discovering a fallen branch gleaming with ruby-red buds atop the snow after a storm. I gather them with reverence, often anointing my lips with a dab of resin—Nature's Lipstick—tingling with vitality.

The scent alone fills me with a deep sense of the sacred. It is no wonder that cottonwood resin has been revered since biblical times. It is a true gift from the forest—a healing treasure offered freely to those who seek it with gratitude.

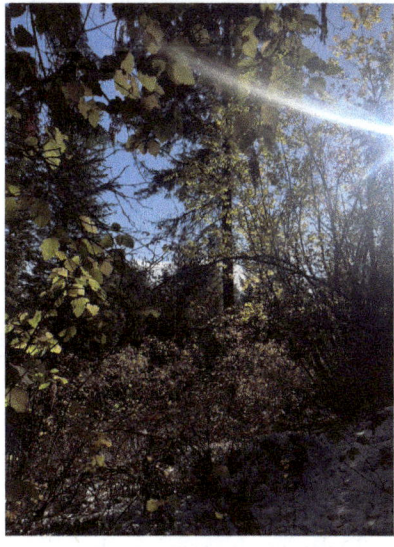

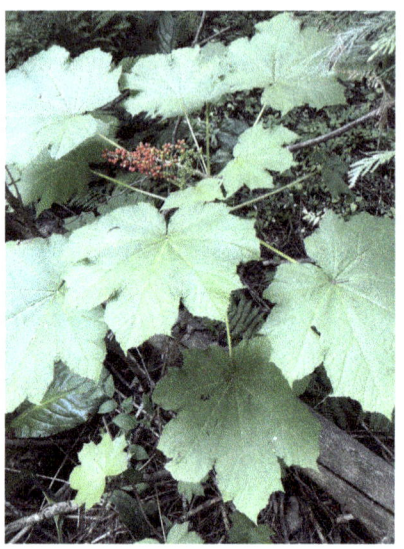

Devil's Club

Oplopanax horridus

Araliaceae (Ginseng) Family

Description: The name alone hints at this plant's fierce nature. Devil's Club bristles with sharp, needle-like spines along its sprawling rhizomes and stout stems—its touch can cause skin irritation if approached carelessly. However, beneath this thorny exterior lies one of the forest's most powerful healers. This erect and imposing perennial unfurls immense, maple-shaped leaves in spring, creating an ancient, almost mythic presence in old-growth forests. Delicate clusters of white flowers bloom in spring, later giving way to bright red berries in mid-to-late summer.

Where it grows: You will find Devil's Club near creeks, springs, and wet forest soils. It thrives in the cool shade of old-growth forests, where its roots help restore the land after logging or soil disturbance—an ecological guardian in its own right.

When and how to harvest: I prefer to work with the roots and rhizomes, harvesting in fall or early spring when the plant enters dormancy. Thick gloves are essential when handling this prickly ally—its spines demand respect.

How to work with it / Medicinal use: The botanical name *Panax* marks Devil's Club as a cousin to both American and Asian ginsengs. Like them, it is rich in adaptogenic compounds that foster resilience, strength, and grounding. The inner bark of the stems and roots contains potent medicine—best prepared as a decoction or tincture — to ease arthritis, aching joints, and chronic coughs, including stubborn respiratory infections such as tuberculosis. Its aromatic essence alone is deeply grounding—breathe it in while wandering through the forest, and you will feel its stabilizing presence.

Among the Inuit and coastal peoples, Devil's Club remains a trusted remedy for Type 2 diabetes. Its saponin compounds help balance blood sugar and aid nutrient absorption, supporting the gut and nervous system, especially after trauma. Indeed, this plant has a healing effect on both physical and emotional levels. Just as its spiny stalks guard its tender core, Devil's Club teaches us to stand firm and protect ourselves while healing deep-rooted wounds and ancestral traumas.

As an adaptogen, it nourishes resilience, strengthening the body's ability to withstand stress and recover from illness or emotional upheaval. Whether taken as a tonic or used topically for joint pain, Devil's Club invites us into greater wholeness.

Healing constituents / Therapeutic actions: Devil's Club is rich in saponins, sesquiterpenes (including equinopanacene), sesquiterpene alcohols (equinopanacol), and acetylenes—potent antifungal and antimycobacterial compounds with promising applications for resistant infections like tuberculosis. Its healing actions include antifungal, antiviral, antibacterial, antimycobacterial, adaptogenic, anti-inflammatory, and immune-stimulating.

Historical connections: For over 30 Indigenous linguistic groups across the Pacific Northwest, Alaska, Canada, and the Inland West, Devil's Club has long been revered as a sacred and spiritual plant. Its traditional uses span at least 34 physical ailments, from diabetes and tuberculosis to arthritis and infections. Coastal tribes crafted fishhooks from their resilient wood and created ceremonial face paint from their bright berries. Shamans used Devil's Club to ward off negative forces and for spiritual protection and purification—a bridge between worlds.

As Nancy Turner (1982) notes in, *Ethnobotany of the Hesquiat Indians of Vancouver Island*, Devil's Club holds a place of deep reverence in Indigenous cultures, both as a physical and spiritual medicine.

Jessica's notes: At first, I was intimidated to work with this plant—its fierce spines make harvesting a challenge, and its energy is equally formidable. You must be ready when you approach Devil's Club, for it does not just heal the body; it reveals what lies beneath the surface—deep emotional wounds and ancestral traumas waiting to be released.

For a time, I sat with this plant, listening and observing. Even its presence is healing. However, lately, I have felt it calling me more strongly, inviting me to engage with it at a deeper level. It is time—for me, for all of us—to heal the traumas of the past and stand rooted in truth, courage, and compassion.

As healers and sensitive souls, we often carry the burdens of others. Devil's Club reminds us to guard our boundaries and stay rooted in who we are. It is a fierce and wise teacher—a faithful ally for the times we are living in.

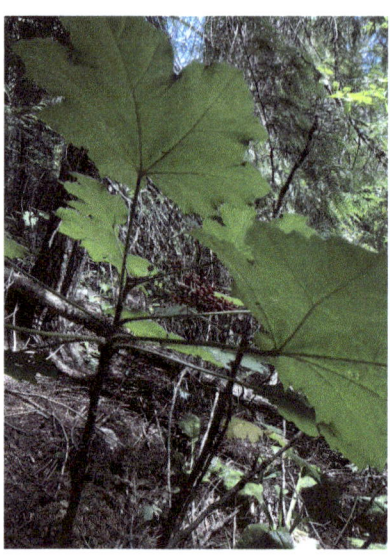

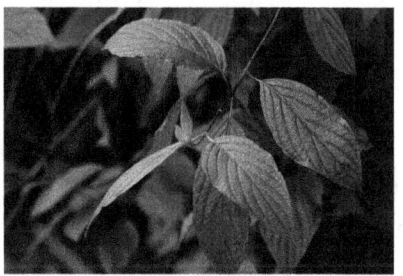

Dogwood

Cornus sericea

Cornaceae (Dogwood) Family
Other common names: Red Osier Dogwood
Description: A large, sprawling mountain shrub, red osier dogwood reaches impressive heights and widths of 10 to 12 feet. One of its most distinctive features is its smooth, red-purple stems, which glow brilliantly against the bare winter landscape—a visual gift in the dormant season. The lanceolate to ovate green leaves are twice as long as they are wide, about 2 to 3 ½ inches in length, with prominent veins, pointed tips, and a lighter, softly hairy underside. In late spring to early summer, the branch tips burst into creamy-white, four-petaled flower clusters, which mature into small, whitish pea-sized fruits. These one-seeded drupes hang in clusters into the fall. Dogwood has an incredible ability to root along its stems, often creating dense, clonal thickets that provide shelter and stabilizing ground co ver.

Where it grows: Look for red osier dogwood along stream banks, wetlands, and other areas with consistently moist soil. It is native across the western Rocky Mountain states and the high country of the Southwest, where it thrives in cool mountain air and riparian corridors.

When and how to harvest: Harvest the roots and lower stems in early spring or late fall when the plant is dormant. Smaller roots can be used whole, while larger roots and lower stem bark can be stripped and dried for teas or tinctures. Dry your harvest well, as the bark can mold if stored too damp.

How to work with it / Medicinal use: Though red osier dogwood has largely fallen out of modern herbal practice, it is a venerable old medicine with much to offer. Traditionally, it was used to support the body during malarial infections and prolonged fevers. Its glycosides have been shown to lower body temperature, making it useful for multi-day illnesses characterized by profound fatigue, chills, and intermittent fever. A cold infusion of the bark is ideal for this purpose; however, a standard decoction will also work effectively. If nausea accompanies the illness, a tincture is preferred, as the taste of the tea can be unpleasant to sensitive stomachs.

As Charles Kane suggests in *Medicinal Plants of the Mountain West*, dogwood medicine is best used during the *ebb* of a fever cycle—not at its peak—offering strength and relief when the body is weak and weary.

Red osier is also a gentle astringent that can help tone the digestive tract, easing diarrhea and loose stools; however, overuse of the tea may cause nausea. Topically, dogwood bark has antimicrobial properties and can be used to make a delicate wash or poultice for stubborn wounds, festering sores, and infections that resist healing.

Healing constituents / Therapeutic actions: Although relatively little modern research has been conducted on the medicinal chemistry of dogwood, it is known to contain glycosides, tannins, and other bitter compounds. Its known actions are bitter, astringent, antibacterial, and antitussive.

Historical connections: Dogwood has served humanity for centuries, both as a medicinal plant and as a material for crafts. The hardwood was valued for making skewers, farming tools, and weaving shuttles—indeed, the name "dogwood" is thought to derive from the Scandinavian *dag*, meaning "skewer."

For many Native American tribes, red osier dogwood was a plant of profound practical and spiritual importance. The bark was steeped into teas to treat coughs, fevers, sinus infections, postpartum bleeding, and liver ailments. The flexible branches were essential for weaving baskets, netting, drying animal hides, and crafting bows and arrows. The bark yielded a red dye, while its inner bark was sometimes smoked ceremonially or used in "kinnikinnick" tobacco blends. In some traditions, dogwood sap was even used to tip arrowheads.

With its strength, resilience, and versatility, dogwood came to symbolize protection and endurance—a guardian shrub standing along the water's edge.

Jessica's notes: How can you tell it is a dogwood tree? By its bark, of course! (I could not resist slipping in this favorite joke.)

For me, dogwood carries a special place in my heart. The very first gift Jason ever gave me was a framed photograph of a dogwood tree in full bloom; a souvenir he bought in the Sierra Mountains. I still have that picture. Whenever I meet a dogwood along my path, I feel a sense of homecoming, a quiet reminder of love, resilience, and the beauty that endures through every season.

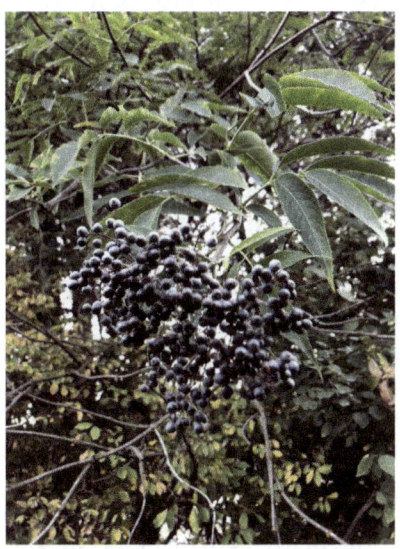

Elderberry

Sambucus nigra- canadensis

Adoxaceae (Moschatel) Family

Description: A statuesque, herbaceous deciduous shrub or small tree, elderberry graces the land with large umbels of ivory flowers in early to late summer, followed by an abundance of deep blue berries ripening through late summer into fall. The blue variety sometimes carries a frosted bloom that dusts the berries in a silvery-white powder. Reddish-brown branches with a soft pith within and a shiny outer layer form many trunks and branches, providing sanctuary for small birds. Elderberry often creates a sheltering grove—a protective presence along the forest edge.

Where it grows: Elderberry thrives at the boundary between field and forest, guarding edges and pathways. True to its nature as a boundary dweller, it wards off unwanted visitors—an example of the Doctrine of Signatures at play. Look for it in riparian areas, along roadsides, moist forest clearings, and country lanes. I often spot elderberry while singing John Denver's *Country Roads*.

When and how to harvest: Harvest the blossoms in late spring and early summer. The berries ripen in late summer through early fall—gather them when fully ripe, always leaving plenty for the birds.

How to work with it / Medicinal use: Modern studies continue to affirm what herbalists have known for centuries: elderberry is a potent antiviral ally. A 2016 clinical study demonstrated that elderberry extract dramatically reduced the severity and duration of colds—within 48 hours, nearly 90% of patients experienced significant relief (Tiralango, Wee, Lea, 2016). Another study in 2004 showed its effectiveness against Influenza A and B, and research continues today, including investigations into its potential benefits for COVID-19. Elderberry also contains the antiviral compound epicatechin, which has been shown to combat HIV.

The berries are rich in immune-boosting nutrients: vitamins A and C, potassium, folate, calcium, iron, bioflavonoids, and anthocyanins. These compounds stain and mark viral and bacterial invaders in the bloodstream, signaling the immune system to take action. A simple decoction of berries combined with raw local honey, cinnamon, ginger, and cloves makes a delicious and effective elixir. My family and community thrive on this remedy—it has shielded us from the chronic illnesses that once plagued us.

Beyond immune support, elderberry promotes skin health through enhanced microcirculation, helps regulate blood sugar by stimulating insulin release, lowers blood pressure, and supports heart health by reducing oxidative stress and uric acid levels (Arulselvan et al., 2016). It also acts as a mild laxative, helpful for constipation and digestive imbalances such as IBS.

The elderflowers, gathered in spring, offer additional healing gifts—high in flavonols (up to 10 times more than the berries), including quercetin, which helps calm allergic responses. Elderflower tea is a classic remedy for sinusitis, colds, flu, bronchitis, and even seasonal allergies. I love making elderflower cordial to brighten up spring drinks, while bees hum happily around the blooms as I harvest.

Elder also lends itself beautifully to the kitchen and craft. Elderberry wine, vinegars, syrups, and fritters (try battering and frying the flower clusters, dusted with powdered sugar) have been enjoyed for a long time. The hollow branches, once stripped of their soft pith, become beads, straws, whistles, and even tools for tapping birch. Elderberries also produce a rich pink dye.

Caution: The seeds, stems, and unripe berries contain hydrocyanic acid. Consuming large quantities can cause diarrhea or, in rare cases, cyanide poisoning. Always strain berries and remove stems before use.

Healing constituents / Medicinal actions: Elder contains polyphenols (including anthocyanins), flavanols (such as quercetin, kaempferol, and isorhamnetin), vitamin C, phenolic acids, and cyanidin derivatives. Traditionally used as a diuretic, antipyretic, and diaphoretic, modern research supports its anti-diabetic, anticancer, and immune-stimulating actions.

Historical connections: Elderberry's place in human history runs deep. Hippocrates, the father of medicine, called it his *"medicine chest."*

Dioscorides praised it in the *Materia Medica*. Elderberry seeds have even been found in 9,000-year-old archaeological sites—a medicine so ancient, it seems written into our DNA.

Native American tribes greatly valued the elder, using elderflower infusions to treat fevers, bark teas for eczema, and fermented berries to alleviate rheumatism and nerve pain. Elder branches were used to craft sacred pipes and musical instruments; the inner bark was used to treat burns and lesions. Leaves were spread around homes to repel insects.

European folk traditions held the elder in deep reverence and awe. Elderflower tea was used for beauty and cleansing purposes, while elderberry wine and syrup were used to treat colds and flu. Elder wood was also woven into magic and superstition. Cradles were not to be carved from elder wood, lest mischievous fairies steal the child. However, on Midsummer's Eve, standing beneath an elder tree might reveal the Elf-King and his court. Elder was also hung in homes for protection and placed on graves to guide the soul's passage.

Elder's botanical classification has a tangled history. Linnaeus demoted it to an "unornamental" oddity, forcing it into a genus that did not fit. However, no classification can diminish elderberry's place in the human heart and medicine chest. It is timeless, tried-and-true.

Jessica's notes: If a dog is man's best friend, then elderberry must surely be humanity's best plant friend. I feel such gratitude for this extraordinary shrub. Since taking elderberry regularly, my family has remained vibrantly well.

I first came to know elderberry as a young mother living in the country. My adventurous son and I would snack on berries from the shrubs lining our dirt road—thankfully, with no ill effects, though I now know to use caution. Later, when my younger son struggled with febrile seizures, I searched for natural remedies and found elderberry again. A family recipe shared by my mother-in-law became the elderberry elixir we still make and share today.

Elderberry is truly a healer of generations, a protector at the edge of the woods. I am grateful beyond words for its presence in our lives.

An Ode to Elderberry
By Jessica Freeborn

The abundant giver of ancient medicine
Found in folklore to teach us wisdom and lessons.
The berries shield us from viral and bacterial strains.
The flowers infused takes away the pain.
A tablespoon of the syrup each day
Shall keep illnesses at bay.

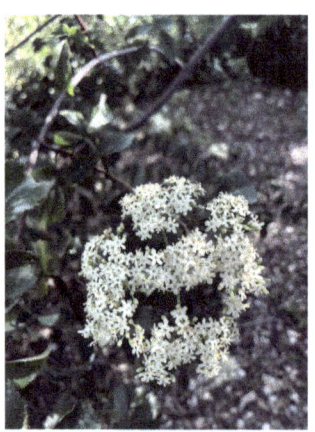

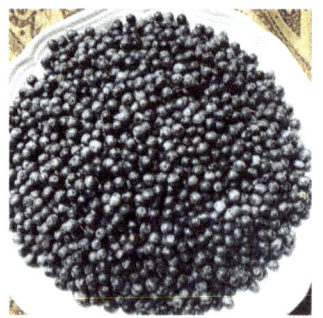

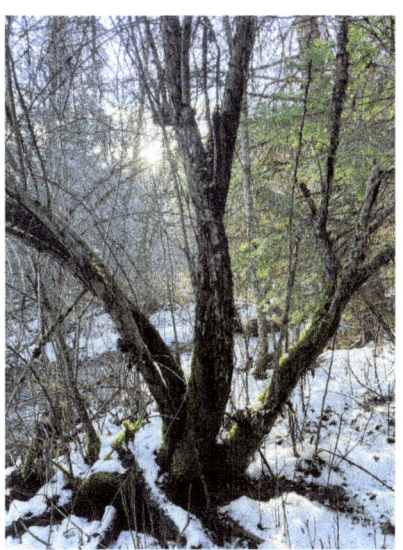

Hawthorn

Crataegus spp.

Rosaceae (Rose) Family
Other common names: English hawthorn, one-seed hawthorn, harthorne, haw, hawthorne

Description: Hawthorn's most striking feature is its ominous, sharp spines—powerful protectors of this ancient tree. It is a deciduous shrub or small tree that can reach heights of up to 50 feet. The crown is often rounded and may have multiple trunks. The bark is dark gray, varying from smooth to grooved or scaly with age. The leaves, about 6 cm long, are deeply lobed and toothed, turning a vibrant yellow in autumn.

In spring, hawthorn bursts forth with flat-topped clusters of highly fragrant flowers—white or occasionally pink—each with five delicate petals. Hawthorn flowers are hermaphroditic, containing both male and female reproductive parts. Once pollinated by insects, these blooms give way to deep-red or bluish-black fruits known as *haws*. The large, pea-sized haws are mealy and semi-sweet, filled with seeds.

Where it grows: Hawthorn can stand alone in fields or prairies, or weave itself into hedgerows and riverbanks. It also grows near springs, creeks, and among other trees, always with a quiet strength, whether solitary or intertwined.

When and how to harvest: Harvest the ripe berries in late summer through early fall. In the spring, gather young leaves and flowers in equal proportions for medicinal purposes.

How to work with it / Medicinal use: Hawthorn is perhaps best known for its gifts to the heart, both physically and emotionally. As a cardiovascular tonic, hawthorn helps prevent heart disease, lowers LDL cholesterol, and regulates blood pressure. Tea or tincture subtly increases coronary artery blood flow, nourishing and oxygenating heart tissue. Like garlic, hawthorn is cardioprotective, guarding against long-term heart disease. Its flavonoids serve as potent antioxidants, preserving cell membranes and enhancing heart resilience.

Hawthorn is also prized for its ability to regulate an erratic heartbeat and lower stress-related blood pressure. It strengthens and supports the aging heart. Herbalist Charles Kane describes hawthorn as one of the best remedies for atherosclerosis, helping to maintain arterial elasticity, stabilize cell membranes, and reduce inflammatory factors.

Hawthorn can also aid digestion when taken as a post-meal cordial. The flavonoids and hyperoxides act as both digestive and cardiovascular tonics.

Beyond its physical effects, hawthorn also mends the emotional heart. It is a gentle nervine that soothes grief, heartache, and stress. "Broken heart syndrome"—a temporary but real cardiac condition caused by grief or shock—can benefit from hawthorn's comforting embrace. A fresh plant tincture offers both emotional and physical support in times of sorrow. Think of hawthorn as an herbal hug—a steadying presence when life feels heavy.

Additionally, hawthorn's flavonoids support venous health, making it useful for varicose veins and other vascular conditions, especially when paired with cardiovascular support.

Caution: Hawthorn should not be combined with pharmaceutical heart medications, especially beta-blockers or drugs for congestive heart failure. Always consult a professional before using hawthorn in these cases.

Healing constituents / Therapeutic actions: Hawthorn contains flavonoids, hyperoxide, vitexin, procyanidins. Therapeutic actions include: anti-inflammatory, antioxidant, nervine, cardioprotective.

Historical connections: The Old English word *haw* means hedge—a fitting name, as hawthorn was traditionally planted to mark boundaries. Its fierce thorns created natural fences, protecting homesteads and fields.

Hawthorn has a long medicinal history in Chinese, Native American, and European traditions, where it has been used for heart and vascular health since Roman times. It was also a symbol of love and marriage in ancient Rome. Hawthorn's flowering in May earned it the names Maythorn, May, and thorn apple. Maypoles for Beltane were traditionally crafted from hawthorn, and the *Mayflower* ship, arriving in America in 1620, was named in its honor, symbolizing hope for new beginnings.

Folklore around hawthorn is rich. Some believed that cutting hawthorn branches brought bad luck, while others hung them to repel witches. Wands and broomsticks were often crafted from hawthorn wood. In the Language of Flowers, hawthorn symbolizes hope, love, intimacy, and marriage.

A delightful bit of folklore claims that if you sleep under a hawthorn tree, you may be transported to the faerie realm, for hawthorn is a guardian of the fae.

Jessica's notes: Hawthorn is the plant said to heal a broken heart. Years ago, while swimming with the Freeborn family in the Spokane River, we stumbled upon red and blue hawthorns along the riverbank. I joyfully harvested the berries, drying them for winter.

One cold, gray winter day, feeling a bit down for no particular reason, I brewed a tea from those hawthorn berries, along with white pine needles and St. John's wort. After a few sips, my mood lifted dramatically—I felt joyful and energized, and soon found myself humming and happily organizing the house.

I am grateful to have wild-harvested hawthorn on hand for those darker winter days. The power of plants, indeed, never ceases to amaze me.

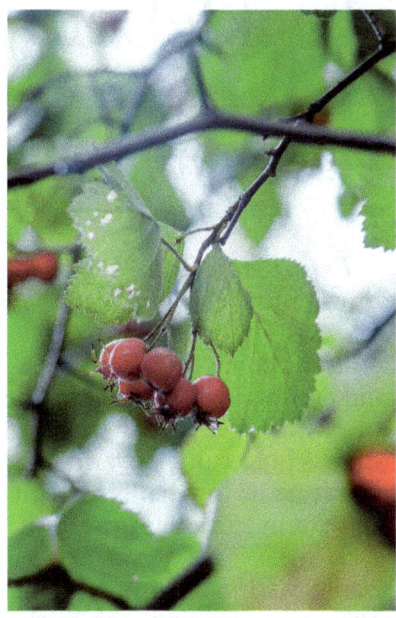

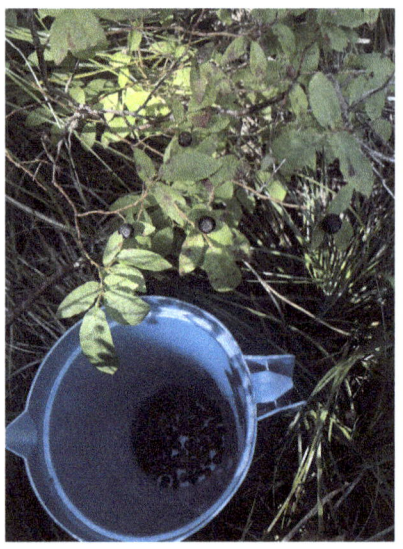

Huckleberry

Vaccinium spp.

Ericaceae (Heath) Family

Other common names: Blueberry, Bilberry, Grouse berry, Grouse Whortleberry

Description: Vacciniums come in various sizes—from ankle-height dwarfs to knee-high and even waist-high shrubs. The larger huckleberries grow as spreading shrubs with ridged branches and light blue-green foliage. Their oval leaves crisscross gracefully, hovering parallel to the ground. These shrubs provide a feast of low-hanging fruit for birds, squirrels, chipmunks, and bears, who in turn help spread the seeds through their droppings.

The smaller dwarf varieties form charming colonies of dark green, tangled branchlets, with younger stems tinged an earthy red. The prized oval berries are deep blue, each marked with a tiny, round, sunken scar at its crown.

Where it grows: Huckleberries thrive in acidic soils, often tucked beneath the protective shade of towering trees where the ground remains moist. The dwarf varieties love the deep, undisturbed shade of old-growth forests, forming sprawling colonies. The larger huckleberries, however, flourish in open spaces after forest clearing, logging, or fires, where new sunlight encourages their growth.

When and how to harvest: Harvest ripe berries in mid-to-late summer, savoring their abundance. Leaves can be gathered in summer through early fall while they remain green and vibrant. To gauge the potency of the leaves, taste a sample—the best medicinal leaves leave a tart, blueberry-tinged aftertaste on the tongue.

How to work with it / Medicinal use: Huckleberries are the jewels of the northern forest—nutritious, immune-boosting, and a true wild delicacy. Unlike cultivated berries, they cannot be farmed; they thrive only in their natural habitat. Both berries and leaves are rich in vitamin C, while the foliage also offers beta-carotene and beneficial carbohydrates. The berries are brimming with antioxidants and resveratrol, supporting immune resilience and overall vitality.

Harvesting huckleberries—especially the dwarf varieties—is a labor of love. I have found the best approach is to settle comfortably on the forest floor and harvest from a seated position. The berries are irresistible fresh from the bush, but those you manage to save can be frozen, canned, or dried for later use.

In the kitchen, huckleberries elevate pies, smoothies, kombucha, lemonade, iced teas, vinegars, fruit leathers, and countless other delights. The leaves, once dried, make a delicious and nourishing tea or tincture that can help flush the bladder and kidneys, soothe urinary tract infections, and support overall well-being. The flavor is bright and pleasant—perfect for sipping anytime.

Healing constituents / Therapeutic actions: Huckleberry leaves: vitamin C, beta-carotene, carbohydrates; actions: astringent, antiseptic, appetite-stimulating. Berries: vitamin C, resveratrol, antioxidants, immunostimulants.

Historical connections: Huckleberries have long captured human hearts. In the Northwest, Native Americans deeply revered this plant. The berries, rich in vitamin C, were dried for winter use and traded among tribes. The Yakama people tell a beautiful creation story about the origin of the huckleberry. In this tale, the Creator made the world from his own body. Realizing the mountains lacked berries, he sacrificed his eyes, planting them in the earth. From the veins of his eyes, roots formed, and the first huckleberries sprouted—gifts from the Creator's very sight.

The name "huckleberry" itself comes from a simple linguistic twist. According to Henry David Thoreau, early European colonists mistook the native berry for their familiar European *hurtleberry*—derived from the Saxon "hart's berry." Over time, *hurtleberry* became *huckleberry*, the name we use today.

Jessica's notes: Huckleberries are a treasured delicacy of the northern forest. Gathering them has become a beloved family tradition. Every late summer, we venture out to fill our baskets, always saving enough to bake a celebratory cobbler. We freeze extra berries, tucking them away like little bits of summer sunshine to brighten the cold months of fall and winter.

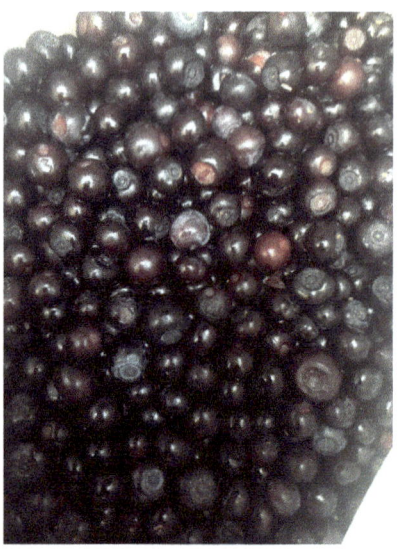

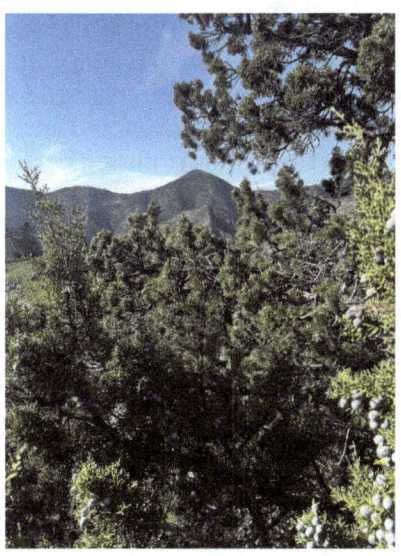

Juniper

Juniperus communis

Cupressaceae (Cypress) Family

Description: Common juniper is an evergreen conifer with remarkable longevity, capable of living up to 200 years. It is a plant of many forms—sometimes growing as a low, sprawling shrub, other times as a stately tree reaching up to 35 feet tall. It is easily identified by its needles, which persist year-round and grow in whorls of three around the ridged twigs. Each needle bears a pale band on top and a greenish-gray underside. The bark is brownish-gray, peeling with age, while young twigs are a reddish-brown.

Juniper is dioecious, meaning it has separate male and female plants. Males produce small yellow globes in the leaf axils, while females bear green structures that, once pollinated, mature into the well-known aromatic berry-like cones—green when young, ripening to deep blue or purple-black over a two-year cycle. These berries are beloved by birds, who aid in their distribution across the landscape.

Where it grows: Common juniper favors rocky, well-drained soils, chalky lowlands, and old-growth pine woodlands.

When and how to harvest: Gather ripe berries in late summer and early fall. Harvest the most fragrant, fresh needles when new growth appears.

How to work with it / Medicinal use: Juniper has a long-standing and well-established reputation for supporting urinary tract and bladder health. Across diverse cultures, it has been used to treat urinary infections and soothe painful urination. Its stimulant and antiseptic properties help eradicate fungal and bacterial strains from the bladder lining. An alcohol extract (tincture) or a berry/needle tea is traditionally used to support urinary function and relieve discomfort associated with chronic cystitis.

Rich in antioxidants and anti-inflammatory compounds, juniper is also an effective carminative. Several ounces of tea or 30-40 drops of tincture can ease indigestion, bloating, and gas. Topically, juniper preparations are soothing for chronic inflammatory skin conditions such as psoriasis and eczema and can help relieve sore muscles and aching joints when used in salves or balms.

In the kitchen, juniper's tannin-rich berries shine. Add them to pickles or fermented vegetables to maintain crispness, or include them in meat brines to deepen flavor. Their bright, piney essence adds a distinctive wild character to culinary creations.

Healing constituents / Therapeutic actions: Juniper contains abundant volatile oils, including monoterpenes (limonene, camphor, beta-pinene), flavonoids, and potent antioxidants. Therapeutic actions include anti-inflammatory, anticancer, antibacterial, carminative, and antiseptic.

Caution: Juniper is not to be used during pregnancy, as its volatile oils can stimulate uterine contractions. Avoid internal use if chronic kidney inflammation is present.

Historical connections: Juniper's medicinal and spiritual value spans millennia. It was revered in Ancient Egypt—juniper berries have been found in tombs, including that of King Tutankhamen. The Romans valued the berries as a substitute for pepper.

North American Indigenous tribes developed a profound connection with juniper. The Apache used it to ease seizures, treat colds and coughs, and aid childbirth. The Cree turned to juniper to reduce fevers, fight lung infections and toothaches, and soothe kidney pain. The Inupiat believed that eating a ripe juniper berry daily could prevent colds and flu. Numerous other tribes, including the Delaware, Cheyenne, Paiute, and Nlaka'pamux, utilized juniper as a gynecological aid to relax muscles, support childbirth, or prevent conception. Traditional uses extended further still, addressing hangovers, stomach pain, STDs, heartburn, vertigo, wounds, ulcers, burns, and even so-called "insanity."

Jessica's notes: Juniper is a beloved ally in my plant medicine chest. The first time I harvested it was a moment I will never forget. Jason and I were exploring the National Forest behind my grandparents' land in Goldendale, Washington, when we stumbled upon a grand old juniper tree, standing tall and alone, having survived a wildfire. Its dark blue berries were abundant, and we joyfully gathered them. At the time, I was perfecting a pickle recipe for Cultured Mama at Pilgrim's Market. Inspired by that juniper tree, I added the berries to my brine to keep the pickles crisp—and it worked! The flavor was incredible. That evening, we brewed an after-dinner juniper tea and shared it with our tribe of cousins, who were astonished that such delicious tea had come from berries we had foraged on their land.

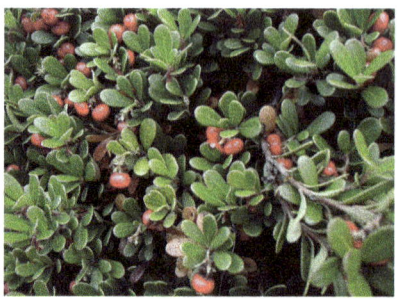

Kinnikinnick

Arctostaphylos uva-ursi

Ericaceae (Heath) Family

Other common names: Uva Ursi, Bearberry, Stone Berry, Meal Berry, Mountain Tobacco, Upland Cranberry, Bear Grapes

Description: Kinnikinnick is an evergreen perennial shrub that forms lush, spreading mats across the forest floor, adding a sense of timeless greenery to the landscape. Its alternate leaves, round-tipped and tapered at the base, grow on twisted stalks along creeping stems. Oval to spoon-shaped, the leaves have a waxy surface that gives them a glossy sheen—dark green on top, lighter green underneath—while tiny hairs line the midrib and edges. In mid-spring through early summer, dainty pink urn-shaped flowers bloom in fuzzy-bracted clusters at the ends of stems, drawing pollinators such as hummingbirds, bees, and butterflies. Come late summer, the plant produces bright-red, miniature apple-like berries that persist through the winter, providing color and sustenance when the forest is otherwise sparse. This dwarf ground cover rarely grows taller than 6 inches. Interestingly, it secretes compounds into the surrounding soil that inhibit the growth of neighboring plants—a natural means of securing its place in the ecosystem.

Where it grows: Kinnikinnick is widespread across North America and commonly found throughout the Inland Northwest. It thrives in rocky soils and exposed areas, often found on dry hillsides and in open pine forests.

When and how to harvest: Gather the evergreen leaves from mid-spring to early fall. Harvest the berries when they are fully ripe, from late summer into late fall.

How to work with it / Medicinal use: Kinnikinnick is a time-honored remedy for urinary tract infections (UTIs). The leaves contain astringent compounds that promote urination, making the bladder environment less hospitable to bacteria such as Escherichia coli, the most common cause of lower urinary tract infections (UTIs). Pairing a leaf tea with a pint of unsweetened cranberry juice is an excellent acute treatment. This combination helps prevent bacteria from adhering to the bladder walls.

For yeast infections or vaginal inflammation, a kinnikinnick-infused vaginal douche can bring relief. Similarly, an afterbirth sitz bath infused with the leaves can prevent postpartum inflammation and reduce bleeding.

Topically, kinnikinnick makes an effective wash for healing cuts, scrapes, and abrasions. In Native American tradition, it is also a ceremonial plant of great importance, often added to smoking blends to purify the lungs and body.

Healing constituents / Therapeutic actions: Kinnikinnick's active compounds include hydroquinone and glycosides, particularly arbutin and methyl arbutin. These constituents contribute anti-inflammatory and antiseptic properties and are excreted through the urine, where they can directly affect the bladder and urinary tract.

Historical connections: The name "Kinnikinnick" is derived from an Algonquin word meaning "smoking mixture." For generations, Native Americans and early pioneers dried and smoked this plant. Merriwether Lewis, in his 1806 journal, called it "tasteless and insipid"—likely because he sampled a fresh

berry, which sweetens when dried.

The Okanogan-Colville tribe utilized the berries more creatively, cooking them with venison and salmon and drying them into cakes for winter storage. Medicinally, Uva Ursi has long been used for urinary tract issues—its reputation as a healing ally is well-deserved and time-tested.

Jessica's notes: I first learned about Uva Ursi working at the health food store. It was often an ingredient in the bladder health supplements we would sell. My customers have reported positive results with Uva Ursi, combined with cranberry extract, in combating urinary tract infections. Another aha moment when I found it growing wild rather than sitting on a shelf in a plastic bottle. Its resilience and evergreen presence remind me that God's medicine is abundant and free.

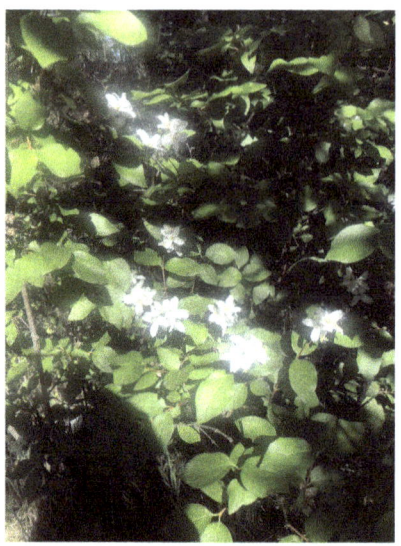

Lewis' Mock Orange

Philadelphus lewisii

Hydrangeaceae (Hydrangea) Family
Other common names: Western Syringa
Description: An elegant, erect deciduous shrub, Lewis' mock orange grows between 3 and 10 feet tall, with arching, spreading branches. Its dark green leaves are opposite, 1 to 2 ¾ inches long, with three prominent veins, fine hairs, and fringed edges. The showy, fragrant white flowers—about 1 ¼ inches across—bloom at the branch tips in clusters of 3 to 11 from May through July. Their sweet scent, reminiscent of orange blossoms, gives this plant its common name, "mock orange." Small woody capsules, about ¼ to 3/8 inches long, follow the flowers and contain the fruit.
Where it grows: Lewis' mock orange prefers well-drained but moist soils and is often found along streams, rivers, and creeks.
When and how to harvest: Harvest the leaves in spring to early summer. Branches can be respectfully gathered from spring through summer.
How to work with it / Medicinal use: Though not widely used in modern herbalism, Lewis' mock orange has a long tradition of medicinal use, especially among Native American peoples. It was primarily valued for topical applications. The fresh leaves were crushed and applied as a poultice

for breast infections and sore breasts. Dried, powdered leaves or charcoal made from the wood were mixed with bear grease or pine pitch to create healing salves for wounds, sores, and swellings.

A tea made from the branches was used to soothe sore chests and respiratory congestion. This same tea also served as a topical wash for eczema and as a remedy to reduce hemorrhoid bleeding.

Mock orange is also a natural soap, rich in saponins, the flowers and leaves lather when crushed with water, providing an effective way to remove dirt and oil from the skin.

Beyond its medicinal virtues, the hardwood of mock orange was traditionally crafted into valuable household items, including combs, knitting needles, cradle hoods, and basket rims.

Though this plant has fallen out of everyday herbal use today, I believe it holds untapped potential and value, one of the many native plants whose wisdom is worth remembering and reviving.

Therapeutic actions / Healing constituents: Philadelphus lewisii contains saponins. Historically, it has been used as an antiseptic, anti-inflammatory, and astringent, though little modern research has been conducted on this American native.

Historical connections: On June 10, 1806, Meriwether Lewis recorded this plant near present-day Clearwater, Idaho, during the westward expedition. At first, he confused it with sevenbark (*Hydrangea arborescens*) due to the similarity of its branches during early growth. However, on July 4th of that year, while observing it in bloom, he correctly identified it as "western syringa" and sent samples back to England. English botanist Frederick Pursh later named the species *Philadelphus lewisii* in honor of Lewis.

The genus name *Philadelphus* is thought to reference King Ptolemy Philadelphus of Egypt (285–246 BCE), a lover of gardens, and fittingly, *Philadelphus* means "brotherly love."

This attractive Rocky Mountain shrub quickly gained popularity as an ornamental in English gardens. For Native American tribes, it was a functional riverside medicine. Easily accessible near water, it served as a practical remedy for treating rope burns, cuts, and scrapes sustained while fishing, canoeing, and traveling by water. Its strong wood was prized for crafting tools and everyday objects.

Jessica's notes: I first discovered *Philadelphus lewisii* by scent on a hot summer day while exploring the Spokane River—land once traversed by Lewis and Clark. The flowers' intoxicating fragrance drew me in. With my well-worn copy of *Edible and Medicinal Plants of the Rockies* by Linda Kershaw in hand, I quickly confirmed that it was indeed Lewis' mock orange. As an American patriot and lover of these wild western lands, the botanical history of this plant resonates deeply with me. It feels fitting that Lewis' mock orange is Idaho's state flower—graceful, strong, and rooted in the history of this place I call home.

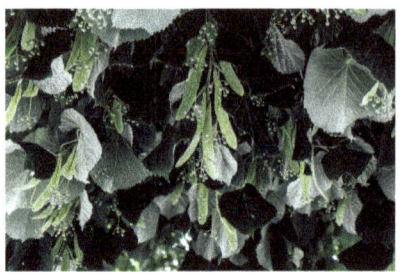

Linden

Tilia cordata

Malvaceae (Mallow) Family
Other common names: Basswood, Lime Tree
Description: The large, beautiful Linden is a slow-growing, long-lived deciduous tree, reaching heights of up to 65 feet and capable of thriving for hundreds of years—some specimens living as long as 1,000 years. Its heart-shaped leaves, coarsely toothed and dark green above with a lighter lime green underside, are typically no more than 3 inches long. In early summer, clusters of fragrant, creamy flowers bloom, filling the air with a sweet scent that often leads the nose to the tree before the eyes spot it.

The small, globular fruits hang beneath narrow leafy bracts, fluttering like ribbons in the breeze. Linden is remarkably resilient, with an impressive ability to regenerate—if the wind breaks its upper limbs, the tree seals the wound and continues to grow.

Where it grows: Linden is a tree beloved by humans—it is often planted in parks, towns, and along streets. Sometimes, it escapes cultivation and grows on the edges of wild places or in the ruins of old settlements, where it was once a community centerpiece.

When and how to harvest: Harvest the leaves and flowers in summer. The bark can be harvested respectfully from spring through summer.

How to work with it / Medicinal use: Linden is a gentle yet powerful medicine for both heart and mind. The leaves and flowers are cooling, moistening, and soothing—ideal for inflamed or overheated tissues. Linden tea or tincture acts as a relaxing nervine, calming the nervous system and easing tension, making it suitable for both children and elders.

As an antispasmodic, Linden helps relax muscles and can relieve stress-induced hypertension and muscle tension. Its demulcent and astringent properties soothe the digestive tract, making it an excellent remedy for diarrhea, indigestion, and stomach upset. It is also helpful for easing painful menstrual cramps.

A warm cup of Linden tea can bring comfort during colds, flu, and fevers, thanks to its ability to promote perspiration and reduce body heat. The flowers, infused in honey, make a delicious throat remedy for sore throats and coughs.

Nutritionally, the leaves and flowers are rich in vitamin C and protein. They can be ground into flour, a common practice during World War II when resources were scarce. The leaves can also be sautéed or steamed as a nutritious addition to a green salad. Linden bark aids digestion, supporting bile flow and fat metabolism. Externally, Linden makes a soothing wash or compress for wounds, cuts, and irritated skin. A calming bath with Linden and red clover is a beautiful way to soothe restless babies and children. Linden also pairs wonderfully with Hawthorn to support cardiovascular health. Beyond its medicinal virtues, Linden wood is strong and versatile, used for many industrial and artistic purposes.

Healing constituents / Therapeutic actions: Linden contains caffeic acid, tannins, volatile oils, flavonoids, polysaccharides, benzodiazepine-like compounds, vitamin C, protein, and mucilage. Its therapeutic actions include antispasmodic, sedative, nervine, vasodilator, and diuretic.

Historical connections: Linden's relationship with humanity runs deep. For millennia, it was planted in village centers, near courthouses, hospitals, and sacred spaces. In Celtic and Germanic traditions, it was known as the "Tree of Justice," under whose shade truth was spoken and disputes were resolved. Eastern cultures also honored it as the Tree of Justice. Pliny the Elder praised Linden bark vinegar for its healing effects on skin ailments more than 2,000 years ago. The bark was also valued for making string, rope, and even the handles of magical wands. Its wood has long been favored for intricate carvings, instruments, and ceremonial objects. In early European villages, Linden trees served as communal gathering places for weddings, spring festivals, and celebrations of life. During the French Revolution, over 60,000 Linden trees were planted as symbols of liberty and hope. Linden flour sustained families during wartime shortages, and Linden branches were once carried to ward off disease. In the Middle Ages, these trees were planted outside hospitals, believed to purify the air. Linden's comforting presence in both rural villages and bustling cities reflects the deep reverence humans have held for it throughout time.

Jessica's notes: Lovely Linden—called the "doctor tree," the tree of love, the feminine tree, and the tree of light—belongs in this book, even if it often grows closer to civilization than in the wild. This tree teaches us how closely humanity depends on sacred plants. We have planted Lindens wherever we have built homes and towns, and even when the ruins of civilization fade, these trees remain, reminding us of our roots. Sometimes, we do not need to venture deep into the wilderness to find food and medicine—often, the ancient Linden grows quietly in an old churchyard or along an abandoned road.

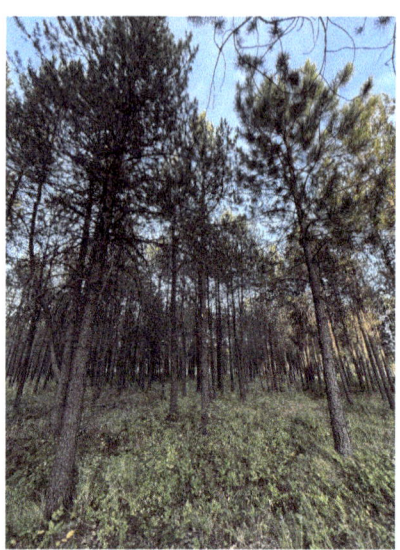

Lodgepole Pine

Pinus contorta

Pinaceae (Pine) Family

Description: A common and stalwart evergreen of the West, lodgepole pine grows up to 80 feet tall. Its brown to blackish bark is thin and scaly, while the tree itself often takes on a twisted, gnarled appearance along lakeshores and windswept ridges—a trait that inspired its botanical name, *contorta*. The needles, which come in pairs, are semicylindrical, twisted, and range in length from 1.5 to 7.5 centimeters. Pinecones, 3 to 5 centimeters in length, cling tightly to the branches, often remaining closed for years, opening only with the heat of summer or wildfire to release their seeds—a reminder of this species' incredible resilience.

Where it grows: Lodgepole pine is one of the most common trees of the West, forming dense stands on rocky ridges, woodlands, and sandy soils. It is among the first to return and reclaim land after forest fires, quickly dominating and restoring the landscape.

When and how to harvest: Harvest the inner bark, needles, pitch, and twigs ideally in the spring, but they can be gathered year-round as needed. When harvesting bark, please remove it from branches rather than the trunk to minimize damage to the tree.

How to work with it / Healing use: Pine offers powerful medicine, carrying antifungal, antimicrobial, and antiseptic properties. The needles and pitch can be prepared as poultices, oils, salves, or creams to heal wounds, cuts, abrasions, acne, eczema, and boils. A wash of pine can soothe sores and aid healing, while liniments or salves ease aching joints and arthritis.

The needles and pitch also make a soothing tea or steam inhalation for respiratory congestion. Their expectorant and camphoraceous qualities make pine valuable for lung infections such as pneumonia, whooping cough, tuberculosis, and croup. A tea made from vitamin C-rich needles and pitch could truly be lifesaving in a survival situation.

The nutrient-dense inner cambium, rich in starch, sugar, beta-carotene, and vitamin C, can be sliced thinly and eaten raw for energy or boiled and added to soups and stews. Pine pitch is also a remarkable splinter remedy—when applied to the skin, it can draw the splinter out.

For culinary creativity, Beverly Gray shares in *The Boreal Herbal* that when she ran out of pine nuts, she used pine inner bark in her pesto instead and loved the result so much that she has never gone back!

Pine, as a flower essence, helps those who are self-critical and burdened by guilt, offering a gentle reminder to release the weight of self-blame and stand tall in their truth.

Beyond its medicinal uses, pine serves countless practical purposes. Its tall, straight trunks earned it the name "lodgepole," as it was historically used for teepee poles and fort-building. Pine needles infused in vinegar or prepared as a decoction make excellent natural cleaners for the home. Diluted, the solution is perfect for floors and furniture, and the aromatic properties of pine can refresh the weary mind and calm nervous fatigue.

If you forget a toothbrush on a backpacking trip, you can even use a small pine twig: peel back the bark and gently scrub your teeth and gums with it—a perfect wild-crafted alternative!

Pine reminds us to remain rooted in truth and stand firm through storms and turbulent times, offering both protection and medicine to the forest and its people.

Healing constituents / Therapeutic actions: Lodgepole pine contains beta-carotene, vitamin C, sugar, and starch. Its therapeutic actions include antiseptic, antimicrobial, antifungal, expectorant, camphoraceous, and aromatic.

Caution: Take pine tea in moderation; the resins can accumulate in the system. Avoid internal use during pregnancy.

Historical connections: Considered a tree of peace, the pine has long been a vital ally to the First Nations and northern tribes. Native Americans relied on *Pinus contorta* for food, medicine, and shelter. They used it to treat ailments such as rheumatism, sore throats, colds, tuberculosis, and gonorrhea, as well as to serve as an emergency food source for both humans and horses. The slender, straight trunks were used for teepee frames, while early European settlers adopted lodgepole pine for lumber, cabin construction, fencing, and firewood.

The great naturalist John Muir once wrote, "Between every two pines is a doorway to a new world."

Jessica's notes: Lodgepole pines were the first to welcome me to Idaho, standing tall in the Welsh Woods on my parents' land. Jason and I spent our first Idaho summer tending to the lodgepoles, cleaning the forest floor. Now, years later, they have grown ever taller and straighter. When life feels scattered and my mind is restless, a walk through these serene woods helps me regain clarity and strength.

I have spent countless hours tending burn piles of lodgepole pine, stewarding the land, and harvesting the gifts these trees offer. Pine provides warmth in our campfires and medicine in our lives—drawing out splinters, soothing a cold, or simply offering the peace of a forest walk beneath their protective canopy. I am endlessly grateful for this mighty and generous tree.

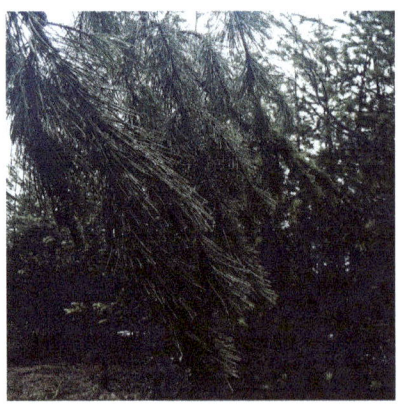

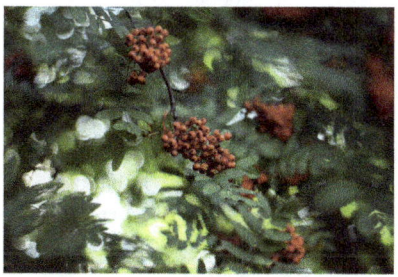

Mountain Ash

Sorbus scopulina

Rosaceae (Rose) Family
Other common names: Rowan, western mountain ash
Description: Mountain ash is a deciduous shrub or small tree, growing up to 20 feet tall with smooth, shiny, greyish bark. The dark green, glossy leaves are pinnately compound, typically with nine to twelve serrated leaflets arranged alternately along slender branches. The Rowan tree bears a resemblance to the elder with its compound leaves and showy clusters of white flowers. However, one can tell them apart easily—Rowan leaves, when crushed, release a distinctly unpleasant odor, unlike the fragrant elder.

As a proud member of the rose family, mountain ash produces brilliant berries resembling tiny apples. The fruits ripen from jack-o-lantern orange to a fiery red that glows against the stark winter landscape. The bright berries remain through the cold months, providing a vital food source for birds and other wildlife when little else is available.

Where it grows: An ally of the old-growth forest, mountain ash favors conifer woodlands, mountain valleys, and foothills. It is a resilient presence among towering pines and firs, thriving in wild and windswept places.

When and how to harvest: Harvest the berries after the first frost. The cold sweetens them, setting the sugars and starches, and making them less sour. The bright clusters can be gathered and preserved for later use.

How to work with it / Medicinal use: These jewel-like berries are rich in vitamins A and C, flavonoids, tannins, and pectin—a wild apple's cousin in both lineage and nutrition. There are many creative ways to enjoy their bounty. After harvesting, the berries can be frozen, used to make wine, or infused into liqueurs. One of our favorite preparations is a wild game chutney made with ginger, orange, hawthorn berries, rosehips, and other wild autumn fruits—a perfect companion to roasted meats.

Mountain ash berries also lend themselves beautifully to jellies, cranberry sauces, tomato-based sauces, and even sweets. In ancient traditions, they were used to craft Turkish Delight, a fitting treat for a berry steeped in enchantment.

Medicinally, mountain ash berries have long been used to ease stomach pain and bleeding. The leaves were historically used to treat sore eyes, rheumatism, asthma, and colds. Though little modern research has been done, the berries' rich tannins and flavonoids suggest antioxidant, astringent, and diuretic properties.

Mountain ash is a hard, elastic wood prized for crafting and historically used for tools and bows—a project I look forward to trying myself someday.

Caution: The berries can cause stomach irritation if consumed in large quantities. Avoid during pregnancy.

Healing constituents / Therapeutic actions: Mountain ash berries contain saponins, vitamins A and C, flavonoids, tannins, and pectin. Their therapeutic actions are likely astringent, antioxidant, and diuretic.

Historical connections: The Rowan tree, as it is called across the British Isles, is steeped in rich folklore and magic. Throughout Celtic and Norse tradition, Rowan was revered as a protector against enchantment and malevolent forces. Its five-pointed, pentagram-shaped flowers and vibrant red berries—considered the color of protection—contributed to its mystical reputation. An old English rhyme tells us: *"Rowan tree and red thread / make the witches tine their speed."* The tree is also beloved in fairy lore and associated with the goddesses. Its tannin-rich leaves were used in the tanning process, and its strong, elastic wood has been crafted into countless tools. In Scandinavia, rowan trees that grow in craggy rock faces—called "flying rowans"—were considered especially powerful and were harvested for the making of rune staves used in divination. In Norse mythology, Rowan saved the life of the god Thor by bending its branches over the river of the Underworld, offering him a lifeline when he was nearly swept away. Truly a tree of resilience and magic. Historically, mountain ash berries were valued as an accompaniment to wild game, much as we still enjoy them today.

Jessica's notes: Mountain ash is a tree of legend, mystery, and resilience—one I always seek out in the fall when the forest begins its slow descent into winter. The clusters of red berries against the bare branches remind me that nature provides nourishment and beauty even in the coldest season. I enjoy watching the birds feast on the bright orange berries and gather greenery for their winter nests. I want to try making a wild chutney with mountain ash berries to accompany our fall harvest feasts. It is always a comforting delight to crack into a jar of wild preserves in the dead of winter.

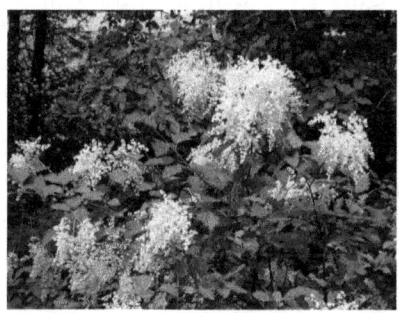

Ocean Spray

Holodiscus discolor

Rosaceae (Rose) Family
Other common names: mountain spray, cream bush, California spiraea, meadowsweet, ironwood

Description: This common forest shrub can grow up to ten feet tall. Copious sprays of white flowers adorn the bush, and as they sway in the wind, they resemble foaming ocean waves—hence the name. The reddish-gray peeling bark is one of Ocean Spray's distinctive characteristics. The light green leaves are soft, plush, and finely haired, slightly lobed with several secondary teeth, and alternate along the stems. The leaves fall to the ground in autumn. Ocean spray blooms from late spring to midsummer, producing cream-colored, five-petaled, tiny flowers arranged in terminal clusters that droop gracefully from the ends of the stems. After pollination, these floral clusters turn brown and often remain on the bush throughout the winter. One-seeded fruits ripen from mid to late summer.

Where it grows: A highly adaptable plant, ocean spray thrives in both sunny and shaded forested areas across western North America. It grows abundantly in the northwest forests.

When and how to harvest: Harvest the leaves and stem bark from mid-spring to early fall. The flowers are best gathered in summer when they are in full bloom.

How to work with it/ Medicinal use: Like other members of the rose family, ocean spray's astringent properties help soothe and tone inflamed or lax tissues. Although seldom used by modern herbalists today, ocean spray holds many valuable traditional medicinal uses. The flowers and leaves can be brewed into tea to help alleviate diarrhea and treat symptoms of the flu and influenza. A leaf poultice can be applied to soothe sore lips and aching feet. A berry tea or seed infusion was traditionally used to support the body in fighting chickenpox and smallpox, as well as for general blood purification. The leaf or bark tea was also used for postpartum care.

Blossom infusions or inner bark teas can serve as gentle eye rinses. Topically, dried and powdered leaves or powdered bark, when mixed with oil, can be applied to burns and wounds. On an emotional level, ocean spray flower essence can help release long-held grief, encouraging one to live with a renewed sense of joy and presence.

The wood of ocean spray is another gift of this plant—dense, challenging, and fire-resistant, it is excellent for crafting tools, walking sticks, and furniture.

Healing constituents/ Therapeutic actions: Although little clinical research has been conducted on ocean spray, its traditional uses suggest that it has therapeutic actions, including astringent, demulcent, and anti-inflammatory properties.

Historical connections: Many Native American tribes had diverse uses for ocean spray. The Lummi tribe of Washington used the blossoms for diarrhea, the inner bark as an eyewash, and leaf poultices for sore lips and feet. The Makah prepared bark decoctions for athletes and convalescents. The Chehalis used seed infusions for smallpox, black measles, and chickenpox. The Navajo and Ramah people used leaf decoctions to treat influenza. The Okanagan-Colville mixed dried and powdered bark with animal fat or oil as a burn dressing, while the Sanpoil used powdered leaves for sores. The Squaxin used the seeds as a blood purifier.

Beyond medicine, many tribes valued ocean spray for its sturdy wood. The branches were used as tongs, for arrows and bows, fishing hooks, digging sticks, walking sticks, drum hoops, toys, teepee post holders, and various tools—a true multipurpose plant of the forest.

Jessica's notes: I hope this book reconnects people to these often-forgotten wild plant medicines and inspires us to work with them in traditional ways once again. Ocean spray is so abundant—it engulfs the low woodlands with a perennial sea of foamy white flowers. Knowing its value in Native American tradition and recognizing its astringent properties as a member of the rose family deepens my respect for this beautiful shrub. Ocean spray wood is tough and practical—Jason has carved walking sticks and other tools from it. Its presence in the forest reminds us that even the most common plants hold ancient wisdom and gifts for those who take the time to learn their ways.

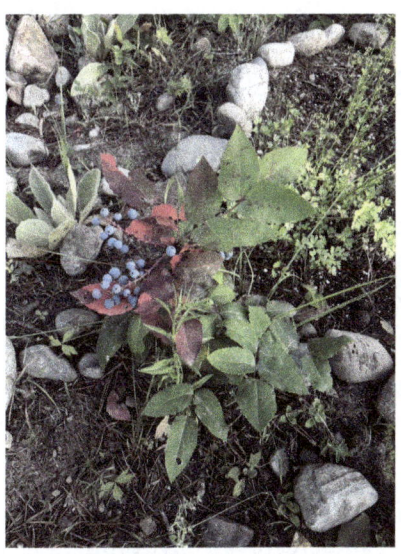

Oregon Grape Root

Berberis / Mahonia spp.

Berberidaceae (Barberry) Family

Other common names: Cascade barberry, dwarf or dull Oregon grape

Description: This spiky-leaved perennial spreads across the forest floor through rhizomes and often forms dense stands. The woody rhizomes grow laterally just beneath the soil's surface. The holly-like leaves are alternately arranged, pinnately compound, and grow in tufts of 9 to 19 leaflets along woody stems. Leaves are glossy, dark green, oval to lance-shaped, with spiny, rough, saw-toothed edges. Bracted, yellow-flowered clusters grow up to 8 inches long and rise above the foliage. Each flower is made up of three greenish-yellow bracts, six brilliant yellow sepals, and six bright yellow, two-lobed petals arranged in five whorls of three. Flowers bloom in early spring, ripening into purplish-blue berries by early summer. The berries, which contain large black seeds, are quite sour. The inner bark of the rhizomes is bright orange-yellow, while the outer bark is yellowish-brown. The evergreen leaves take on shades of orange to red in the fall.

This entry includes all species of *Mahonia* commonly found in the mountain states. Some, such as *M. aquifolium*, grow taller and larger, while dwarf varieties like *M. repens* remain closer to the ground.

Where it grows: Oregon grape is shade-tolerant and typically found in mixed evergreen forests, often growing under pine trees.

When and how to harvest: Harvest the rhizomes from non-flowering plants from mid-spring to late summer. The ripe berries are ready to gather in summer.

How to work with it/ Medicinal use: The roots, stems, and leaves of this plant contain high levels of berberine, a bright yellow, bitter alkaloid known for its potent antimicrobial properties. Both ancient and modern herbalists prize Oregon grape as a powerful aid for fighting infection, used both topically and internally. Berberine also stimulates bile production, making this an effective remedy for liver and digestive disorders. Oregon grape is an excellent, sustainable alternative to goldenseal, a threatened species due to overharvesting.

Prepare a decoction or tincture for respiratory support—Oregon grape is safe for children and works wonderfully in a cough syrup. It helps remove waste from the blood and creates an environment less hospitable to bacteria and pathogens in the microbiome. Oregon grape tincture can be used to treat internal infections such as Giardia, Staph, and Salmonella. It also stimulates the liver, purifies the blood, and removes damp heat. Take the tincture for food allergies, grogginess upon waking, or a sluggish, stagnant liver—conditions that often manifest as skin problems, such as psoriasis, eczema, acne, or fungal infections like athlete's foot, ringworm, and jock itch.

In line with the Doctrine of Signatures, the yellow, bile-colored inner rhizome signals its ability to stimulate digestive juices and support bitter tonic actions. Taken before meals, Oregon grape can help improve digestion, aid in breaking down fats and oils, and enhance nutrient absorption.

Topically, it can be used as a balm, ointment, or oil infusion to treat fungal infections and itchy skin conditions—making it excellent for diaper rash, athlete's foot, and jock itch. Though the berries are extremely sour, they can be combined with other wild berries to create vinegars, wines, or jellies.

Healing constituents/ Therapeutic actions: The primary bioactive constituents in Oregon grape root are isoquinoline alkaloids. Alongside the primary yellow alkaloid, berberine, the roots and foliage also contain berbamine, oxyacanthine, and oxyberberine, as well as additional compounds such as canadine, mahonine, magnoflorine, and jatrorrhizine. Therapeutic actions include hepatotropic, bitter tonic, and blood cleanser.

Historical connections: On February 12, 1806, Meriwether Lewis documented "Mountain Holly," now identified as *Mahonia aquifolium*, after gathering a sample near the Columbia River Gorge. Native American tribes used Oregon grape for food, medicine, and fabric dye. The Blackfoot used the root to treat rheumatism, purify the blood, and for infant care. The Flathead tribe crushed the root and applied it to wounds. The Apache used it for gum ailments, while the Nitinaht, Sanpoil, and Miwok used it to treat tuberculosis. For centuries, Northwest Indigenous people have turned to Oregon grape for bacterial infections, digestive disorders, inflammatory skin conditions, and fevers.

Jessica's notes: Oregon grape brings me and the forest students so much joy! The kids call the berries "dare bombs" and love daring one another to eat the tart, sour berries during our forest walks. They also make perfect natural face paint and "fake blood" for imaginative play. It feels like a magic trick every time I pull a rhizome from the earth and shave off the outer layer to reveal that vivid yellow core. When I explain how this bitter medicine aids digestion, just like bile in our bodies, the kids are always amazed—and they love that it is such an easy plant to identify in our forests.

Jason and I were once hired to remove Oregon grape from a client's yard. Naturally, we took the roots home and made potent medicine from them. It is incredible how many people do not realize the powerful healing plants growing right around them, or do not care to learn about them. In the wild, these evergreen colonies of Oregon grape form beautiful, lush collars around the mighty pine trees. They are steadfast allies of the forest and the people.

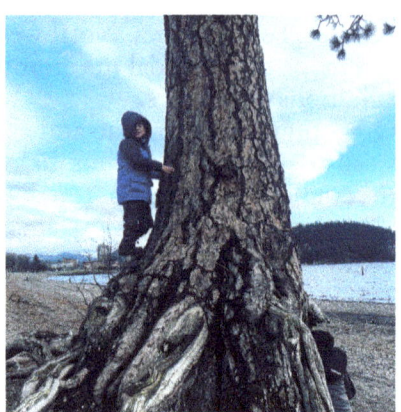

Ponderosa Pine

Pinus ponderosa

Pinaceae (Pine) Family

Other common names: bull pine, yellow pine, rock pine, western yellow pine

Description: A forest giant conifer with straight trunks, 4-5 feet in diameter, growing 90 to 200 feet tall with a tapering crown of thick, heavy limbs. The bark is easily identified: cinnamon-brown, with thick bark that chips off in jigsaw-like plates. The yellowish green needles are in clusters of three, 4-10 inches long, and are the longest of all the conifers found in the northwest. Deep reddish-purple, egg-shaped seed cones turn reddish-brown as they ripen in their second year and then transform into a solid brown cone. Each cone scale has a sharp, outward-facing prickle at the tip. Ponderosa pines can live to the ripe old age of 300- 600 years.

Where it grows: It is found in grasslands, sunny slopes, and dry valleys. Ponderosas grow abundantly in the Northwest. They are drought-tolerant but shade-intolerant, and mature trees are fire-resistant.

When and how to harvest: Harvest the new growth needles in early spring. This is also a good time to remove thick lower branches, cut strips of bark, and set them to dehydrate. Remove chunks of dried pitch year-round. Avoid harvesting from a fresh wound, as this impedes the tree's ability to seal and heal an injury. Gather pine pollen on male cones when they are actively producing from early to late spring and tincture while still fresh.

How to work with it/ Medicinal use: Ponderosa's needles, bark, and pitch are warming, drying, and restorative. Tea, tincture, or steam from the needles or bark can open up the nasal passages and break up hard, stuck phlegm. The vitamin A- and C-rich pine needle tea can be drunk to help clear phlegm, soothe a sore throat, and resolve respiratory infections. The tea can also be used as a gargle for sore throats and a nasal wash. Pine tea and tincture can help reduce excessive mucus flow with their drying properties. Chewing on a chunk of pitch will release the aromatic oils in the lungs. Finding the right consistency will take some practice. Too hard, it cracks and sticks; too soft, and it will get stuck in your teeth, which may require filling a cavity, but it will taste bitter. Vitamin C-rich needles will help clear a urinary tract infection. Pine pitch salve has been made for centuries to heal wounds and prevent infection. Warmed pine pitch can draw out splinters and any embedded objects. Pine pollen tincture can help boost immunity, testosterone levels, and endurance. These mighty pines provide food in a survival situation. The inner cambium can be cooked and eaten, providing a source of carbohydrates and nutrients. Pine seeds can be gathered for protein and essential fatty acids. We enjoy pickling the young tender seedlings of early spring or eating them as a trail snack. The resin can be dried in droplets and burned like incense for a ceremony.

Healing constituents/ Therapeutic actions: Pine contains oleoresins, antimicrobial volatile oils, vitamin A and C complexes, phenolic compounds, and chlorophyll (in needles). The pine pitch and resin are antimicrobial and antiseptic, and the needles and bark are warming, drying, and restorative.

Historical connections: In 1826, botanist David Douglas misidentified the tree in Washington state as Red Pine. He named it *Pinus ponderosa* due to its heavy, reddish-brown bark. In 1836, Scottish nurseryman Charles Lawson formerly classified the name as we call it today. Native Americans utilized ponderosa for food, medicine, shelter, and ceremonial purposes. Various tribes used it as a gynecological aid and for the same modern-day uses. Pine pitch was used to create a waterproof and airtight coating for water vessels. In Scotland, pine was a survival food during famine. Pine has been an important plant for people since the beginning of time.

Jessica's notes: Ponderosa pine provides significant protection, whether from invisible enemies such as viruses and harmful bacteria or shelter from the elements and forest fires. These mighty forest giants make me feel strong and capable of walking under their grandiose canopies. One day, the family and I were taking our neighbor's dog on a hike because he was in the hospital, and we were caring for his animals. Behind his property, we discovered the largest ponderosa pine I have ever seen in the National Forest. My eyesight could barely reach the top of the canopy. Its presence was awe-inspiring and ephemeral. I went to take a photo only to realize that I had left my phone in the car!

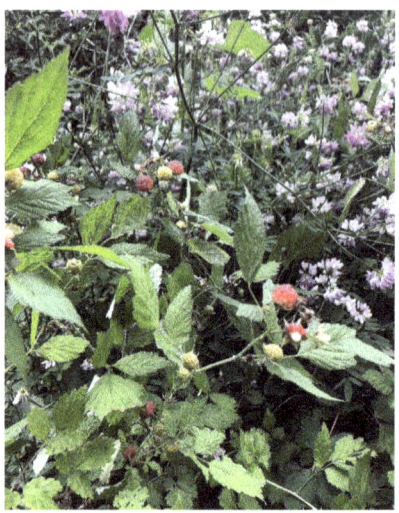

Red Raspberry

Rubus idaeus

Rosaceae (Rose) Family

Description: Red raspberry is a perennial, deciduous, erect shrub with a biennial two-year growth cycle. In the first year, it produces long, unbranched stems called "primocanes," which bear dark green, pinnately compound leaves composed of three to seven serrated leaflets. In the second year, as a "floricane," the stems develop several side shoots that bear three to five smaller leaflets. The white flowers bloom in spring on short racemes at the tips of these side shoots, each with five petals. By mid-to-late summer, the plant produces its well-loved red fruit. Technically, the fruit is an aggregate of many juicy drupelets clustered around a white central core. When picked, the drupelets detach from the core, leaving the fruit hollow.

There are hundreds of wild berry varieties, and they often hybridize, which can make it tricky to distinguish wild raspberry from blackberry, especially when the plant is not fruiting. Fortunately, both are edible and rich in nutrients, so there is no need to worry if you misidentify them.

Where it grows: Red raspberry is a widespread plant found throughout North America and much of the world. It thrives along stream banks, in moist open woodlands, and near rivers and lakes.

When and how to harvest: Harvest the leaves in early spring through summer. Always dry them thoroughly before use; wilted leaves can cause digestive upset. The ripe berries are ready for harvest in mid-to-late summer.

How to work with it / Medicinal use: Red raspberry leaf is a beloved woman's tonic that supports the female reproductive system through all phases of menstruation, pregnancy, postpartum, and breastfeeding. Its astringent and mineral-rich properties tone the uterus, bladder, and reproductive system. A tea or infusion can ease cramping and nausea during menstruation. For smoother cycles, drink the tea starting a week before and during menstruation, steeping it for at least 15 minutes.

During pregnancy, red raspberry leaf tea is traditionally consumed in the second and third trimesters to help tone the uterus and prepare the body for labor and birth. It also makes an excellent postpartum sitz bath thanks to its astringent qualities. Rich in minerals, this tea is perfect for breastfeeding mothers and helps support healthy lactation. However, it is not just a woman's herb—this is a gentle, everyday tea for the whole family! The flavor is mild and reminiscent of black tea, making it enjoyable both hot and cold. On warm days, I love to add a squeeze of lemon and chill it for a refreshing summer drink.

The berries themselves are nutritional powerhouses, packed with antioxidants, fiber, and minerals that benefit heart and skin health.

Healing constituents / Therapeutic actions: Raspberry leaf contains flavonoids (rutin, isoquercitrin, caffeic acid derivatives, and phenolic acids), as well as vitamins C and B, magnesium, calcium, iron, and phosphorus. The berries offer antioxidants (anthocyanins and anthocyanidins), vitamin B6, fiber, potassium, manganese, zinc, selenium, omega-3 fatty acids, calcium, vitamins A, E, and K, as well as a B-complex. Therapeutic actions include astringent, anti-diarrheal, and anti-inflammatory properties.

Caution: Wilted leaves can be toxic. Always use either completely dried or freshly harvested leaves.

Historical connections: The Latin name *idaeus* is derived from Mount Ida, where raspberries grew abundantly. In Greek mythology, these berries were beloved by the gods of Olympus. *Rubus* translates to "red" in Greek, so the full name *Rubus idaeus* means "bramble bush of Ida."

According to legend, the berries were originally snow white until Ida, a nursemaid to baby Zeus, pricked her finger while picking them, staining the berries red forever. Raspberry canes have been found near Neolithic caves across Europe, indicating that humans have enjoyed these berries for thousands of years. By the European Middle Ages, raspberry leaf was widely used as a woman's tonic.

In Native American tradition, red raspberry was used similarly to support women's health.

Jessica's notes: Raspberries have always been one of my favorite fruits. I first began drinking raspberry leaf tea as a teenager while exploring holistic ways to balance my hormones. I loved the taste then and still do! I drank it throughout my pregnancies and credit raspberry leaf—along with other herbs traditionally used by women—for helping me experience healthy and easy births.

Finding this familiar and comforting herb in the wild never fails to excite me. Wild raspberry leaves have a much stronger flavor than store-bought versions. Moreover, stumbling upon ripe berries while foraging is truly a trail snack fit for the Greek gods!

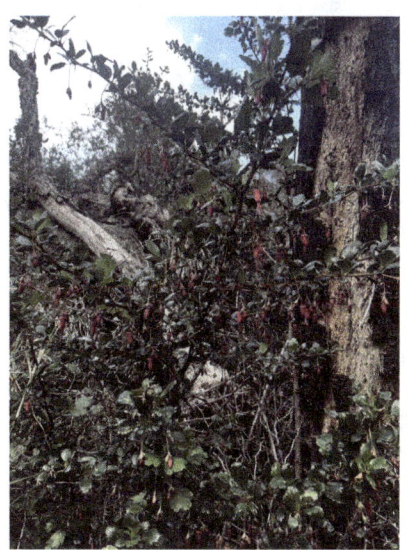

Ribes

Ribes L.

Grossulariaceae (Currant) Family
Other common names: Gooseberry, Black Currant
Description: The genus *Ribes* includes over 60 species of shrub-forming perennials. These shrubs display small, maple-like leaves that are alternately arranged, palmately lobed, and prominently veined. Depending on the species, stems may be smooth or covered with spines or bristles. The flowers vary in form—some are tubular, while others are squat with flared openings. When mature, the fruit develops into smooth or bristly berries that may be orange, red, or deep purple-black in color. Some species produce berries that remain green even when fully ripe. Each berry contains several small seeds.
Where it grows: Throughout the Pacific Northwest, particularly in North Idaho, various *Ribes* species thrive "where the wild things grow." They prefer moist soils, sunny slopes, and open woodlands.
When and how to harvest: In spring to early summer, snip 1–2 inches from the tender, leafy branch ends and place them in an open basket or breathable bag. Once the leaves have dried, strip them from the branches and store them for later use.

How to work with it / Medicinal use: The leaves of *Ribes* offer mild astringent properties, similar to other members of the rose family. A strong decoction of the leaves can be used as a gargle for sore throats, inflamed gums, and mouth sores. Internally, the same preparation helps relieve diarrhea, gastric distress, and inflammation in the urinary tract, making it helpful in flushing the bladder and soothing irritated tissues.

Out in the field, the crushed fresh leaves can be applied as a quick poultice to scrapes, cuts, and sunburns. European *Ribes* species are well-documented for their anti-inflammatory and pain-relieving properties, particularly in the treatment of arthritis. Given that our native North American species also contain phenolic acids, they likely share these healing properties. Black-fruiting varieties are especially valued for their higher content of anti-inflammatory compounds.

The berries themselves are edible and rich in vitamin C. They can be enjoyed fresh or used to make jams, jellies, and preserves.

Healing constituents / Therapeutic actions: The leaves contain phenolic acids, flavonoids, quercetin, and kaempferol. The fruits are rich in ascorbic acid (vitamin C), flavonoids, anthocyanins, and anthocyanidins. Therapeutic actions include anti-inflammatory, astringent, and anti-diarrheal properties.

Historical connections: Native American tribes valued *Ribes* as an important wild fruit. English settlers brought black currants to the Massachusetts Bay Colony in 1629, and they were cultivated widely across North America. By 1899, more than 12,000 acres of black currants were under commercial cultivation, primarily in New York.

However, in 1911, the U.S. government banned the cultivation, sale, and transport of currants to protect white pine trees from the devastating white pine blister rust, a disease introduced on infected seedlings from France in 1910. The disease required a secondary host, such as gooseberries and currants, to spread. Although the federal ban was lifted in 1966, much damage had already been done to white pine populations. Since then, organizations such as the U.S. Forest Service have worked to restore white pine forests.

Jessica's notes: Ribes shrubs make a strong impression when you encounter them along the trail. Their sharp thorns and unusual flowers always catch my eye, inviting a closer look. I often use gooseberry bushes as natural landmarks to help me navigate, as they tend to grow in prominent places where the forest seems to need a post or protective shield.

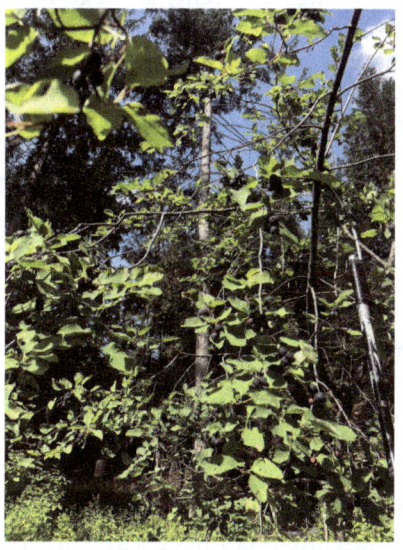

Serviceberry

Amelanchier alnifolia

Rosaceae (Rose) Family
Other names: "Sarviceberry," Saskatoon, Juneberry
  Description: Serviceberry is a tree-like shrub that grows from 4 to 25 feet tall, often forming small thickets or colonies through underground parallel stems. Its bark is smooth, dark gray to dark brown. The simple, alternate leaves have rounded tips and sharply toothed margins. In the spring, clusters of white flowers appear, each with five petals measuring 5–14 mm in length. By late summer, the shrub produces juicy, blackish-blue berries.
  Where it grows: Saskatoon prefers open woodlands, sunny slopes, and moist soils. It often grows near mountain springs and creeks, thriving among elderberries and mountain ash trees.
  When and how to harvest: Harvest the leaves from early spring through early summer. The pomes (berries) are best gathered when fully ripe in summer. Alternatively, unripe berries can be harvested for their astringent qualities to help with diarrhea.
  How to work with it / Medicinal use: Serviceberry truly serves both people and wildlife with its nutrient-dense berries and durable wood. Like

other members of the rose family, its leaves are astringent. They can be used to tone inflamed tissues internally and externally, while also helping to reduce excess mucus in the lungs.

The berries and leaves carry a subtle almond-vanilla flavor due to their cyanogenic compounds—eating the raw berries in large quantities may cause diarrhea, but cooking the leaves and berries neutralizes this compound. The berries offer a wealth of vitamins and minerals that help reduce inflammation and oxidative stress. Compared to other wild berries like strawberries or huckleberries, Saskatoon berries provide higher levels of usable energy and nutrients, including three times the iron and copper found in raisins. With their nutritional richness, they also exhibit antiviral properties.

There are countless creative ways to enjoy serviceberries: ripe berries can be frozen, cooked into syrups, or used in Saskatoon pies, pastries, jams, jellies, and preserves. They can also be dried like raisins or pureed into fruit leather.

The dried leaves can be brewed into teas to help prevent diarrhea, soothe urinary tract infections, and reduce excess mucus. As a flower essence, Saskatoon can help individuals connect with their higher self, promoting mental clarity and concentration.

In addition to its medicinal qualities, the shrub's thorny branches are strong and can be crafted into walking sticks, furniture, and other valuable items.

Healing constituents / Therapeutic actions: Serviceberry is a nutrient-dense food, containing vitamins C, calcium, copper, iron, magnesium, manganese, potassium, phosphorus, sulfur, protein, fat, and fiber. Therapeutic actions include anti-inflammatory, antiviral, and antioxidant effects.

Historical connections: First Nations people have a long history of using Saskatoon as both food and medicine. Traditionally, the berries were boiled to make a juice that was used to relieve diarrhea and digestive ailments. The berries were sometimes combined with inner bark and roots to help prevent miscarriages, stop excessive menstrual bleeding, and support women transitioning through menopause. After childbirth, the juice and inner bark were used to ease pain and act as a blood tonic. The berries were also used to treat eye and ear infections.

Jessica's notes: Saskatoon bushes are abundant throughout the Northwest, and I love snacking on their ripe, blue berries while foraging. Their flavor—a delicious blend of almond, vanilla, and tart blueberry—always delights me. Birds adore them, too, and I often find myself harvesting alongside flocks of feathered friends, who dance and sing in celebration of this abundant wild berry.

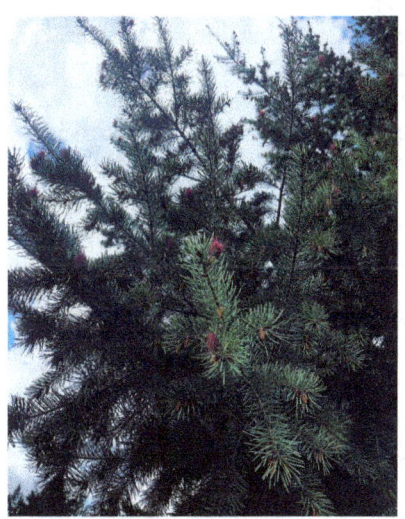

Spruce

Picea spp. (including Picea engelmannii, Picea pungens)

Pinaceae (Pine) Family

Other common names: Engelmann Spruce, Blue Spruce (*Picea pungens*), White Spruce, Mountain Spruce, Silver Spruce

Description: Spruce species are towering coniferous evergreens, often an iconic choice for Christmas trees. In the wild, they can reach heights of up to 180 feet, with trunks nearly 5 feet in diameter. Blue Spruce can be identified by its bluish-green needles, which are coated with a whitish bloom. The needles are somewhat flexible, aromatic when crushed, and can be blunt or pointed at the tips. They grow on all sides of the twig, which features a rhombic cross-section. Each needle measures between ¾ inch and 1 1/8 inches long.

In spring, conical purple cones (about 1 cm) appear, releasing yellow pollen through wind dispersal. The non-resinous buds have rounded scales and adorn the pine-laden branches. The cones mature into light brown after 4 to 7 months. Seeds are small, black, and winged for dispersal. The bark is thin, reddish, and scaly, flaking off in round, disk-like pieces. Young trees feature conic crowns that mature into cylindrical tops.

Caution: The Yew tree is sometimes mistaken for Spruce—be certain of your identification when harvesting.

Where it grows: Spruce is moderately shade-tolerant but not as much as subalpine fir. It depends on occasional forest fires to outcompete other species, though its thin bark and shallow roots make it somewhat vulnerable to fire. It thrives in moist, rich soil and can be found in mixed stands with lodgepole pines, western hemlock, and subalpine fir across a range of forest habitats.

When and how to harvest: Harvest young tips in late spring. Pitch can be gathered year-round from healthy trees, and young male catkins can be harvested in late summer.

How to work with it / Medicinal use: Spruce tips are rich in vitamin C and possess antiseptic, antifungal, and antimicrobial properties. Interestingly, freeze-drying the tips increases vitamin C content by 30% (Jysky et al., 2020). They also contain vitamins A and E, as well as essential minerals such as potassium and magnesium.

These tender tips emerge in spring, perfect timing for helping the body detox after a long winter. Spruce medicine strengthens the immune system and supports balance and vitality. A tea made from young tips soothes sore throats, relieves coughs, and speeds recovery from colds and respiratory infections. The aromatic needles can also be used in steam inhalations to loosen chest congestion. A tincture made from the needles is another option for short-term immune support.

Culinarily, spruce tips can be integrated into a variety of dishes and drinks. A naturally fermented soda made from young tips is a fun way to enjoy their flavor, and they can also be added to sauerkraut or fermented vegetable blends.

Spruce resin is antifungal and antimicrobial—its role in protecting the tree translates to human use as well. Traditionally, spruce resin was used to make throat lozenges. The pitch can be applied directly to cuts and scrapes as a natural bandage to prevent infection, or it can be made into antiseptic salves, liniments, or oils.

Spruce pulp and wood have many industrial applications. Native American tribes used spruce resin as a waterproofing agent for canoes and vessels. The wood's exceptional resonance makes it ideal for crafting musical instruments, such as guitars, violins, pianos, and soundboards.

Healing constituents / Therapeutic actions: Spruce tips are especially rich in vitamin C, magnesium, phosphorus, and potassium. The young shoots also contain high levels of secondary metabolites, including flavonoids (kaempferol, quercetin, isorhamnetin, and myricetin), condensed tannins, stilbenes, and terpenoids. These compounds contribute to the plant's antioxidative and immunomodulatory properties. Spruce resin is antimicrobial and antifungal.

Historical connections: Though spruce is not commonly used in modern clinical herbalism, it remains an important folk remedy rooted in Native American traditions. Native peoples used spruce in various ways:

decomposed wood was ground into powder to treat diaper rash and fungal skin conditions, the roots of young trees were used to make cordage for canoes, and resin served as a chewing gum or a waterproofing agent.

Early settlers also learned to use spruce—brewing beer from the young tips or crafting gum from the resin. During World War II, spruce's strong yet lightweight wood was used in the construction of airplanes. For centuries, spruce has played a role in both wartime and peacetime, serving as a source of medicine, food, and fine musical craftsmanship.

Jessica's notes: The first time I worked with spruce was many moons ago during a foraging adventure with the Freeborn family in a dense, shaded forest. Jason pointed out the vibrant, lime-green young tips, and we eagerly harvested a basketful. We nibbled on a few as we worked, noting their tart, vitamin C-rich flavor.

Then inspiration struck: I could ferment them! I combined the tender tips with green cabbage and sea salt, leaving the mixture to ferment for two weeks. The result? A unique, exciting flavor—though next time, I think I will try making a carbonated fermented beverage instead of sauerkraut!

For me, food is medicine, and it is great fun to integrate wild, foraged ingredients into traditional recipes and folk remedies. Spruce is a joyful ally to work with, offering both nourishment and healing to those who seek it.

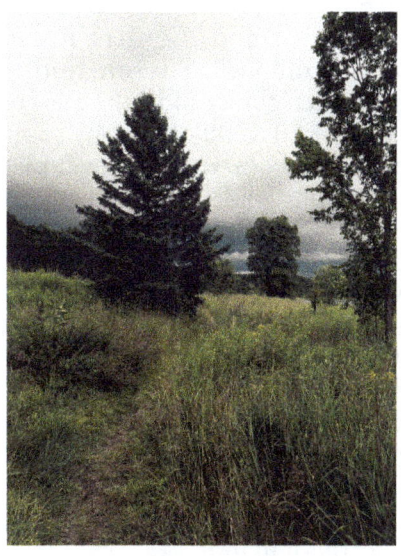

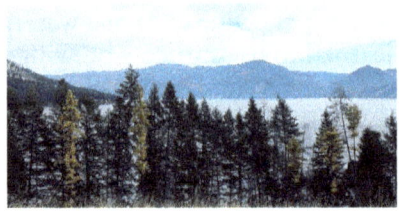

Tamarack

Larix occidentalis

Pinaceae *(Pine) Family*
Other common names: Western Larch, Mountain Larch, Hackmatack, Montana Larch

Description: A slender giant of the forest, Tamarack can reach heights of up to 200 feet. Uniquely among conifers, it sheds its needles in fall. Tamarack stands out in autumn when its soft, feathery needles turn a brilliant yellow, creating a golden glow amidst the evergreens. The flat, flexible needles grow in clusters of 10 to 20 on stubby spur branches. In spring, new needles emerge in a bright Granny Smith apple green, maturing to a soft blue-green before turning golden and falling to the ground in autumn.

The crown of the tree typically comprises only one-third to one-half of its height, leaving a tall, clear trunk that can extend 60 to 100 feet in length. The cinnamon-brown bark is marked with shallow, smooth ridges. Thanks to its fire-resistant, insect- and disease-tolerant dense wood, Tamarack can live for more than 800 years. After death, it returns to the forest as a "nurse tree," providing shelter and nutrients for new growth.

Where it grows: Tamarack grows in coniferous stands, competing for sunlight with Douglas firs and ponderosa pines. Though shade-intolerant, it is fire-resistant and often among the first trees to regenerate after a wildfire. It commonly grows along lake shores and in wet, old-growth forests throughout Northern Idaho.

When and how to harvest: Harvest young leaves in early spring and bark year-round. Exercise care when harvesting resins, as improper harvesting can harm or kill the tree.

How to work with it / Medicinal use: Western Larch is an ancient Native American medicine that has since been validated by modern science for its efficacy. The inner bark contains *Larch arabinogalactan*, a powerful prebiotic fiber that nourishes beneficial gut bacteria and acts as an immunomodulator. It can support the immune system, aid digestion, and help regulate autoimmune responses. Clinical studies have also demonstrated arabinogalactan's anticancer properties, affirming the historical Native American use of Tamarack for cancer treatment (D'Adamo, 1996).

Though herbalists today seldom use other parts of the tree, Tamarack has a rich history of medicinal use among Indigenous peoples and early settlers. Leaves and stems were traditionally used as appetite stimulants and blood purifiers. Decoctions, both internal and external, were employed in cancer care to nourish and support emaciated patients. Like other conifers, the inner resin can be applied to cuts, scrapes, and bruises as an antiseptic wound dressing. Bark tea can be used to soothe a sore throat.

Healing constituents / Therapeutic actions: Western Larch contains *arabinogalactan*, a potent prebiotic starch. The leaves and stems have antirheumatic, antiseptic, and appetite-stimulating properties. The inner bark is an immunostimulant.

Historical connections: Native Americans recognized the power of Tamarack long before modern science confirmed its benefits. Decoctions of the stem tips were used both internally and externally to treat arthritis. Gum from the inner bark was applied to wounds, while bark infusions helped alleviate colds, coughs, and tuberculosis. Strong decoctions were also used as wound washes, and the sap was chewed to soothe sore throats (Moerman, 1998).

Maude Grieve includes Tamarack in her classic *Modern Herbal* (1931): *"The bark used as a decoction is laxative, tonic, diuretic, and alterative, useful in obstructions of the liver, rheumatism, jaundice, and some cutaneous diseases. A decoction of the leaves has been used for piles, haemoptysis, menorrhagia, diarrhoea, and dysentery.— Dosage: 2 tablespoonsful of the bark decoction."*

Jessica's notes: Tamarack is one of those mighty trees that inspires me deeply. Each fall, as the forest begins to quiet and darken, Tamarack does the opposite — it bursts into radiant golden light, as if to remind us to shine when everything around us is dimming. There is such wisdom in that. Tamarack teaches me that even when life feels heavy or uncertain, I can choose to glow with my inner light.

I often find myself walking beneath their golden boughs in late autumn and simply standing in their presence, soaking up their quiet strength. The resilience of this tree — fire-resistant, long-lived, and nourishing the forest even after it has fallen — mirrors the kind of resilience I strive for in life. Working with Tamarack reminds me that strength and beauty often lie in how we weather life's seasons and how we shine in the darker times.

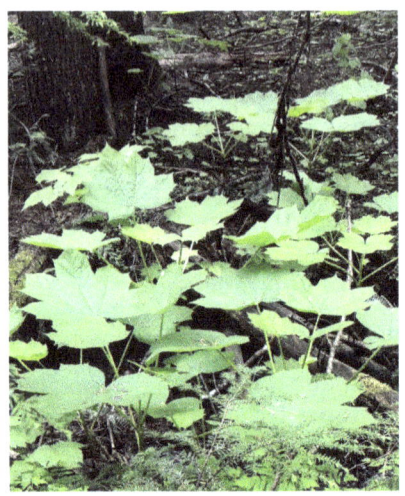

Thimbleberry

Rubus parviflorus

Rosaceae (Rose) Family

Description: Thimbleberry is a dense shrub that spreads by underground rhizomes, forming large clumps. The canes can grow up to 8 feet tall and are about ½ inch in diameter. Unlike many other rose family members, thimbleberry has no thorns or prickles. Its large, palmate, soft, fuzzy, dark green, maple-shaped leaves can reach up to 20 centimeters across, typically with five lobes. The name perfectly describes the berry's shape: once plucked, the hollow fruit resembles a thimble, with tiny indentations like those used to press a sewing needle. Similar in flavor and color to raspberry, the berries are softer and smaller, composed of more delicate drupelets. The five-petalled, slightly crinkled white flowers resemble large strawberry blossoms and grow in clusters atop the maple-shaped leaves.

Where it grows: Thimbleberry thrives in thickets near springs, babbling brooks, and dense forest understories.

When and how to harvest: Harvest the ripe berries from mid to late summer. Leaves can be gathered while they are still green, from spring through early fall. Tender young shoots are sweet in early spring.

How to work with it / Medicinal use: Thimbleberries are nutrient-dense, like many wild berries. Because they are very soft compared to raspberries, they are best enjoyed fresh, dried, or preserved in jams and jellies. They are rich in vitamins A and C, fiber, and carbohydrates—an ideal trail snack.

Thimbleberry leaves contain tannins and can be boiled into a tea to help alleviate stomach issues and stimulate the appetite. Out in the wild, the large, soft leaves make an excellent natural toilet paper and can also be added to herbal baths to soothe inflamed skin. Crushed leaves can be applied as a poultice to treat wounds, burns, pimples, and blackheads.

The young shoots, harvested in spring, can be eaten raw or cooked like asparagus and offer a good source of vitamin C. The canes can be made into a tea and used as a diuretic. Additionally, the large leaves are excellent for use as natural food wraps—for cooking, steaming, preserving, or serving meals.

Healing constituents / Therapeutic actions: Thimbleberries are rich in vitamins A and C, fiber, and carbohydrates. The leaves contain tannins. Therapeutic actions include anti-inflammatory and diuretic.

Historical connections: Thimbleberries were a significant dietary staple for many Native American tribes. The First Nations of British Columbia valued them greatly—the delicate fruits were eaten fresh and pressed into cakes for storage. On Vancouver Island, West Coast peoples harvested canoe-loads of sweet, juicy spring shoots, peeling and eating them raw, much like sugar cane. The Okanagan people lined steam-cooking pits with thimbleberry leaves. The Shuswap and Carrier First Nations crafted small carrying baskets from the leaves to separate different berries during gathering. The Cowlitz of present-day Washington State boiled thimbleberry bark to make a natural soap.

For a bit about botanical etymology: "*Rubus*" means red and traces back to an ancient Roman name for a plant in this family. "*Parviflorus*" means "small-flowered," though ironically, thimbleberry's large white blossoms are bigger than those of many other berry vines!

Jessica's notes: One sunny afternoon, the family and I were having a picnic and barbecue in the backcountry along Hayden Creek. I had forgotten to pack paper plates, so I channeled my inner mountain medicine mama. I gathered four clean pieces of cedar bark near the creek and layered them with thimbleberry leaves to make the perfect plates for our burgers. We even garnished them with wild violets, miner's lettuce, and sautéed morel mushrooms! (Can you guess what time of year we were foraging?) It reminded me how adaptable and generous the wild plants are—always providing what we need if we pay attention.

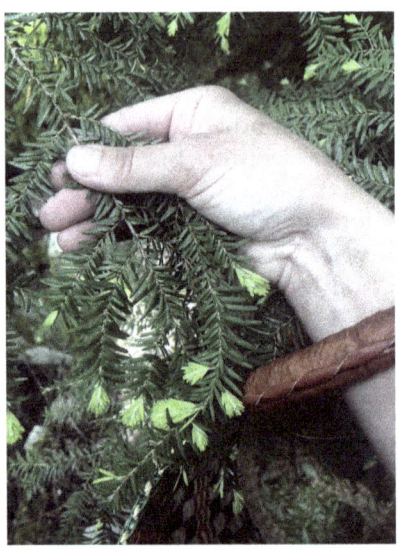

Western Hemlock

Tsuga heterophylla

Pinaceae (Pine) Family
Other common names: West Coast Hemlock, Pacific Hemlock, Coast Hemlock

Description: Western Hemlock is a graceful tree with a distinctive, narrow, drooping crown that seems to bow with humility. This tall, evergreen conifer can reach heights of 90 to 200 feet. Its short-stalked, flat, finely toothed needles grow from 5 to 20 millimeters in length. Young bark is smooth and reddish-brown, while mature bark darkens and becomes deeply furrowed, forming flat-topped, flaky ridges. The ovoid seed cones are short-stalked, brown, and hang elegantly from the ends of twigs, with thin, papery scales.

Where it grows: A shade-tolerant species, Western Hemlock thrives in the understory of coniferous forests, often growing alongside other shade-loving trees. It is commonly found near springs, creeks, and streams. Hemlock plays an integral role in maintaining the ecological balance of the Inland Northwest, forming thick stands that support diverse forest communities.

When and how to harvest: The pitch can be harvested year-round. Bark and pitch must be gathered sustainably—never cut around the entire girth of a tree, and when harvesting bark, cut in vertical strips to avoid girdling.

How to work with it / Medicinal use: Though rarely used by modern herbalists, the medicine of Western Hemlock remains alive through traditional knowledge and folk use. Like other conifers, its young tips are rich in vitamins A and C and can be brewed into a refreshing, immune-supportive tea. The flavor pairs beautifully with wild mints.

The pitch can be applied as a field poultice for itchy insect bites or rubbed into the hair to treat head lice. When mixed with fat (such as deer tallow) or prepared as a salve, it can be applied to the chest to ease colds or used as a natural sunscreen. Powdered bark can be used to treat foot odor, as a baby powder, and for fungal skin issues.

A decoction of pounded bark has traditionally been used to treat hemorrhages and tuberculosis. The bark's astringent properties also make it a diuretic and diaphoretic. An infusion of the twigs can soothe sore throats and is used for bronchitis, asthma, and whooping cough. Though little scientific research backs these traditional uses, this wisdom has been passed down through countless generations.

High in tannins, the bark also produces a beautiful red dye and has long been used for tanning and painting.

Healing constituents / Therapeutic actions: No clinical studies are currently available for the healing constituents of *Tsuga heterophylla*. However, traditional wisdom suggests that its needles are rich in vitamins A and C, and that the tree offers immunomodulating, diuretic, and diaphoretic effects.

Caution: Do not consume during pregnancy. As with all conifer needles and resins, consume in moderation and for short periods—resins can accumulate in the system and may stress the kidneys.

Historical connections: For centuries, Native Northwest peoples have used Western Hemlock as a tanning agent, dye, pigment, and cleansing solution (Pojar & MacKinnon, 1994). Coastal Salish tribes used the red dye to stain goat wool, basket materials, facial cosmetics, and even as a hair remover. Hemlock's durable wood was carved into children's bows, spoons, combs, roasting sticks, dip net poles, and more.

The Mainland Comox people used hemlock boughs for drying meat and fish, as well as for lining steam pits. Among the Kwakwaka'wakw, ceremonial dancers adorned themselves with hemlock headdresses, and young women would dwell in huts made of hemlock boughs during the days following their first menstruation. Hemlock pitch was chewed like gum, and both bark and needles were used medicinally in the folk ways still practiced today.

One Coastal Salish legend teaches a lesson in humility: When the Creator distributed cones to the trees, Western Hemlock was not paying attention and ended up last in line. As a result, it received the smallest cone of all. Its characteristically bent top is said to reflect this humble nature.

Jessica's notes: I have always been drawn to the humble energy of Western Hemlock. Its drooping top reminds me to remain grounded and grateful, no matter how tall or strong we may grow. It is a tree of quiet strength, supporting the forest and its creatures without fanfare. When I sip tea made from the tender spring tips, I feel a deep connection to this gentle wisdom. It reminds me that healing comes not only from bold action but often from quiet presence.

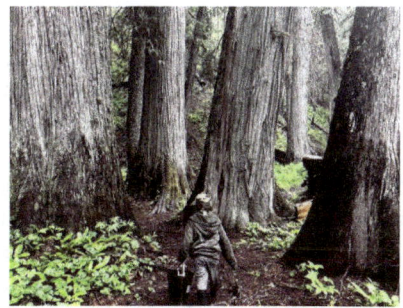

Western Red Cedar

Thuja plicata

Pinaceae (Pine) Family

Description: A distinctive, towering evergreen with a broad, buttressed base, Western Red Cedar can grow to truly gargantuan proportions. The bark is fibrous, ribbed, and ranges from cinnamon brown to gray. Its J-shaped branches often create natural seats or handy places to set up shelter. The greenish-yellow, flat leaves form in pairs, arranged in opposite scales. In summer, small, round flowers bloom, giving cedar a golden hue. When in bloom, clouds of cedar pollen fill the air, dusting everything in a fine golden powder. The seed cones, shaped like tiny brown rosebuds, have 8 to 12 scales, each engineered like a miniature wind turbine to funnel pollen. The largest cedar trees can soar to 200 feet tall with diameters of up to 19 feet, and they can live for over 1,000 years.

Where it grows: Cedar prefers moist environments and is often found along alpine creeks, springs, wet meadows, and mountain slopes.

When and how to harvest: The leaves can be harvested year-round, but are most aromatic in early summer. Bark is best harvested in spring when the sap is running. Cedar roots can be carefully harvested in fall, spring, or summer, though they are labor-intensive to gather.

How to work with it/ Medicinal use: Cedar is a powerful antimicrobial, containing essential oils that resist mold, fungi, bacteria, and insects. Reflecting the damp forests where it thrives, cedar's aromatic oils provide protective medicine against external threats.

Topically, cedar leaf preparations are effective in treating fungal infections. A foot soak of cedar leaf tea soothes athlete's foot and nail fungus. Simply steep a generous handful of fresh or dried leaves in approximately

10 cups of hot water, then let it cool before soaking your feet for at least 10 minutes.

Cedar tea or tincture can help promote immune function by increasing white blood cell activity, breaking down cancer cells, and clearing bodily debris. To preserve the delicate oils, a cold infusion is ideal—soak about one tablespoon of cedar leaves in 1 cup of cold water for several hours or overnight.

For respiratory infections, cedar steam inhalation, done several times daily, can help loosen phlegm and clear congestion. An infused oil or salve made with cedar leaves is effective for treating fungal skin conditions.

Cedar's aromatic oils also repel moths and biting insects. Burning cedar or using it as incense purifies the air—a traditional practice used to clear viruses from the home after illness and to dispel negative energies.

Beyond its medicinal uses, cedar has been prized for centuries for its rot-resistant wood, used to craft canoes, waterproof baskets, durable clothing, cordage, and grand longhouses.

Caution: Cedar contains thujone, a potent volatile oil that can be toxic in large doses. Cedar medicine should be used only for short periods and avoided during pregnancy and in individuals with compromised kidney function.

Healing constituents / Therapeutic actions: Western Red Cedar contains volatile oils, including Athantol, Atlantone, Fenchone, and Thujone, as well as flavonoids, glycosides, resveratrol, proanthocyanidins, resins, tannins, and terpenes. Its therapeutic actions include antifungal, antimicrobial, anti-inflammatory, expectorant, and analgesic.

Historical connections: Cedar is sacred to many Indigenous cultures across North America. The Salish People call it *Grandmother*, *Long Life Maker*, and *Rich Woman Maker*. They held special ceremonies for the felling of cedar trees. Coastal Native Americans relied on cedar for joint pain remedies (both internally and externally), for coughs and tuberculosis, and chewed the pitch as gum. Cedar bark was used to make longhouses, clothing, and baskets—a practice still alive today.

In Irish folklore, cedar represents strength and durability. A Mi'kmaq tale warns of being careful what one wishes for: A man asked the fabled Glooskap for immortality, and in response, Glooskap turned him into a cedar tree, granting him a life longer than any man's.

A Potawatomi story recounts the tale of seekers who approached the Sun for gifts. One asked for immortality and was transformed into a cedar tree. This symbolizes the use of cedar and stone in sweat lodge ceremonies.

In Judeo-Christian tradition, cedar symbolizes protection and strength. It was used to build Solomon's temple, and medieval lore holds that the cross of the crucifixion was made from cedar, making it both revered and taboo. Planting a cedar tree was considered good fortune, while naturally sprouting ones were viewed with superstition.

Jessica's notes: There is nothing quite like standing in a cedar grove—one of the most healing experiences nature offers. The spicy, earthy aroma makes me feel alive, grounded, and protected. At Forest School, if the insects are particularly bothersome, I love to rest against a cedar during storytelling. Somehow, it always seems to ward off the pests!

I have long been intrigued by the *Ringing Cedars* tradition of Russia and how cedar is revered as a sacred tree for humanity. It is easy to see why cedar offers us so much: protection, medicine, and connection to the wisdom of the forest. I believe this mighty tree plays a vital role in the health and balance of both the land and its people.

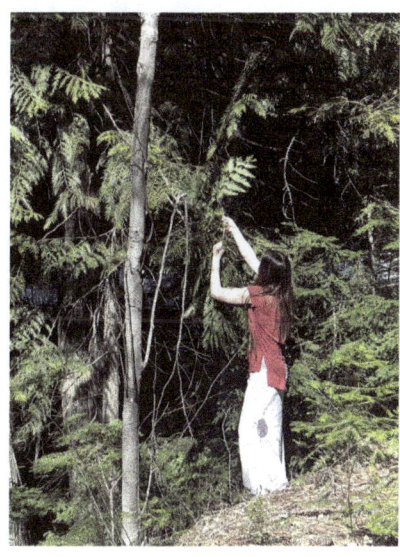

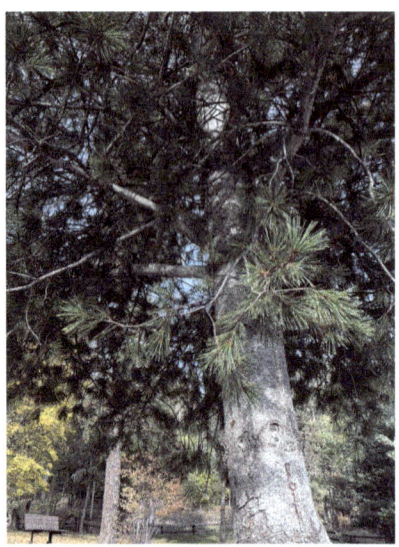

Western White Pine

Pinus monticola

Pinaceae (Pine) Family
Other common names: silver pine, California mountain pine
   Description: Needles of five—you have found white pine! The slender, evergreen needles grow in bundles of five, each measuring 3 to 5 inches in length. The stalked cones grow straight and range in length from 5 to 15 inches. Western White Pine has a tall, straight trunk, and its mature bark is gray-white, broken into rectangular plates that flake off in chunks. These mighty giants can soar over 200 feet tall, with most averaging between 90 and 150 feet in height.
   While related to the Eastern White Pine (*Pinus strobus*), the Western White Pine boasts longer cones, needles with a longer lifespan (2–3 years), and more prominent stomatal bands.
   Where it grows: Western White Pines prefer deep, porous soils and gentle slopes. Once the dominant tree of old-growth forests, their numbers have diminished due to the introduction of white pine blister rust, over-harvesting, and fire suppression. Blister rust arrived in 1910 via ornamental French white pines and devastated native populations. Without regular

fire to clear shade-tolerant competitors, species like cedar and fir have overtaken many areas once ruled by white pine.

In recent decades, restoration efforts have introduced rust-resistant varieties into national forests and parks. These fast-growing trees, shooting up 1 to 2 feet per year, are a hopeful sign of resurgence. The tallest known white pine, measuring 219 feet, is located near Elk River, Idaho.

When and how to harvest: Harvest the evergreen needles year-round. Young spring tips are especially flavorful, but white pine offers medicinal benefits throughout all seasons. Resin can be collected by making minor, vertical cuts—always harvest with great respect and caution.

How to work with it/ Medicinal use: Western White Pine offers warming, healing, and stimulating aromatics. The vibrant green needles are rich in chlorophyll and aromatic compounds that stimulate the body's endocannabinoid system. High in vitamins A and C and loaded with antioxidants, white pine makes a bright, tangy tea—perfect for boosting immunity and fighting off harmful bacteria and viruses during the winter months.

Pine tea supports respiratory health, helping to alleviate symptoms of colds, flu, and even tuberculosis. It is helpful for both wet and dry coughs, although pairing it with a moistening herb, such as mallow, is particularly beneficial for dry coughs. Infused with honey, white pine makes a soothing and effective cough syrup.

Externally, pine resin is a powerful antiseptic and healing agent. It can be applied to wounds, burns, boils, and skin infections. Salves and balms made with pine pitch have a long tradition of treating severe infections and stubborn wounds. A drop of dried resin can even be applied to seal cavities and prevent further decay. Pine resin is also excellent for drawing out splinters and infections.

Steam inhalation with pine can help loosen phlegm and aid in detoxification. The needles can be added to bath salts for an invigorating winter soak or used to make an immune-boosting body scrub.

Healing constituents/ Therapeutic actions: Pine needles are rich in vitamin C and antioxidants. Resin-derived turpentine is antiseptic, diuretic, rubefacient, and vermifuge.

Historical Connections: "There is no finer tree," wrote American naturalist and activist Henry David Thoreau in his journal in 1857. The white pine has long held a place of honor in both the natural and cultural history of North America. Chosen as the state tree of Idaho in 1935, it is a tree deeply woven into the fabric of the American story.

Among the Haudenosaunee (Iroquois) Confederation, the white pine symbolized peace and unity as far back as the 15th century. According to legend, five tribal chiefs buried their weapons beneath a great white pine, whose five-needle bundles came to represent the unity of the Mohawk, Oneida, Onondaga, Cayuga, and Seneca nations.

For generations, white pine offered both nourishment and medicine to Native peoples and later to European settlers. During the American Revolution, it emerged as a potent symbol of independence; its towering trunks, once reserved for the British crown's navy as the so-called "king's pines," became emblems of resistance. Revolutionary flags bore its image, and the 1772 "White Pine Riot" stands as one of the earliest acts of rebellion that helped spark the Revolution.

From the 1600s through the Civil War, white pine was often referred to as "the tree that built America." It is straight, resilient lumber that provided the beams and planks for barns, homes, bridges, churches, and ships, shaping the very architecture of a young nation.

Though its numbers were later decimated by disease, invasive pests, and overharvesting, the white pine is now making a hopeful recovery, thanks to the efforts of forest stewards, restoration projects, and those who continue to honor and protect this noble tree.

Jessica's notes: White pine reminds me that resilience is possible even in the face of hardship. Even in the face of blister rust and centuries of felling, this tree shoots toward the sky, reclaiming its place in the forest. I love sipping a bright pine needle tea in the cold months—its citrusy tang and warming aromatics feel like a blessing in a cup. Moreover, when I harvest the resin to make healing salves, I feel a deep connection to the ancient peoples who also honored this sacred tree.

"The pine stays green in winter... wisdom in hardship." — *Norman Douglas* (1868–1952)

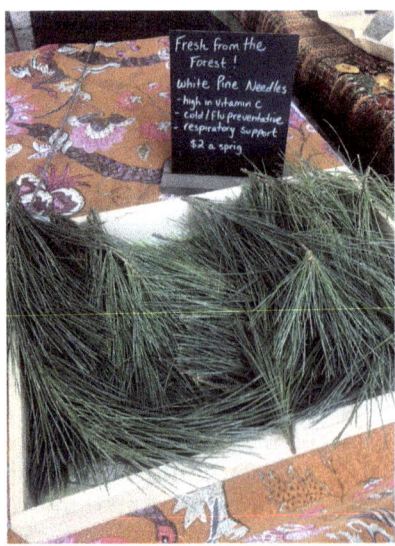

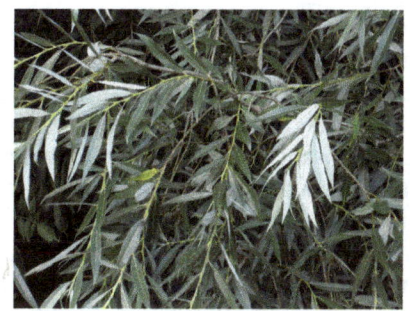

White Willow

Salix alba

Salicaceae (Willow) Family

Description: White willows are graceful, deciduous trees that reach heights of 10 to 30 feet, with trunks up to 1 foot in diameter and irregular, often leaning crowns. The bark is grayish-brown and becomes deeply grooved as the tree matures. The slender, oval leaves are dark green on top, with a silvery underside covered in fine, silky white hairs.

In early spring, the tree produces catkins—soft, elongated flower clusters that insects pollinate. White willow is dioecious, meaning male and female catkins grow on separate trees. Male catkins measure 4–5 cm long, while female catkins are 3–4 cm at pollination and lengthen as the seeds mature. Each catkin holds numerous capsules containing tiny seeds coated in silky hairs, which help them drift on the wind.

Where it grows: If there is water, there will be willow! White willow thrives along riverbanks, creeks, and springs, often in mixed stands of conifers. Wherever moisture is present, this adaptable tree is likely nearby.

When and how to harvest: Harvest the inner bark in early spring, when the sap is running and the bark peels easily.

How to work with it/ Medicinal use: White willow is known as "nature's aspirin," thanks to its pain-relieving compound, salicin—the natural precursor to modern aspirin. Numerous studies confirm that willow bark's analgesic properties are especially effective for treating rheumatic conditions, lower back pain, and general inflammation.

Unlike synthetic aspirin, willow bark is gentler on the liver and digestive system. The medicine lies in the inner bark, but instead of stripping mature trunks, it is best to harvest young spring shoots, peeling the bark into strips. These can be used fresh, dried for tea, or made into a tincture. If you prefer not to use alcohol, infusing the bark in apple cider vinegar creates an excellent tonic.

Externally, willow makes a powerful liniment, salve, or oil infusion to relieve rheumatoid arthritis, tennis elbow, sports injuries, and sore muscles. The entire plant is edible in a survival situation, although it is very bitter.

Beyond its medicinal gifts, willow's supple limbs have long been used to craft furniture, fencing, baskets, and even forts. Its flexibility is legendary.

Healing constituents/ Therapeutic actions: White willow bark contains salicin, salicylic acid, flavonoids, and tannins. Therapeutic actions include analgesic, antipyretic, and anti-inflammatory.

Historical Connections: White willow is one of humanity's oldest known remedies for pain—an ally that has walked beside us for millennia. Ancient healers from China, Egypt, Greece, and Rome all turned to willow to ease suffering. The earliest known mention of its medicinal use dates back to ancient Mesopotamia around the 20th century BCE. By the 16th century BCE, Egyptian physicians were writing of willow on papyrus scrolls, blending its leaves with myrrh to create soothing, pain-relieving preparations.

In the classical world, great physicians such as Dioscorides, Galen, and Hippocrates praised willow bark for its ability to relieve pain, reduce fevers, and ease the pains of childbirth. Across the ancient Mediterranean, willow extracts were a trusted remedy for swelling, fever, and various types of discomfort.

Centuries later, in the 18th century, English cleric Edward Stone famously used powdered willow bark to treat malaria and fever. His observations helped spark scientific interest in the plant's healing powers. By the 19th century, chemists were working diligently to isolate its active components. In 1828, German pharmacist Johann Buchner extracted "salicin" from willow bark. Soon after, Italian chemist Raffaele Piria transformed it into salicylic acid, though its harsh side effects inspired the search for gentler forms.

That breakthrough came in 1897, when Bayer chemist Felix Hoffmann synthesized acetylsalicylic acid, the form we know today as Aspirin. Though Bayer's marketing helped turn aspirin into a household name, its roots lie in the simple grace of the willow tree.

While modern aspirin can irritate the stomach lining, the whole bark of the willow, when used as nature intended, remains a gentle and highly effective remedy. In my view, it is time we return to these ancient, time-honored methods of safe and natural pain relief.

Jessica's notes: I have so much respect for Willow. This tree is both graceful and strong, flexible enough to bend without breaking, and deeply rooted in the ancient wisdom of herbal healing. I always think of it as a compassionate tree, soothing our aches and easing our suffering. When I brew a tea or make a salve from its bark, I feel connected to the generations of healers who came before me. Why rely on a synthetic pill when nature has provided us with this gentle ally for thousands of years?

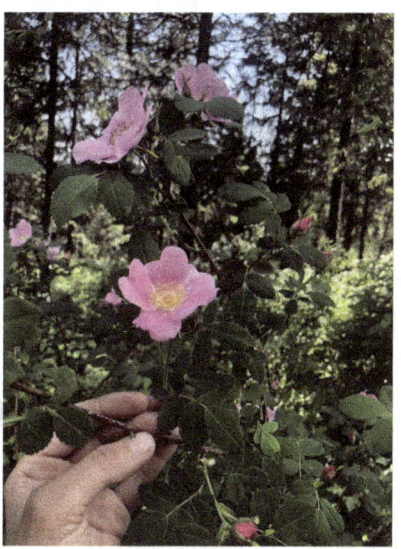

Wild Rose

Rosa carolina, Rosa palustris

Rosaceae (Rose) Family

Description: Wild rose is a deciduous shrub that can grow up to six feet tall. Some species form large, bushy thickets, while others send arching limbs to climb over fallen trees and neighboring shrubs. Each plant takes on a unique form, shaped by its environment. The stout upper branches are mostly smooth, with just a few scattered thorns—these are stout, curved, and slightly flattened at their base. The shiny green leaves are compound and divided into 7 or 9 dark green leaflets, oblong to oval in shape, with coarse, toothed margins. The flowers, typically pink but occasionally white, are five-petaled, with many yellow stamens in the center. Each blossom, measuring 5 to 8 centimeters across, has gently heart-shaped petals. Wild rose plants do not bear fruit in their first year. In later seasons, the rose's center develops into a bright ruby-red fruit known as the rosehip. This fleshy fruit contains numerous seeds covered in fine, sticky hairs.

Where it grows: Wild roses thrive in hedgerows, mixed conifer stands, and near springs and creeks. You can also find them reclaiming abandoned homesteads and old town sites, in dry ditches, or along roadsides. They are one of nature's reminders of beauty returning to forgotten places.

When and how to harvest: Harvest leaves in spring and summer, and rose petals from early to late summer. When gathering petals, leave the flower center intact so it can mature into rosehips come fall. Harvest ripe rosehips from late summer through late fall. Roots can be gathered in early spring or fall.

How to work with it/ Medicinal use: The wild rose offers a threefold medicine—leaves, petals, and hips—each with its gifts for supporting skin health, capillary strength, blood building, and cardiovascular wellness. Rose petals bloom twice a season—once in late spring, and again in a second, late-summer flush. Petals can be dried for teas, infused into honey, skin oils, balms, and salves, or used to create rose water—a beloved ingredient in Asian and Indian culinary traditions. Rosehips arrive in late summer and fall as vitamin C-rich, ruby-red jewels. Although their inner seeds are covered in irritating hairs and time-consuming to remove, much of their medicinal value resides in the skin. I typically dry them whole for use in teas or infuse them into syrups and jellies. Rosehip seed oil is deeply nourishing for the skin and excellent for supporting the healing of scar tissue. Rosehips are packed with bioflavonoids, vitamin C, and carotenoids—powerful antioxidants that exhibit both antiviral and antibacterial properties. Rose leaves, with their astringent tannins, can soothe diarrhea and inflammation of the mucosal lining. Furthermore, let us not forget their culinary delight: rosehips can be used to make tart jellies or added to wild berry jams for both flavor and health.

Healing constituents/ Therapeutic actions: Roses contain citric acid, flavonoids, fructose, malic acid, sucrose, tannins, vitamins A, B3, C, D, E, and P, along with calcium, phosphorus, iron, and zinc. Their therapeutic actions include astringent properties (leaves), as well as antiviral and antibacterial properties.

Historical connections: The rose has been cultivated for over 3,000 years and has long been honored as the "queen of flowers," used in perfumes, cosmetics, and ritual. In Christian tradition, it is said that roses grew without thorns in the Garden of Eden, only sprouting thorns after the Fall to symbolize humanity's loss of innocence. In ancient Greek mythology, the rose was a symbol of love and devotion, strongly associated with the goddess of beauty, Aphrodite. Closer to home, on September 5, 1804, Meriwether Lewis recorded the wild prairie rose in his journal, adding it to his plant collection during the expedition.

Jessica's notes: Wild rose is true medicine for the heart. My dear herbal mentor and wise friend, Sandy Anderson, often refers to it as "the remedy for a heart that has been broken again and again." When grief weighs heavily or my heart aches from loss, I blend a tea of rose petals, rosehips, hawthorn flowers and berries, and St. John's Wort. This comforting infusion feels like a familiar herbal hug—it never fails to bring solace to a tender heart.

Afterword

As we come to the close, having journeyed through the stories, traditions, and medicines of 109 plants, I hope you feel both inspired and deeply connected to the living world around you. Each of these plants offers more than medicinal properties—they are teachers, companions, and reminders of the wild wisdom that surrounds us.

In learning their names, their gifts, and their ways of growth, we rekindle an ancient relationship between humans and the plant world. This relationship is essential not only for our healing but also for the healing of the land and our communities.

My intention in sharing these plant profiles is not only to provide helpful knowledge, but to encourage reverence. May you approach each plant with curiosity, humility, and gratitude. May you remember that when we gather a leaf, a flower, a root, we are stepping into a reciprocal dance—one where giving thanks and giving back are just as important as receiving.

Above all, let this be an invitation to go out and meet the plants, where the wild things grow: to forage through forest and meadow, to kneel beside creek and hedgerow, to smell, to taste, to feel, to listen. May you find yourself at home among them.

Moreover, may the wisdom of the wild continue to guide your heart, your hands, and your healing path.

— Forest TEAcher, Jessica Freeborn

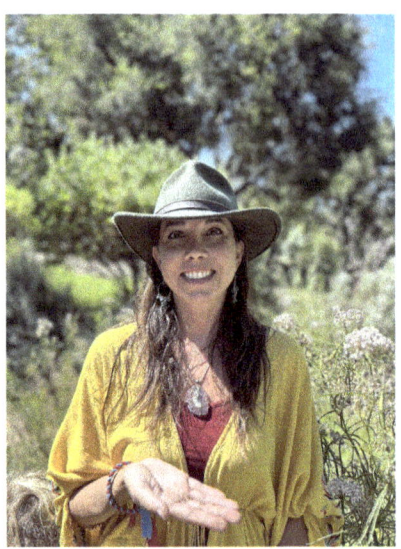

About the author

Jessica Freeborn is a self-taught herbalist, forager, creative writer, and nature educator who has spent the last 18 years learning directly from the wild. She is the founder of *Freeborn Family Forest School*, where she teaches children and families to connect with the land through hands-on experiences in foraging, folk medicine, and earth-based wisdom.

Jessica lives with her husband and two sons on Figueroa Mountain, where her family stewards the land, grows medicine, and crafts herbal remedies. Her work is rooted in reciprocity, reverence, and a deep love for the healing plants that have walked with her through every season of life.

Where the Wild Things Grow is her debut book—a heartfelt collection of stories, field wisdom, and plant teachings gathered over nearly two decades of walking with the wild. She hopes it will inspire others to return to the plants, rekindle ancestral knowledge, and remember the medicine that lives all around us.

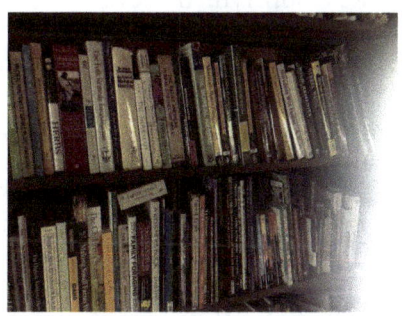

Bibliography

And suggested reading

Books

Apelian, N., & Davis, C. (2019). *The lost book of herbal remedies: The healing power of plant medicine*. Global Brother.

Bennett, R. R. (2014). *The gift of healing herbs: Plant medicines and home remedies for a vibrantly healthy life*. North Atlantic Books.

Boutenko, S. (2013). *Wild edibles: A practical guide to foraging, with easy identification of 60 edible plants and 67 recipes*. North Atlantic Books.

Coles, W. (1657). *Adam in Eden*. London.

Culpeper, N. (1975). *Culpeper's Complete Herbal: Consisting of a comprehensive description of nearly all herbs with their medicinal properties and directions for compounding the medicines extracted from them*. W. Foulsham.

Eggleston, E. (1901). *The transit of civilization from England to America in the seventeenth century*. D. Appleton and Company.

Elpel, T. J. (2013). *Botany in a day: The patterns method of plant identification* (6th ed.). HOPS Press.

Gladstar, R. (2012). *Rosemary Gladstar's medicinal herbs: A beginner's guide: 33 healing herbs to know, grow, and use*. Storey Publishing.

Gray, B. (2011). *The boreal herbal: Wild food and medicine plants of the North*. CCI Press.

Grieve, M. (1931). *A modern herbal: Volume I & II*. Dover Publications.

Kane, C. W. (2017). *Medicinal plants of the western mountain states*. Lincoln Town Press.

Kloos, S. (2017). *Pacific Northwest medicinal plants: Identify, harvest, and use 120 wild herbs for health and wellness*. Timber Press.

Meredith, L. (2016). *The forager's feast: How to identify, gather, and prepare wild edibles*. The Countryman Press.

Moerman, D. E. (1998). *Native American ethnobotany*. Timber Press.

Moore, M. (1993). *Medicinal plants of the Pacific West*. Red Crane Books.

Rose, B. (2022). *Knowledge to forage: Wild edible &medicinal plants & trees*. Independently published.

Schofield, J. J. (2002). *Discovering wild plants*. Alaska Northwest Books.

Sumner, J. (2004). *American household botany*. Timber Press.

Sumner, J. (2022). *Plants in the Civil War: A botanical history*. McFarland.

Sumner, J. (2000). *The natural history of medicinal plants*. Timber Press.

Thayer, S. (2006). *The forager's harvest*. Forager's Harvest Press.

Thayer, S. (2017). *Incredible wild edibles: 36 plants that can change your life*. Forager's Harvest Press.

Turner, N. J. (1982). Traditional use of devil's club (*Oplopanax horridus*; Araliaceae) by Native Peoples in Western North America. *Journal of Ethnobiology*, 2(1), 17–38.

Turner, N. J., & Efrat, B. S. (1982). *Ethnobotany of the Hesquiat Indians of Vancouver Island*. British Columbia Provincial Museum.

Turner, N. J., Thompson, L. C., & York, A. Z. (1990). *Thompson ethnobotany: Knowledge and usage of plants by the Thompson Indians of British Columbia*. Royal British Columbia Museum.

Journals, Articles & Studies

Al-Snafi, A. E. (2015). The chemical constituents and pharmacological effects of *Capsella bursa-pastoris* – a review. *International Journal of Pharmacology and Toxicology*, 5(2), 76–81.

Bate-Smith, E. C. (1968). Chemotaxonomy of *Nuphar lutea Phytochemistry*, 7, 459.

Blanco-Salas, J., Hortigón-Vinagre, M. P., Morales-Jadán, D., & Ruiz-Téllez, T. (2021). Searching for scientific explanations for the uses of Spanish folk medicine: A review on the case of mullein (*Verbascum*, Scrophulariaceae). *Biology*, 10(7), 618. https://doi.org/10.3390/biology 10070618

Ebeling, S., Naumann, C., Pfützner, W., Kinzinger, M., Lenschow, C., & Korting, H. C. (2014). From a traditional medicinal plant to a rational drug: Understanding the clinically proven wound healing efficacy of birch bark extract. *Planta Medica*, 80(13), 1118–1125. https://www.ncbi.nlm.nih.gov/pmc/articles/PMC3899119/

Emrich, E., Domogalla, M., Fritz, H., et al. (2022). Antimicrobial activity and wound-healing capacity of birch, beech and larch bark extracts. *Molecules*, 27(9), 2817. https://www.mdpi.com/1420-3049/27/9/2817

Furuyashiki, A., Tabuchi, K., Norikoshi, K., Kobayashi, T., Oriyama, S., & Kobayashi, M. (2019). A comparative study of the physiological and psychological effects of forest bathing (*Shinrin-yoku*) on working age people with and without depressive tendencies. *Environmental Health and Preventive Medicine*, 24, 46. https://pubmed.ncbi.nlm.nih.gov/31228960/

Goun, E. A., Petrichenko, V. M., Solodnikov, S. U., et al.(2002). Anticancer and antithrombin activity of Russian plants. *Journal of Ethnopharmacology, 81*(3), 337–342.https://doi.org/10.1016/S0378-8741(02)00116-2

Grosso, C., Ferreres, F., Gil-Izquierdo, A., et al.(2010–2011). Chemical composition and biological screening of *Capsella bursa-pastoris*. *Revista Brasileira de Farmacognosia*, 21(3), 493–500. https://www.scielo.br/j/rbfar/a/mqHRWn4bzgcr7smph5RwLzS

Jyske, T., Hytönen, J., Venäläinen, M., et al. (2020). Sprouts and needles of Norway spruce (*Picea abies* (L.) Karst.) as Nordic specialty—Consumer acceptance, stability of nutrients, and bioactivities during storage. *Foods, 9* (10), 1397. https://www.ncbi.nlm.nih.gov/pmc/articles/PMC7570650/

Park, J. Y., Yuk, H. J., Ryu, H. W., et al. (2012). Diarylheptanoids from *Alnus japonica* inhibit papain-like protease of severe acute respiratory syndrome coronavirus. *Biological and Pharmaceutical Bulletin, 35*(11), 2036–2042. https://www.jstage.jst.go.jp/article/bpb/35/11/35_b12-00623/_pdf

Tiralongo, E., Wee, S. S., & Lea, R. A. (2016). Elderberry supplementation reduces cold duration and symptoms in air travelers: A randomized, double-blind placebo-controlled clinical trial. *Nutrients,8*(4), 182. https://www.ncbi.nlm.nih.gov/pmc/articles/PMC484865

Wesolowska, A., Nikiforuk, A., Michalska, K., Kisiel, W.,& Chojnacka-Wójcik, E. (2006). Analgesic and sedative activities of lactucin and some lactucin-like guaianolides in mice. *Journal of Ethnopharmacology, 107*(2), 254–258. https://pubmed.ncbi.nlm.nih.gov/31137691/

Zakay-Rones, Z., Thom, E., Wollan, T., & Wadstein, J.(2004). Randomized study of the efficacy and safety of oral elderberry extract in the treatment of influenza A and B virus infections. *Journal of International Medical Research, 32*(2), 132–140. https://pubmed.ncbi.nlm.nih.gov/15080016/

Online Resources
Acornherbschool.com
Britannica.com
Chestnutschoolofherbalism.com
Eattheweeds.com
Ediblewildfoods.com
Feralforaging.com
Herbalacademy.com
kingjamesbibleonline.org
Practicalplants.org
Practicalselfreliance.com
Wildfoodmedicine.com

Index

www.ingramcontent.com/pod-product-compliance
Lightning Source LLC
Chambersburg PA
CBHW070612030426
42337CB00020B/3769